THE NUCLEAR HEALTH SERVICE

THE NUCLEAR HEALTH SERVICE

Weapon of Mass Compassion
1948–1968

GEORGE E SCOTT

New Generation Publishing
London

Published by New Generation Publishing in 2015

Copyright © Dr George E Scott 2015

First Edition

The author asserts the moral right under the Copyright, Designs and Patents Act 1988 to be identified as the author of this work.

All Rights reserved. No part of this publication may be reproduced, stored in a retrieval system or transmitted, in any form or by any means without the prior consent of the author, nor be otherwise circulated in any form of binding or cover other than that which it is published and without a similar condition being imposed on the subsequent purchaser.

www.newgeneration-publishing.com

 New Generation **Publishing**

To my grandchildren, Polly and Charlie

May they never stand in fear of a nuclear war

CONTENTS

Tables ii

Maps ii

Illustrations iii

Abbreviations vi

Preface vii

Introduction 1

1. Atomic Reactions 8
2. Cold Comfort War 40
3. Surgical Spirits 61
4. Facade Fatigue 89
5. Admission Impossible 112
6. Body Language 141
7. Nursing Numbers 167
8. Alternative Medicine 197
9. Which Doctors 224

References 251

Appendices 282

Bibliography 294

Index 315

LIST OF TABLES AND MAPS

Table

1.	Mobile First Aid Unit Support to Civil Defence Regions	30
2.	Blood Donors and Donations 1949 to 1956	42
3	Gamma Radiation Effects	142
4.	National Hospital Service Reserve Recruitment	168

Map

1.	Hospital Evacuation Areas	x
2.	Regional Hospital Boards	xi
3.	Civil Defence Regions and Zones	xii

ILLUSTRATIONS

Front cover

NHSR personnel simulate the treatment of a casualty burnt by an atomic heat flash, London, 1952 (Keystone Pictures USA/ZUMAPRESS.com)

Cover design by Katherine Scott

Plates

1. Aneurin Bevan (Getty Images)

2. Leaflet announcing the start of the NHS (Bath Record Office)

3. Outpatients attend an East London hospital April 1949 (Getty Images)

4. Sir Ernest Rock Carling (The National Portrait Gallery, London)

5. Sir Alexander Hood (The National Portrait Gallery, London)

6. The Civil Defence Staff College, Ascot, Berkshire (Bath Record Office)

7. Staff College atomic bomb lecture in progress (Bath Record Office)

8. Atomic bomb target map of Bristol (The National Archives, HO 357/3)

9. Recruitment poster for the Ambulance Section (Bath Record Office)

10. 1950s recruitment poster for the Ambulance and Casualty Collection Section (Bath Record Office)

11. Vote counting at BMA House regarding participation in the NHS (Getty Images)

12. Dame Enid Russell-Smith (The National Portrait Gallery)

13. Rescue and first aid exercise on a Bath bomb site (Bath Record Office)

14. Army Training ground for Civil Defence (Bath Record Office)

15. MFAU demonstration outside the Ministry of Health HQ (Corbis/Keystone Press)

16. MFAU packed van (Bath Record Office)

17. Civil Defence Ambulance with stretcher racking (Bath Record Office)

18. Civil Defence stretcher loading exercise (Bath Record Office)

19. Ambulance team stretcher demonstration (Author's Collection)

20. Ambulance team stretcher demonstration (Author's Collection)

21. London County Council Civil Defence ambulances (Author's Collection)

22. Bath Civil Defence ambulances (Bath Record Office)

23. Auxiliary Fire Service water relay exercise (Getty Images)

24. Cartoon (The National Archives, MH 55/998)

25. Radiation detection exercise (Getty Images)

26. Blood bank at a London hospital (Getty Images)

27. Nurses in prayer before starting a shift (Getty Images)

28. EXERCISE RELIANCE. (Bath Record Office)

29. EXERCISE RELIANCE. (Bath Record Office)

30. EXERCISE RELIANCE. (Bath Record Office)

31. EXERCISE RELIANCE. (Bath Record Office)

32. Experimental Coffin. (National Records of Scotland, HH 51/277 E)

33. Experimental Coffin. (National Records of Scotland, HH 51/277 F)

34. Experimental Coffin. (National Records of Scotland, HH 51/277 D)

35. Police first aid competition (Bath Record Office)

36. Children participate in a Civil Defence exercise (Bath Record Office)

37. Civil Defence open day on a London estate (Getty Images)

38. Carnival float. (Bath Record Office)

39. Headquarters Section staff. (Bath Record Office)

40. Mayor of Bath inspects the Ambulance and Welfare Sections (Bath Record Office)

41. Sir Winston Churchill inspects a wartime group of auxiliary nurses (Keystone Pictures USA/ZUMAPRESS.com)

42. Ministerial inspection of the NHSR (London Metropolitan Archives, City of London, ref. HA/NW/E/03/030)

43. NHSR baby care shop window display (The National Archives, MH/984)

44. NHSR hospital bed shop window display (The National Archives, MH/987)

45. The Minister's Cup Competition final (Getty Images)

46. WVS food support to an exercise (Author's collection)

47. WVS field kitchen (Bath Record Office)

48. NHSR poster for trained nurses (The National Archives, BN 10/204)

49. NHSR help your local hospital (The National Archives, BN 10/203)

50. The author as a Senior Scout in 1963 (Author's Collection)

51. BMA poster 1965 (Bath Record Office)

52. Civil Defence radiation monitoring demonstration (Getty Images)

ABBREVIATIONS

AEC	(US) Atomic Energy Commission
BMA	British Medical Association
BRCS	British Red Cross Society
CAT	Category
CD	Civil Defence
CDJPS	Civil Defence Joint Planning Staff
CND	Campaign for Nuclear Disarmament
CNR	Civil Nursing Reserve
CMWC	Central Medical War Committee
CWD	Civilian War Dead
DTC	Defence Transition Committee
EMS	Emergency Medical Services
FMAU	Forward Medical Aid Unit
GP	General (Medical) Practitioner
GZ	Ground Zero
HDR	Home Defence Review Committee
LA	Local Authority
LCC	London County Council
MO	Medical Officer
MOH	Medical Officer of Health
MP	(British) Member of Parliament
MFAU	Mobile First Aid Unit
NATO	North Atlantic Treaty Organisation
NHSR	National Hospital Service Reserve
NMC	National Medical Committee
NNR	National Nursing Reserve
PF	Protective Factor
RAF	Royal Air Force
RAMC	Royal Army Medical Corps
RCN	Royal College of Nursing
RHB	Regional Hospital Board
SAMO	Senior Administrative Medical Officer
TB	Tuberculosis
UK	United Kingdom
WVS	Women's Voluntary Service

PREFACE

Something I shall always remember is the Cuban Missile Crisis of 1962 as the Americans conducted their naval blockade to prevent long-range Soviet rockets being sited on the island. During some of those tense moments, when the world edged toward nuclear war, I stood with friends in the playground of my old school, John Fisher (on the outskirts of South London) and we huddled around a small transistor radio smuggled in against all the rules to hear what our chances were of surviving the day. Living with the bomb always had a subconscious feeling of possible annihilation, but this event heightened that sense of impending catastrophe as never before. I also recollect that there were two ways of looking at the situation if it did go nuclear. The pessimistic scenario meant the entire school succumbing to vaporisation within seconds and no possible escape. Conversely, the optimistic view suggested there would be many survivors at the periphery of a nuclear explosion. If the worst came to the worst, government policy promised the NHS would deliver medical salvation as a stretched version of its peacetime counterpart. In the Senior Scouts, I had even been involved in civil defence exercises with the medical services and although these were part of the nuclear regime of reassurance, I must admit my thoughts still turned towards total annihilation being the only possible outcome.

Many years later, after retiring as a Chartered Surveyor, I followed a passion for history developed at school thanks to one of those incredible teachers who, unusually for that time, brought the subject out of its dreary routine of just learning dates. During the course of my surveying career, I had dealt with all kinds of disasters that involved buildings including bombs, fire, floods, as well as the oil crisis, which drew me to the study of the legislation introduced to protect property during the Second World War. Later this became the subject of a Master's dissertation, which in turn provided useful background when I decided to extend my interest to the Cold War and the civil defence services of that era that had promised my generation the nuclear safety net described. A decision to pursue the subject through the rigours of a doctoral thesis could not have been more propitious. The *Freedom of Information Act 2000* provided exactly the right conditions for unmasking some of the innermost government secrets that otherwise may never have seen the light of day. Peter Hennessy (Lord Hennessy, Attlee Professor at Queen Mary University of London) had begun the process in his book *The Secret State, Whitehall and the Cold War* (2000). Crucially this exposed the civil defence system as a socio-political deception, but where the concept of 'deception' was transferred from the realms of subjective conspiracy theory to the objective side of the historical equation defined by government itself and not the historian.

The completion of my doctorate in October 2006 reflected that exceptional opportunity, as secret papers were uncovered with an exhilaration akin to the archaeologist dusting off the precious artefacts for the first time. During the research process, I brought to light several documents of national importance and on one occasion received an invitation to review these at the Cabinet Office before their dispatch to The National Archives. A particular aspect which tantalisingly appeared was that the National Health Service had not only become part of the overall deception, but also the biggest player on the welfare side because of its promise to deliver mass compassion to millions. Whilst my academic work identified the main strands of that proposition, this clearly represented only the tip of an iceberg of social manipulation, which in the inner sanctum of Whitehall had been baptised as 'the facade' of civil defence.

The idea of a book to reveal more about the medical involvement appeared an appropriate way forward. However, the initial enthusiasm of discovering a new historical landscape seemed at risk of falling victim to the researcher's nightmare of losing the historical trail through gaps in primary sources. Unfortunately, the departmental papers of the Ministry of Health held at The National Archives suffered from a good deal of thinning out. Unlike the meticulous retention of Cabinet papers, the records dealing with the medical profession were not just patchy, but provided only a fraction of its history. Breathing life into the project meant extending the base research to the National Records of Scotland. Not only did the country put into place its own medical defence systems, it often did so through joint committees and meetings with the Ministry of Health that dealt with England and Wales. Along with closing the missing links, by adopting this methodology, other considerable benefits resulted by gaining a broader understanding of the issues involved. A fortunate by-product especially arose through the different approaches of the two countries to medical planning which caused many tensions to occur and conveniently illuminated areas of policy that might have otherwise remained hidden from the prying eye of the inquisitive historian.

For certain, the process came with the bonus of concluding not just an amorphous history of the British medical civil defence system, but also the very distinctive history of the Scottish involvement, particularly through the interplay between the philosophies north and south of the border. The British Medical Archive at BMA House in London added a further vital dimension through their minute books which recorded the essential decision making process of the medical profession. A nuclear agreement for mobilising and controlling general practitioners, agreed in principle by the BMA after years of wrangling, was a notable find. This particularly ranks as a landmark document in the history of the NHS and its rightful context assured reflecting an episode that threatened to tear the National Health Service apart in peace, whilst preparing for nuclear war. Discoveries of this kind do so often rely on the support of archivists and I am most grateful for the considerable assistance that the BMA provided to complete the history in all its various facets.

Echoing those sentiments, Colin Johnston, Principal Archivist at Bath Record Office, deserves a special mention for his unstinting support and I am indebted to his generosity in allowing the use of photographs from the archive's extensive civil defence collection. Bath, located next to Bristol, one of the prime targets for Soviet attention, became a city highly committed to civil defence with some of the most important medical exercises of national significance conducted in the immediate region. My thanks also go to the staff at the National Records of Scotland in Edinburgh who were magnificent in preparing many files before my visit to ensure it was as productive as possible. The National Archives at Kew, as well as many other archives have been similarly accommodating in helping to provide the breadth and depth of research material so essential to creating a work almost entirely dependent on primary sources. Certainly, the sum total of that support has enabled many important aspects of the NHS and its recent past to be revealed for the first time. Collating charts and maps takes a special aptitude and I am indebted to historian John Penny for his help in this time consuming and intricate endeavour. Finally, is the enormous debt of gratitude I owe to my academic mentor, Associate Professor Kent Fedorowich at the University of the West of England, Bristol. As a leading Imperial and Commonwealth historian, he has provided me with advice and support for many years. But the list of thanks does not end there because, of course, behind some writers there is a patient wife and in my case Valerie has been no exception. I thank her for being stalwart in suffering my despair when things did not go right and delighted when everything went well.

George Edward Scott
Bath

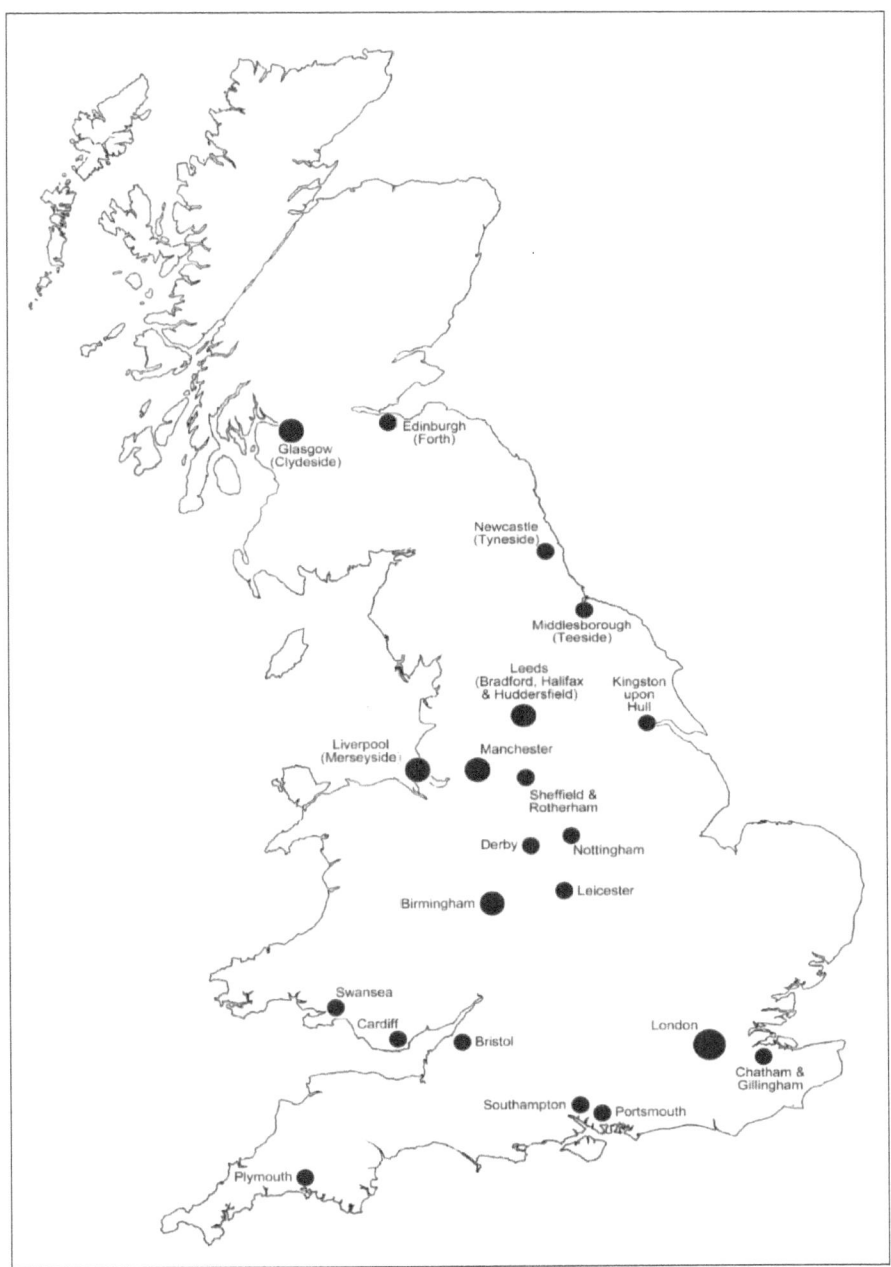

MAP 1: Hospital Evacuation Areas.

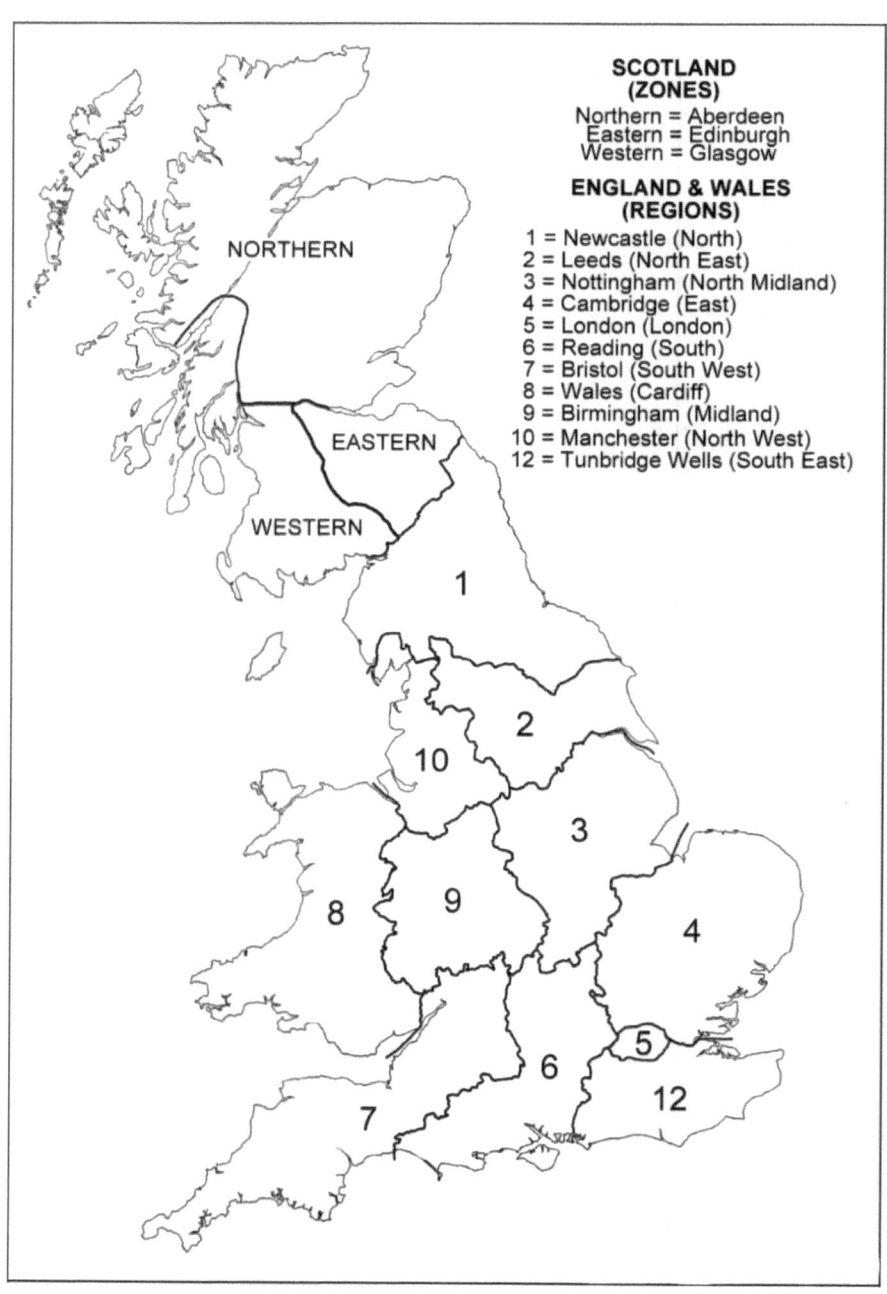

MAP 2: Regional Hospital Boards.

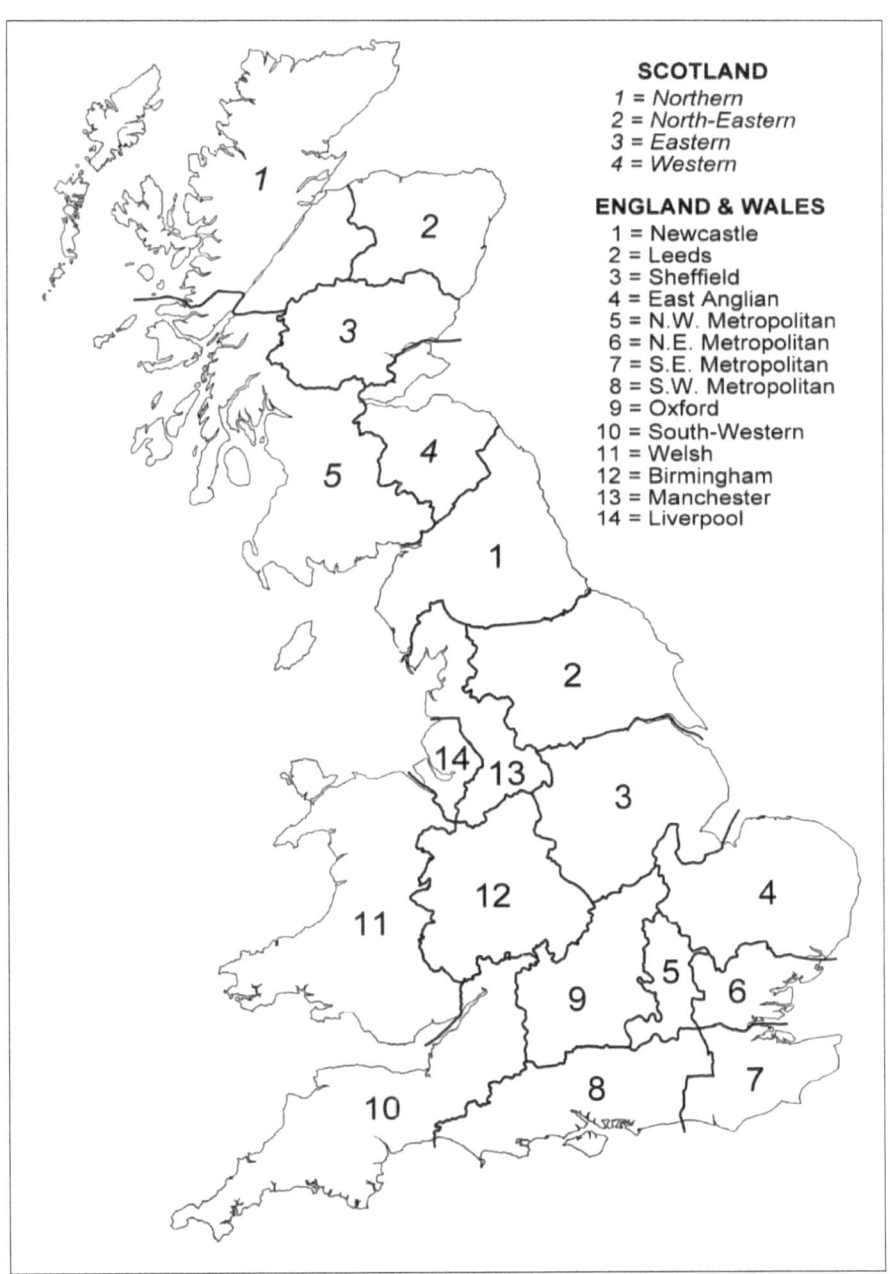

MAP 3: Civil Defence Regions and Zones.

INTRODUCTION

1948 was a year whose events affected Britain to a degree that their political legacies still very much resonate in our own age. On the 12 May, a Parliamentary announcement disclosed the country's atomic weapons programme for the first time.[1] Probably of greater interest to most people, the second event followed shortly afterwards: the foundation of the National Health Service. This came into being on 5 July, 1948. Known as 'the appointed day', the service gave some fifty million people a right to access a common structure of medical care provided by the state, particularly by the poor, the elderly and the unemployed. Then, just weeks later, the Berlin Blockade by the Soviets provided a harsh reminder of what the Cold War might bring and threaten a third world war. Little wonder that the political heat generated during 1948 caused a fusion of some consequence to take place. A secret metamorphosis started, which involved the NHS becoming an integral part of deterrence policy by turning into the antidote for the effects of mass destruction that had begun perilously to face the nation.

Conceptualising mass casualties into diagnosable and treatable entities became a propaganda struggle against seemingly impossible odds. The NHS required stretching to provide new ethically acceptable space where each individual received treatment, particularly the seriously injured. Signification of individuality within the nuclear holocaust was not without difficulty. John Hersey, in writing *Hiroshima* (1946) had discomfortingly highlighted the personal suffering extricated from indeterminate terms such as 'mass casualties' or innocuous optimism denoted by 'the survivors' that had begun to obscure the face of nuclear war in post war polemics. A particularly distressing scene that met Father Kleinsorge, a Catholic priest, remains one of the iconic images of those caught in the heat flash of an exploding atomic bomb:

> When he had penetrated the bushes, he saw there were about twenty men, and they were in exactly the same nightmarish state: their faces were wholly burned, their eye sockets were hollow, the fluid from their melted eyes had run down their cheeks – their mouths were mere swollen, puss covered wounds, which they could not bear to stretch enough to admit the spout of a teapot. So Father Kleinsorge got a large piece of grass and drew out

> the stem so as to make a straw, and gave them all water to drink that way.²

Always vulnerable to evocative pictures such as those described, civil defence in general and the medical services in particular had to purge such absolute hopelessness, magnified millions of times, with counter-statements of hope. At a very early stage such an exercise began to cause the policymakers a troublesome dilemma. The way ministers responsible for civil defence reacted when considering the format of the first manual *Atomic Warfare,* also to go on sale to the public at His Majesty's Stationery Offices around the country, illustrates just how problematic marketing atomic survival was turning out to be:

> Discussions turned on the general form of the manual. There was no doubt that it would receive much publicity – more perhaps if an attempt were made to restrict its circulation to instructors than if it were made generally available. It was, therefore, desirable, while having strict regard for the truth, to avoid giving an unnecessarily horrific impression to the casual reader, or an opportunity to make alarmist selections for propaganda purposes. Some of the descriptions of the effects of an atomic explosion were perhaps unnecessarily detailed and grim. Certainly the descriptions by themselves, gave a worse impression than they would if each were followed immediately by a statement of the protective measures available. Admittedly, there were difficulties in doing this, and the result might sometimes be to show how little were the protective measures possible. Nevertheless, it was agreed that the pamphlet should be re-arranged on these lines.³

This debate, conducted in March 1950, and the nature of its uncomfortable circularity between producing transparency and reconciling the effects of an atomic bomb with some means of protection exposes the propaganda burden which the new era of mass destruction had brought to the political table. Indeed, the real imagery continued to haunt Whitehall, the degree of discomfort even reaching the prestigious Civil Defence Staff College in Ascot, Berkshire. The college library hid Hersey's little 'Penguin'-sized book from its shelves and attendees were advised in the course notes that they could borrow it, but only 'on application to librarian'.[4] From that inherent fear within the government about the management of public fears over the bomb emerged the only possible answer. The problems associated with nuclear survival and their solutions simply had to be in harmony with each other, or, as the language of the day put it - possess the vital ingredient of 'logic'. Expressed another way, it meant producing new realities, but these of necessity had to be supported by organisations which could add the element of trust to the message. But if, as postulated in the preface the government adopted such a policy of deception, secretly known as 'the facade', it begs the question as to how the NHS, as one of the country's most ethically-principled institutions could have been placed on the nuclear chessboard on those terms.

An important contributory factor undoubtedly stems from the timeline under review that provided a climate of acquiescence in a number of ways. During the Cold War that lasted between 1947 and 1991 several kinds of survival regimes had been introduced, each with different names such as *Emergency Services* or propagandist titles that included the *Protect and Survive* era, promoted by Margaret Thatcher's government. The period between 1948 and 1968, however involved arrangements where nuclear survival was projected through a uniformed volunteer service, which had many similarities with the rescue and welfare services established during the last war. Moreover, during that time Britain still remained a country where institutional trust, deference to authority and patriotic duty shaped by two world wars were still out there ready to be soaked up into an ideological formwork favourable to propagandising nuclear survival. Representing a package of emotions, values and experiences, these were also used to create a medical belief system that, for the purposes of the book is called 'the nuclear health service'. In many respects the episode developed into an organisational stress-test of epic proportions as the potential for friction increased with the advancement of nuclear weapons and the need to adapt 'the facade' to sustain its contrived logic and believability. With that in mind, the nature of the environment the manipulative process faced is appropriate to outline since it emphasises both the difficulties encountered and the nature of the achievement of keeping the ideology in place.

At the heart of the propaganda problem was the way the destructive power it faced developed exponentially. Momentous changes occurred to every aspect involved in the business of mass destruction. Weapon delivery systems developed from bombers to guided missiles and finally nuclear submarines, all of which impacted the element of surprise and collapsed preparation times for the new Home Front to react to just two or three days. Weapons grew into hideously unimaginable monsters. Sending a warning to the West, the Soviets detonated the 'Tsar bomb' possessing a yield of some 58 megatons that could be ramped up to 100 megatons without further tests.[5] All this had started with the modest Hiroshima-size atomic bomb of twenty kilotons of TNT and its comparatively limited capacity to destroy houses up to the three-eighths of a mile from ground zero. In stark contrast, a hydrogen bomb with a ten-megaton warhead could produce a destructive power five hundred times as great and create a total damage ring up to three and a half miles in just seconds.[6] Moreover, the possible attack scenarios increased from a handful of Hiroshima-size bombs, aimed at mainly civilian targets, to strikes involving over 300 hydrogen bombs directed at multiple targets that included cities, government bunkers and military bases.[7] What then really added to the horrors came with the radiation problem. The Hiroshima bomb, though awful, generated radiation mostly lethal to those near the burst, but in the new science of the hydrogen bomb, radiation delivered by dust particles and spread over vast distances added a new dimension on an unprecedented scale.

The possible obliteration of Britain on this progressive trajectory of doom engaged Whitehall with the predicament of how to externalise a medical policy that could transfer the image of universal care the NHS provided in peace and stretch it into a nuclear healthcare safety net predicated on the same terms. Assuring the public they would not end up becoming an amorphous entity of so-called 'mass' casualties meant each and every person needed to be confident of receiving medical attention without the fear of abandonment. The challenge this represented not only related to its sheer audacity, but because of the inherent danger of actually destroying the National Health Service itself so shortly after its establishment. While the organisation might have seemed a perfect solution to the projection of mass compassion, it also had the potential to turn into a horror story with serious consequences.

The positives were particularly underwritten by new legislation. The NHS appeared not only as a cohesive organisation, but also flexible in ways unimaginable in previous wars because of the *National Service Act 1946* in England and Wales under which it had been founded. Scotland enjoyed its own legal arrangements to fit in with the circumstances of the country, but for the purposes of reaching the same national objective little difference existed. Overall, the hospital service worked through 14 Regional Hospital Board areas in England and Wales and 5 in Scotland, providing beds supported by a whole range of medical professionals including surgeons, house doctors, nurses, radiologists, physiotherapists and blood transfusion units. Having said that, in addition to those responsibilities, the medical estate extended into other areas which included hospitals that catered for the mentally ill, tuberculosis hospitals as well as isolation units.[8] Secondly, a total of 146 Local Health

Authorities were run by councils through their Medical Officers of Health. These provided domiciliary, maternity and child welfare services; ambulance services; public health management; the after care of the sick and importantly, the provision of health centres offering a range of medical, dental and welfare facilities under one roof, a defining symbol of community care. Finally, the new medical package included the general practitioners and dentists who practiced outside the hospital or local authority spheres through their own surgeries. Executive Councils represented their interests in the area of each Local Health Authority and it was the duty of these ECs to arrange for the provision of medical services determined by local needs.[9]

Additional to those layers of peacetime medical establishments, another sector of public and civic support came about through the *Civil Defence Act 1948*. Because of this legislation, local authorities were required to establish operational controls in bunkered accommodation. Their intended occupants involved a headquarters staff consisting of councillors and civic officials including town clerks, borough surveyors, medical officers of health, plus science teachers acting as scientific advisers on radioactive fallout. Collectively these would direct the volunteer civil defence organisation, known as the Civil Defence Corps, much in the same way as in the Second World War. Within that Corps, which included wardens, rescue and welfare units, the Ambulance Section was to supplement the ambulance service run by the councils that would convey casualties out of the scenes of atomic devastation. Hospitals themselves, if they had over two hundred beds, were to encourage non-medical staff to mirror that national pattern within their own walls by joining the 'Industrial Civil Defence Service'. In this way they could, the propaganda suggested, protect their immediate community and provide a link to external aid should this become necessary.[10] Volunteer organisations were also established to augment other peacetime services, including the Auxiliary Fire Service and Special Constabulary. Even the hospitals became beneficiaries of this expansion principle and the National Hospital Service Reserve created with the aim of bolstering the nursing resources by attracting qualified nurses that had retired or left and training members of the public as auxiliaries.

However robust the system might have looked from the outside, underneath it all history had created a honeycomb of instability. Combining all these elements into 'the nuclear health service' entailed reshaping a system beset by its own anxieties. Each element did not exist as a passive organisational entity but embodied complex domains of power and self-interest very much influenced by the recent past. The country's medical organisation had undergone a radical and painful overhaul in the formation of the Emergency Medical Services specifically to cover the medical needs of the Second World War. Under the arrangements made that in many ways became a forerunner of the National Health Service, the best of the voluntary and municipal hospitals entered into a pooling system primarily to support civilian and service war casualties. Then the war itself created psychological divisions between those medical professionals who regarded war as a medical challenge and willing to transfer that interest into the atomic dimension, whilst for others any involvement in a nuclear game remained a complete anathema. Some were even veterans of the First World War where the same considerations applied and the horrors of that experience not far removed from the landscape of nuclear war.

The construction of the National Health Service itself had caused a sense of discouragement in several sectors, particularly the Local Health Authorities. Many actively attempted to manage the deficiencies of the medical services before the introduction of the NHS only to see their hospitals and specialist clinics pass to the Regional Hospital Boards. As for the personal effects of the changes, Medical Officers of Health working in the Local Health Authorities sphere lost much of their old power and prestige. The devaluation of their status must have seemed especially demoralising. They had been behind the planning of much of the wartime medical organisation, involving the setting-up of the casualty hospitals, dealing with public health matters due to crowded shelters or the evacuation of children, as well as arranging emergency maternity homes. Doctors and surgeons also suffered. Formerly able to pick and choose their patients and build up lucrative practices, they now had to contract to a regime of universal medicine. General practitioners, in particular, obsessed about the possibilities of state medicine impinging on their medical independence.

So both the creation of 'the nuclear health service' and the way it was sustained to continuously reflect the caring state and its morality became a dynamic that needed to ride out both the complex environment of change and cultural sensitivity. That meant deconstructing the National Health Service and reconstructing it in ways to ensure that domain interests within the system did not generate organisational friction capable of damaging the image of cohesion. Added to those difficulties, the visualisation of commitment to nuclear healthcare was not immune to succumbing to the economic ills of the country that narrowed the possibilities of marketing the promise of mass compassion to the public. With Britain building up the welfare state whilst at the same time rebuilding the ravages of war and rearming with nuclear hardware, it meant that funding the illusion of mass compassion became increasingly problematic, especially in the economic downturns that occurred on a cyclical basis.

The nine chapters of the book follow that process to illustrate how the result added up to an extraordinarily resilient mythology as it grappled to overcome those seemingly impossible obstacles. A measure of just how the overall facade of civil defence had crystallised into a perceptible belief system is evident in the reaction to civil defence by the Campaign for Nuclear Disarmament, founded in 1958, which felt the need to challenge the contrived idealism of the concept head-on. The disarmers acknowledged that in the General Election of 1959 they had not been in a position to make any impact on the issue. Their strategic plan *Telling Britain,* prepared for the 1963 General Election, by contrast, sought to reveal the insidious connections of civil defence with the bomb more directly. Activists were to follow the 'Croydon questionnaire' and raise pertinent issues at important pre-election meetings. Consisting of a list of ten questions, the last represented a rhetorical statement aimed directly at the facade. It asked, 'Do you see civil defence as a rescue operation in a nuclear war, or would you justify its continued existence on the grounds that its abandonment would worry the population unduly and thus set off a questioning of this country's nuclear strategy?'[11]

The very reaction of CND shows the facade of civil defence was not possible to dismiss out of hand as an irrelevance. Their highly-focussed and considered attack reflected the fact government had planted a propaganda knotweed pernicious by nature and exceptionally difficult to eradicate. The rhetorical question itself answered the reason for the propaganda whereby successive administrations felt a need to deploy a system of emotional management to protect deterrence policy. An essential ingredient in that endeavour was the requirement to harness the NHS to create the mask of a caring and moral state, behind which it was possible to fight the Cold War in the most dangerous circumstances the world has ever faced. With that in mind, a need for the book arises to underscore the fact that in the gesturing of the super powers, a social history of some consequence was also in the making. Using the NHS meant that it became a heavyweight player in the psychological regime with the result that its propaganda invaded everyday life through hospital waiting rooms, high streets, cinemas, and even football matches to project the promise of medical attention to every potential nuclear casualty. In other words, the NHS took on a secret purpose to nurse the bomb, which affected ordinary people in some extraordinary ways.

Chapter 1

ATOMIC REACTIONS

The Cold War could at times involve living with a distinct feeling of both hope and hopelessness and during 1951, those two emotions were played out very publicly. On the one hand, the Festival of Britain promised the British people a new age of science and ingenuity. On the other, the outbreak of the Korean War sent out a blunt reminder about those same aspects of modern life being combined for more destructive purposes if the conflict erupted into a global war. However, another event was supposed to nudge the pointer towards 'the hope' side. The Ministry of Health announced its plans as to how the National Health Service would provide a healthcare safety net for every citizen in the event of the country experiencing saturation bombing on the scale and weight delivered on Dresden or through an attack by atomic bombs. The care promised could not have been more extensive, being described as 'An expanded Hospital Service which would not only deal with civilian air raid casualties and the acute sick, but also with casualties and acute sick from the Armed Forces, including those brought home from overseas, so far as the Armed Forces own hospitals cannot handle them.'[1]

Everything in the plan promised prompt attention being given to as many casualties as possible, especially the seriously injured. To fulfil its obligations the NHS planned to increase bed numbers considerably but still offer a high level of treatment. In England and Wales the staffed bed capacity for 'the normal sick' amounted to 150,000 beds and was to be expanded into a complement of 450,000 beds. On top of that, a further commitment appeared relating to 300,000 'special' beds supporting TB, maternity, and children's establishments, as well as the institutions for the mentally ill that accounted for the greater part of the category. Included in that new deal, most of the patients in these units were in line for transfer to alternative accommodation if situated in target areas. The policy signified a gesture of immense importance by confirming the mentally and chronically sick would be supported by the caring state and were not expendable, even in atomic war.[2]

The Times newspaper gave over much copy to the civil defence plans and in a special report particularly praised the medical proposals for combining new initiatives with established procedures. Under the headline of 'Victims of Mass Bombing, A Plan for the Civil

Defence Casualty Service,' it saw the exercise as a denouement of manageable proportions and gave its blessing: 'As in the last war, hospital staffs would have to provide visiting teams for surgery, medicine and resuscitation, besides manning the special centres that must be re-established and multiplied, and their mobility will need organisation. All that has been done before, but the scale would be greater'.[3] Reassuring as such overtures were, they amounted to no more than an illusion of hope and for the NHS its 'cold comfort war' had begun in earnest.

Treatment Spaces

The journey taken by the NHS in its parallel nuclear life began, of all days, on 5 November, 1948 (Bonfire Night) when a small group of five medical men held their first meeting to consider how the fledgling National Health Service should fit into Britain's new civil defence organisation. Certainly, no suggestion of 'gunpowder, treason or plot' could be laid at the door of the august body which had been named the Working Party on Medical Aspects. The mission of the group was to formulate medical policy as part of the greater plans under preparation by the Civil Defence Joint Planning Staff established to create a new civil defence scheme for the protection of the United Kingdom. Involved in the venture were some of the most distinguished medical professionals of the day. They included the chairman, Sir Ernest Rock Carling, an eminent surgeon and radiologist, Sir Claude Frankau, Consulting Surgeon at St George's Hospital, London and Lieutenant-General Sir Alexander Hood, formerly of the Royal Army Medical Corps, later to become Governor of Bermuda.[4] Like so many men of their generation, they had served with distinction in a medical capacity during the First and Second World Wars and were now ready to bring their vast experience of conflict and medicine to the atomic battlefield. Sir William Scott Douglas, Secretary of the Ministry of Health, (entrusted by Aneurin Bevan to establish the NHS), had given them a brief which was 'To consider ways and means of disseminating information about the diagnosis and treatment of atom bomb casualties and the planning of measures which may have to be taken to expand the normal hospital and blood transfusion services in order that they may cope with such casualties'.[5]

In addition to that long-term agenda came another, more pressing problem highlighting the enormity of the task that lay ahead. Just weeks after its introduction, the NHS faced its first crisis of the Cold War. The Foreign Office had issued a statement, in the light of the blockade of Berlin by the Soviets, confirming the British Government's intention to maintain their position in the city and as the diplomatic language of doom put it, 'there could be no question of yielding to Soviet pressure'. Underlining the potentially flammable situation, instructions raised the stakes that if barrage balloons went up to prevent the planned airlift of supplies into the city, then they were to be shot down.[6]

The threat of another war so soon after the last took on an ominous and depressing picture in contrast to the joy of the victory celebrations only a few years earlier. A status report prepared by the Ministry of Health reflecting on the outcome of a sudden attack illustrated just how far the dismantling of the country's civil defence systems had gone. Caught in the middle of a hospital organisation virtually run into the ground by war and in the throes of reorganising to meet the needs of the NHS, the hospital side of things looked very bleak indeed. Hospitals were already 80% full and casualty plans would require a high degree of improvisation with patients simply placed onto mattresses laid on the floor. Outside the hospital, the prospect of makeshift preparations also highlighted the lack of resources. Collecting and transporting casualties would fall to the worn out fleet of ambulances belonging to local authorities and commandeered vehicles, with the supply of stretchers described as woefully inadequate. After the first bombing, a clearance of patients out of hospitals needed to take place to make way for others, but with no ambulance trains and ambulance buses the wartime patterns of casualty transfer out of the frontline were simply impossible to achieve.[7]

Two years later when the Berlin situation subsided and the nuclear hospital plan was in the course of preparation, this also seemed in danger of entering the realms of hopelessness through certain doubts delivered by the country's most prestigious medical journal. Published in February 1950, a leading article in *The Lancet* under the heading of 'Atomic Defence' delivered a cautionary message about approaching the medical consequences of an atomic attack with any kind of optimism. It referred to American studies as to the medical resources which might be involved if the treatment of casualties on the scale of destruction delivered by the Hiroshima and Nagasaki bombs became necessary. These had killed some 99,000 people, but the two explosions also left an estimated 94,000 casualties with serious injuries of which 34,000 constituted severe burns cases due to the phenomenon of heat flash. Considering the problem this posed for mass compassion, the article suggested it could take 170,000 'professional persons' involving doctors, nurses and technicians, and some eight thousand tons of medical supplies (enough to fill a Liberty ship) at a cost of ten million dollars just to deal with one aspect of treatment. Adding to the impossible balance sheet, a further study concluded a single bomb of the Hiroshima type would create a need – within the first twenty-four hours – for 300 first-aid teams, 500 stretcher-bearer teams, 400 casualty-collection points and 24 neuro-psychiatric centres. *The Lancet* warned any idea of establishing a medical system to cope with that kind of casualty problem could not be seriously entertained and counselled that whilst deterrence policy might be designed to prevent war, 'it is as well that everyone should realise what is involved in the 'atomic defence' of which some politicians speak so glibly'.[8]

In a riposte to that conclusion, Sir Ernest Rock Carling admonished *The Lancet* for making so much of the American arguments. According to his view, they amounted to defeatism. He argued good preparations such as the introduction of shelters and dispersal plans, plus the fact British buildings offered better protection would all help in reducing the casualty list to manageable proportions.[9] Carling's persuasive powers were considerable. A testament as to just how much so could be gauged in the way *The Lancet* in its December 1950 edition had by then done a complete somersault and agreed the medical profession were capable of leading the country to nuclear salvation. Caught in the spirit of optimism the medical journal had just months before precisely warned against, it now conceded: 'Man's tolerance of adversity is always greater in the event than in the forecast; during the last war civilians in Britain – and in other countries as well – shouldered calmly a far greater burden of anxiety and hurt than had been thought possible without disintegration of the social structure. No doubt the same would happen in the even more dangerous conditions of a new war'.[10] From a timing point of view, the about-turn could not have been more opportune because it coincided with the setting-up of the 'the nuclear health service' across the United Kingdom.[11]

Factoring the National Health Service into the 'adversity' circumstances mentioned by *The Lancet* must have appeared more easily manageable by comparison to the medical preparations of the last war. On the face of it, the organisation had all the right makings of a convenient entity capable of rollout to provide a highly-efficient wartime service. Not only did it now have the benefit of common management structures, a crucial change had also occurred to the way first aid services were to be organised. During the Second World War local authorities had been in charge of setting up first aid posts as part of their Home Front preparations. They scattered these around target areas manned by volunteer doctors and nurses to ensure swift support for casualties wherever they might occur. Subsequently, under the *Civil Defence Act 1948*, the responsibility for all aspects of first aid passed to the National Health Service, which enabled the working party to impose their own ideas on the hospital side without becoming involved in the inevitable wrangles that local politics could otherwise bring.[12]

Given this new level of planning latitude, the only question remaining concerned how much of that was going to affect the plans, particularly when the NHS was still very much in the process of its physical formation.

Notwithstanding the atomic bomb age had arrived, the timeline for facing its possible consequences looked comparatively leisurely. The Chiefs of Staff had declared the atomic threat not to be immediate and confidentially decreed the Soviets would need some time before they could develop a Hiroshima-type bomb and manufacture it in sufficient quantities to mount a war against the West. Three phases were set, one might say in strategic stone, which the Home Office, as the lead Ministry on civil defence distributed to all other Whitehall departments for planning purposes. Phase I, fixed between 1949 and 1951, assumed a possible attack by high-explosive and incendiary bombs on the same scale experienced during the Second World War, with guided missiles of the V-1 type used after two months of war. Mustard gas still appeared as a possibility, but the threat of biological war regarded as improbable. During Phase II, reckoned to be between 1951 and 1955, the prospect of mass destruction weapons being employed could not be ruled out. But the critical line came in Phase III, beginning from 1957 onwards, when mass destruction weapons would be available to the enemy in 'adequate quantities' and it was essential for full atomic readiness to be in place.[13]

Though history soon consigned the prediction to the outrageously optimistic, at the time relief over the breathing space offered was palpable. Most Whitehall departments simply brushed off their last war plans to comply with the initial stage. Throughout World War II, hospitals in areas thought to be at risk from bombing evacuated their chronically sick and other patients, but the exercise did not occur primarily to conserve medical resources. Rather it reflected the operational objective of the day to ensure casualty beds were always available close to the scene of attacks and enable the provision of treatment without undue delay. Heavy civil defence precautions appeared, including sand bagging, protecting windows with wire to prevent glass splinters and using asbestos sheeting in roof areas against incendiary bombs. Despite the fact that clearance of upper floors took place, the essential idea of immediacy always remained.[14] Special arrangements applied in London. Hospitals in the capital were evacuated adopting a segment based plan that fanned out into the countryside.[15] Nonetheless, in all these plans the principle prevailed that casualties would receive care at a hospital situated near to the scene of destruction and their transfer arranged only sometime after.

Based on past practice the working party could, therefore, have quite reasonably revived such protocols thereby leaving the atomic attack problem closer to 1957 to resolve. In 1949, postponing the inevitable must have seemed a highly tempting proposition rather than wrestling with the more distant prospect of mass destruction by atomic bombs and the sheer scale of complexity and upheaval involved. The decision the subcommittee took reflected a clarity of thought rarely encountered in

Whitehall during those early years. Instead of ignoring the atomic threat, they chose to deal with the situation by adopting the 1957 perspective that meant imposing the circular ring of territorial destruction produced by an atomic bomb of the Hiroshima-type as their foundation for planning purposes. Phases I and II were then to be managed within that geographical ring until the full atomic Phase III conditions were necessary to accommodate.[16] Therefore the way forward very much depended on deciding how much phasing should be undertaken within that circle both in staff numbers, patients and equipment.

Unhappily, the position the subcommittee faced seemed viciously unforgiving, even in the use of conventional weapons. These had acquired a vocabulary such as 'de-housing' or 'carpet bombing', referring to the underlying objective to destroy civilian morale and not just industry. Moreover, conventional weapons were taking on a new dimension and no longer simply assessable against the destruction experienced by Britain during the last war. The sense of frustration encompassing the working party is evident in their view about the term 'killed'. This could be easily defined, but the description 'seriously injured' had become more blurred because of so many complicated medical cases expected to occur as a result of surprise attacks by the successors to the German rockets or through the increased weight of bombs likely to be used in the way described.[17]

Eventually, the Ministry of Health itself suggested a figure of 300,000 casualty beds would meet the circumstances of Phase I and allow a suitable margin. Admitted to be 'necessarily speculative', the number did actually possess a historical pedigree of some consequence.[18] During the early stages of the Second World War, the Emergency Medical Services in England and Wales had planned to provide up to a total of 500,000 hospital beds of which 300,000 were reserved specifically for casualties.[19] Those numbers necessarily represented a pessimistic set of medical mathematics that reflected predictions about a possible massive onslaught by the Germans which would result in 52,000 casualties a day, of whom at least 22,000 would need hospitalisation. Providentially, the expected attacks on the scale initially envisaged never materialised and the casualty beds reduced at the end of 1940 by nearly 100,000.[20]

Notwithstanding the Ministry's view founded on experience, the working party itself remained sceptical any kind of finite figure was possible to regard as adequate. Britain had stood up to conventional warfare during the Blitz by the spacing of bombardments that allowed for recovery time, but the new forms of mass destruction, especially the atomic dimension created an unforgiving situation on an unimaginable scale. The prospect of thousands of casualties created in seconds effectively extinguished the luxury of 'recovery time' altogether.

Furthermore, the impact of immediate radiation added an almost impossible dimension. A team of specialists had visited Japan to study the atomic bomb explosions and report on the distribution and types of casualties produced by the new weapon. If applied to the medical problem in Britain, their findings indicated casualty plans would need radical rethinking. On a densely populated area the gruesome reckoning suggested a Hiroshima size bomb would cause at least 30,000 fatalities instantly and a further 50,000 casualties, of which roughly one third would eventually die. Although the estimate of the number of atomic bombs the United Kingdom might have to face remained unclear, considered opinion suggested even a small number would be catastrophic for the UK health services. The inescapable fact thus emerged that hospital bed numbers and atomic warfare no longer held any kind of valid relationship and the situation would depend on the medical resource which was there and capable of being brought into operational use quickly.[21]

Caught in a situation where the future looked impossibly horrific, whether conventional weapons or atomic bombs were dropped on the UK, it led the medical subcommittee to the inescapable observation 'the total number of beds needed by casualties would never be available in existing hospitals, even if they were expanded at a satisfactory rate'.[22] Exasperated as to the prospect of ever coming to grips with the problem, their difficulties increased with the unexpected Russian explosion of an atomic bomb on 29 August 1949, made possible by the espionage activities of Klaus Fuchs.[23] At first, the event seemed to answer the question that planning for any kind of conventional war had no further validity. Despite that the timescale demanded by the Home Office held fast, even though a revised estimate by the Chiefs of Staff overlaid the original assessment with a greater destructive potential during May of the same year. A total of 10,000 tons of bombs had been dropped on Britain during the peak attacks of September 1940, but the new projection, disconcertingly considered 30,000 tons, might be used in the first month of a war rising to 40,000 tons in the second month, with even the possibility of 'a few atomic bombs' being used.[24]

Against this ever-growing uncertainty, the working party began their examination of just how much stretch capability existed in the National Health Service. The task of putting together the first ever assessment fell to a Scottish doctor, also a member of the subcommittee. Dr John Smith had recently joined the Scottish Health Department after a war career that included writing the medical plans for the D-Day Landings.[25] Having put his mind to the problems of the new and intimidating battleground, Smith dispatched his ideas to London during May 1949. He declared no bed numbers at this stage since the NHS was very much in its early days of formation, but did outline some basic principles for consideration. Three fundamental elements came into his submission built up from the support 'the general surgeon' could provide. Following an extensive study of military and civil practices, the most promising answer to the mass casualty problem appeared in the structure used by the military Field Surgical Teams. These consisted of one surgeon, one anaesthetist, plus theatre staff, designed to cover 12 operations per 8-hour shift. Observing they dealt mainly with gunshot wounds, which might turn out to be relatively minor or more major, Smith considered the procedure capable of translation into civil defence practice to conduct at least one operation per hour. The equation thus allowed some reserve potential if a high proportion of cases were relatively minor. Secondly, and key to stretching the surgical and medical resource, the maximum sub-unit within a hospital capable of supervision by a single whole time surgical or medical specialist was to be 150 beds. Adopting this as a base figure, Smith proposed an ideal hospital unit should consist of 300 surgical beds and 150 medical, the latter to deal with non-surgical issues such as radiation or chemical injuries. The third element included building in flexibility across the new structure by requiring hospitals to prepare mobile surgical units and mobile transfusion teams so that these could be hived off to provide support to hard-pressed areas, should that become necessary.[26] Although mobile surgical units had appeared operationally in limited numbers during the last war, adopting them as a Cold War tactic envisaged their use as a means of taking over an operating shift in the form of a relief unit rather than additions to the numbers operating per shift, which had been their original intent.

Smith argued that with all these features knitted together and shift patterns for 24-hour surgery introduced by increasing the number of theatre tables, a workable system could be devised. Critically, the package was intended to leverage limited resources to save as many lives as possible within the 'golden hour' by the application of basic surgical techniques. The radical nature of the proposal is evident in the way his suggested cover allocated to one surgeon raised the eyebrows of the team's two most eminent specialists. Both Sir Ernest Rock Carling and Sir Claude Frankau initially considered the support one surgeon could give might be only in the region of 120 beds rather than the 150 proposed. Accordingly, they requested Smith to seek further advice on this point by approaching two surgeons who had experience of large hospitals during the last war. Notwithstanding that referral, the original calculations prevailed and upheld as the most efficient use of this critical resource.[27]

For all the logic the new operational patterns might have possessed to deliver an increase in hospital beds any hopes that this would provide a significant game-changing solution soon disappeared. Smith's principle that the system should still provide a high level of medical expertise at the operating table and adopted as the critical path was turning into a medical chimera. When provisional estimates suggested there were to be about 2,500 general surgeons in England and Wales, plus 300 in Scotland, Smith applied this to his working model. Combined with specialists, registrars and anaesthetists he considered that on the ratio of 2 acute beds to 1 medical bed, it would be possible to staff 200,000 surgical beds and 100,000 medical beds south of the border and 24,000 and 12,000 respectively in Scotland.[28] Not surprisingly, the result came as a blow and greeted with complete dismay since it offered little more than the casualty bed numbers proposed at the start of the Second World War.

More bad news was not far behind. Smith also had to warn his colleagues of the possibility that the bed numbers might suffer further reductions as the Armed Forces grappled with their medical requirements in the new era of mass destruction weapons. At first, the medical working party reacted by deliberating whether any alteration or extension of the peacetime training programme for 'specialists' required consideration. Several ideas came in for discussion including the possibility of specialists receiving training for a dual function, one more valuable in peace than war and the other the opposite way around.[29] Just when the National Health Service 'stretch' factor seemed impossibly limited, Sir Alexander Hood intervened and questioned whether the operational conclusions actually represented the complete picture. Whilst acknowledging the capacity of the NHS might only provide for a core of 300,000 casualty beds in England and Wales, Hood noted this depended on the supervision of a surgeon covering 150 beds. Drawing on his own experience, he expressed doubts whether a patient needed to have no more than 10 or 11 days under such direct attention and suggested the pattern of support, albeit already diluted, was capable of further stretch at this point. Patient transfers to recovery beds within ten miles of acute hospitals, Hood felt, could be 'staffed by newly qualified housemen or elderly doctors not physically capable of more strenuous duties'. Based on such an arrangement, with specialists then having to make only periodic visits to the recovery units, the NHS, according to the General, could expand casualty beds to a total of 450,000 or more.[30]

With everything riding on this further step into radical territory, another serious disappointment seemed in prospect. The average wartime stay in hospital involving seriously injured casualties suggested Hood's figure was seriously optimistic. For civilians the average had amounted to 35 days and 30 days in respect of Service patients. On this occasion, Sir Claude Frankau came to the rescue pointing out that many civilians, though suffering trivial injuries, had also been put into the chronically sick category and could not be discharged quickly. (No doubt a reflection of the pre-NHS era) With military battle casualties, transfers to convalescent homes had often not been necessary because there was no pressure on hospitals to free up space and it was more convenient to keep them in situ. Taking these and other circumstances into account, Frankau concluded that the length of stay assumption could be accepted.[31] So, with this last hurdle overcome, the Ministry of Health accepted the 'stretch' thesis in its entirety. In order to adhere to the phasing principles linked to the Chiefs of Staff attack assumptions the Department also considered the idea of prioritising the evacuation of beds, patients, and staff to keep disruption to a minimum until the full atomic Phase III position arrived. Under this arrangement, each target would be ranked against its risk of being attacked from 1 to 3 and the evacuation completed partially or fully according to the factor applied.[32]

Having tested out the theory of partial evacuation, however, the proposal appeared highly problematic in maintaining the operational efficiency of hospitals under a reduced staffing complement. Consequently, the Ministry of Health took a decision of enormous importance and discarded approaching the phasing strategy in that way. In other words, the plan now proposed the evacuation of the entire hospital service in all zones designated potential targets and in just a single step. The Ministry clearly regarded the change as their crucial stress test of organisational capability; a view recorded when a junior civil servant remarked with some concern that the revision involved a 'formidable task'. Very much confirming that sentiment, Under-Secretary Sydney Wilkinson responded: 'Thank you. I agree the Senior Administrative Medical Officers will have a formidable task. But we cannot reasonably set the ceiling any lower – for Phase III it will probably have to be raised. It is as well that everybody should face the problem right at the start.'[33]

The only consolation in respect of the immense task that awaited RHBs was that to put the plans in place, Hospital Groups could appoint professional Civil Defence Officers in a similar way local authorities also relied on such appointments for coordinating their civil defence services. Badly paid, the job usually attracted ex-military men who wished to supplement their Service pensions. Amongst their chief attributes to do the job were adaptability and a personable presence especially to gain the confidence of hospital staff at many levels, particularly matrons. At first appointments of this kind were mandatory, but later made compulsory.[34] Whilst a small gesture in itself, the move firmly embedded the Whitehall propaganda machine into the hospital system. As senior officers, they would have attended the new Civil Defence Staff College established at Sunningdale, near Ascot in Berkshire, its purpose being to provide training and study into the higher direction of civil defence. Signifying the centre of excellence, reflected by a classical building constructed in the 1830s with grounds to match, it became the hub of much development of medical nuclear tactics in the rarefied atmosphere of deferential duty the edifice exuded.

Atomic Compassion

When the planning blueprint was ready, 'the nuclear health service' started to be built circular by circular. These orders told Regional Hospital Boards how they were to prepare for evacuating everything out of the designated target areas and stretch their hospital resources according to the Carling plan. Behind the project, however, the vital point remained that the medical aspects team had created a comparatively high level treatment service, until it faced a full atomic attack. After that the plan would inevitably default to a resource allocation service for casualties or as Carling's team had succinctly put it, 'that proportion representing the maximum number which can be treated by the available doctors'.[35] Under those conditions, the proposals did anticipate the eventual problem of abandonment, the deficiency only possible to mitigate by a greater number of doctors and surgeons applied to the problem. However, this difficulty must have seemed rather in the nature of a distant issue, particularly with more pressing concerns over a war in Southeast Asia looming in the background.

Delayed by the General Election, the 'formidable task' dropped into the laps of the Regional Hospital Boards on 23 May 1950 just days before the start of the Korean War. Obviously, the situation added an incredibly sensitive dimension with the danger of the hospital plan receiving its baptism of fire sooner rather than later. No direct reference to that prospect appeared, but the way secrecy prevailed, no doubt to avoid panic, the possibility must have been at the forefront of the Ministry's mind. Marked 'Strictly Confidential', only Chairmen, Senior Administrative Medical Officers, Treasurers and Secretaries of Regional Boards received the instruction for attention and Chairmen and Secretaries of Boards of Governors for information. Although the circular described the project as a long term strategy, it still contained distinctive hallmarks of a mobilisation crash plan with certain steps requiring action 'without delay'. These included the grouping of hospitals within each Regional Hospital Board for operational purposes, the designation of Group Officers and the choice of new wartime headquarters where necessary.[36]

On the day of issue, the instructions still attached a high degree of optimism the plan represented only the initial phase where the full treatment potential of the hospital service could be relied on, a matter expressed in the following crucial narrative:

> As the weapons that could be used in the enemy air attack become more destructive the potential need for casualty beds will steadily increase. Ultimately the number of beds that could be provided will be limited by the number of doctors and nurses available. Before that limit is reached, however, the determining factors would be the amount of accommodation that could be set aside and equipped for hospital purposes and the number of beds it could contain. The present aim is a total of 450,000 acute, sick and recovery beds in England and Wales outside the central zones of the target areas. This provision would be for both civilian and Service casualties and for the sick. It is exclusive of, and additional to, the number of beds required for the chronic sick, tuberculosis, maternity, fever, mental and mental deficiency patients.[37]

Whilst this simple statement should have been a matter of routine intent, fate turned it into a defining moment of just how unpredictable planning for the Cold War was turning out to be. On the very same day as the hospital memorandum went out to the RHBs with its comforting overtones, Cabinet Ministers responsible for civil defence received the news that the attack appreciation of the Chiefs of Staff had profoundly changed since their last phasing assessment. In the period up to the end of 1951, hitherto called Phase I, they considered there could no longer be any guarantee of immunity from a significant attack by atomic bombs. The statement ended with the sobering thought: 'In the very worst possible case sufficient atomic bombs might be launched against the United Kingdom to cause widespread devastation'.[38]

Suddenly the new realities meant the hospital plan involved the means to take good care of the few at the expense of the countless many. There were boundaries the planners had simply been unwilling to cross in the dilution of medical care. While the proposals assumed a high turnover of casualties, they still envisaged specialist support of all kinds somewhere within the system, a fact very evident in the way Smith had approached the stretch issue. Strategically, the objective remained to investigate radiation injury, cover orthopaedics, neuro-surgery, thoracic surgery, ophthalmology, and all manner of other medical provision.[39] The only possible give in the system was rather left to the realm of informality which might involve choosing to treat casualties at the expense of the sick or simply by abandoning certain classes of casualty altogether. However, not a jot of that prospect appeared in a codified form because it would have meant breaching the all-important mantra of substantive care for all. The Phase I plan, thus conveniently mutated into the full atomic plan, not to mention a grand illusion, which would become the object of staunch defence over the next few years.

Carling's 'nuclear health service', of course, provided the perfect vehicle to follow that route, though even its basic principles were equally becoming a monument to wishful thinking. When Regional Hospital Boards received their instructions about the atomic framework part of the plan under a separate and 'secret' Defence Memorandum these did everything to provide every reassurance possible. It advised RHBs that the bomb did not represent the absolute terror weapon able to destroy everything in one explosion. Atomic bombs were still based on the technical jargon of 'the nominal' bomb with a power of 20 kilotons as used against Hiroshima and Nagasaki. Accordingly, the memorandum piled on the comfort that despite their terrible consequences, they did not possess the power to destroy the larger British cities at a single stroke and the area of intense damage would be contained within a circle of one mile in radius drawn from ground zero. Further encouragement to prevent despondency came with the information atomic bombs were difficult and costly to make and therefore their use would be limited. On that basis, the choice and extent of 'key areas' likely to suffer an atomic attack reflected the need of an enemy to maximise damage either through hitting economic targets or dense population to undermine morale, or both.[40] So given these working assumptions, the key areas were those indicated on Map 1.

Following agreement on the target plan based around the GZ points chosen, wartime hospitals were to receive a designation according to their risk exposure to blast and heat flash and post attack operational use. Those premises situated inside the damage ring faced closure with patients discharged or transferred to establishments in safer areas, along with their staff and equipment. Some on the fringes of the ring of destruction would be designated *Casualty Transit Centres* to deal with street, factory, railway and other accidents as well as acute cases, where a delay in transportation outside the target zone might be dangerous to the patient. Centres of this kind had to operate in parts of the building that provided protection such as in basement areas supported by medical teams taking shifts and necessarily risking their lives in that process if they ended up at the unit when the bombs fell.[41]

Allowing for the power of the bomb and potential error in Soviet bomb aiming, *Cushion Hospitals* caution suggested, required a location of not less than 4 miles from ground zero to receive immediate casualties and idealistically give a continuing service to the acute civilian sick. Urgent surgical resources to save life would be provided, but in order to free up beds for other casualties as quickly as possible patients requiring prolonged specialist treatment were to be transferred further back to *Base Hospitals*. Rules for their siting recommended a distance of not less than 15 miles from the target area allowing some to be organised with special centres offering neurosurgical, thoracic and orthopaedic facilities. Underlining the completeness of these units, they were to be fully equipped with rehabilitation facilities to support long stay cases with convalescent and recovery hospitals included in the package.[42]

Using that specification, Regional Hospital Boards had to conduct a desktop exercise by 31 July 1950 and detail the numbers of beds, supported with plans and data, they could individually contribute towards the national objective.[43] To find bed spaces for those lost in the evacuation of target areas, hospitals outside were to make up some of the difference by discharging up to 50% of their acute patients and crowding the bed complement in wards by 10%. In an expansive statement of intent, the Ministry of Health provided a list of potential long and short-term measures aimed at bringing together the new premises resource:

Expanding in advance suitable existing hospitals

Converting, or using beds in fever, chronic sick, tuberculosis and mental hospitals and mentally deficient hospitals

Converting to hospital use convalescent homes and large nursing homes

Converting other suitable buildings such as ex-American hospitals, large boarding schools and holiday camps

Reducing admissions of civilian sick, and shortening the period of stay in hospital

Increasing the number of beds in staffed wards[44]

Once all the results of the study were gathered in, Senior Administrative Medical Officers and their deputies received orders to attend a course at the Civil Defence Staff College on the wartime hospital and first aid service, followed by a conference at the Ministry of Health in London. Records of the event reveal the administrators took the opportunity to protest about the large amount of wartime planning involved given that they were in the throes of establishing the NHS itself.[45] Well may they have complained. The level of detail amounted to an astonishing catalogue of information needing conversion into operational plans around the objective of saving staff and patients together with as much equipment as possible. Regional Boards had already conducted surveys to ascertain the storage potential for items scheduled to be removed. They were then also required to make returns of the equipment, staff and patients due for transfer so that a detailed assessment could be made of the total transport requirements across the entire country. At the beginning of 1952, the overall picture suggested that taking an average profile of patient categories at least 52,400 patients would need evacuation on stretchers and 17,660 sitting cases. The staff complement scheduled for evacuation amounted to 70,060 personnel along with a lorry requirement to transport some 11 million cubic feet of equipment, high on the list being any portable X-ray equipment capable of movement elsewhere.[46]

The woes of hospital administrators did not end with that assignment and another problem arose due to the numbers of 'special patients' sited in target zones requiring transfer, but with little prospect of alternative accommodation being immediately available. A glimpse of just one such example is in a request made by the Senior Administrative Medical Officer of the North East Metropolitan Hospital Board in Southern England to the Senior Administrative Medical Officer of the Eastern Regional Hospital Board in Dundee during December 1950. The Metropolitan SAMO set out very persuasively the predicament that in his densely-populated area, finding enough space had become impossible. Using the medical categories of the day he asked whether 7,000 mental patients, 2,000 tuberculosis patients, 1,500 mental defectives, 4,000 chronics, and 500 epileptics could be evacuated to Scotland.[47] Unfortunately, the moral vision of mass compassion supporting the mentally and seriously ill also had a particularly difficult impact north of the border. Many mental institutions were located inside target areas and in Glasgow, the incidence of tuberculosis added to the complications of finding alternative space. Special attempts followed to secure accommodation in single units for TB patients and avoid splitting up what were termed respiratory and non-respiratory units. Gleneagles, the Scottish golf club resort came into the frame as the preferred location for this purpose. It was just one example of many that really pointed to the kind of problem areas being encountered in the north, which meant taking on those south of the border simply remained out of the question.[48]

All these complications required urgent resolution with the final objective of constructing the new hospital framework itself and even this side of planning had its own special problems. Economies of scale were important in terms of gaining the fullest benefit of the surgical support Carling's team had laid down as the standard. Instructions confirmed the minimum hospital unit was to be 450 beds made up of three 150 sub-units or more. In addition, further resource capability had to be squeezed out of the system, given mass destruction weapons meant the demise of recovery time for dealing with the enormous number of casualties that would occur with indecent speed. Based on the highly optimistic assumption attacks would not occur on every designated target with the same ferocity, or at all, each hospital unit needed to have a mobile surgical team available that could be peeled off and support harder-pressed areas, if necessary. To accommodate those additional teams, frontline acute hospitals were to provide two, or if possible, three, operating tables that would allow the surgical challenge to be met head-on.[49]

In the order of medical battle, cushion hospitals on the periphery of the target zones would receive the first wave of casualties with resident surgeons dealing with that influx. If they found themselves at breaking point, then the mobile teams would play their part to alleviate the situation. Attaining a high level of casualty throughput was deemed absolutely essential which involved the transport of patients to base hospitals as soon as they were fit enough to be moved. Regional Hospital Boards initially received orders to maintain 150,000 acute beds in cushion hospitals on the front line to undertake the quick primary surgery and site the remaining 300,000 beds in base hospital areas. Then, during October 1950, that frontline capability came in for a review and drastically reduced it to 75,000 acute beds, a change that demanded 375,000 beds of all kinds, from recovery to acute being located much further back. The instruction claimed this allowed a more comprehensive spread of secondary treatment in the chain, but in reality it probably reflected the distribution of hospitals and that a great many acute units were simply not conveniently available next to the edge of the target zone.[50]

By its very nature the plan placed a huge reliance on inter-hospital transfers to process patients in the numbers envisaged. A great deal of appropriate iconography appeared to secure the operational validity of the scheme, particularly using 'ambulance coaches' which had strong resonance with the last war. Supporting that idealistic aim involved requisitioning most of the country's fleet of single-decker Greenline coaches and racking them out to carry eight stretchers. As a result, 1,270 of these vehicles were scheduled to be stationed across England and Wales and 130 in Scotland.[51] Also, in the halcyon days of rail, before the 'Beeching cuts' emasculated the network, hospital trains also still carried much symbolic value. Plans were prepared for 47 to operate in the United Kingdom each equipped to carry 284 casualties with 40 allocated to civilian needs, compared to the 30 used in the last war and 7 reserved for Service patients. Agreement regarding the design of the train was reached during 1953 that allowed for a capacity for 284 patients and a staff of 37 including the medical and nursing support, but not the train crew. In the prevailing belief a long warning period would still be available, the proposal also came with an understanding the actual conversion of railway rolling stock into ambulance trains would not be undertaken before the threat of war. The Railway Executive nevertheless requested detailed plans be prepared in advance, estimating it would involve 10,000 man-hours and translated the project in terms of requiring 11 men over six months, costing about £2,000 to complete.[52]

To throw a greater number of doctors at the atomic problem, the Ministry of Health commissioned a study to look at the possibilities of importing surgeons and doctors from overseas. But when completed, the exercise proved to be a catalogue of negativity. The report noted that although 300 Irish medical students finished their medical training in Great Britain every year, they left the country before becoming liable for National Service. In any event, the paper wryly concluded, few would be prepared to give their support to the UK. Referring to the chances of securing American doctors the report expressed the view levels of pay were not attractive enough to make it a tempting proposition. It caustically added wartime experience had shown that generally those who had not been able to make good in their own country had been allowed to practice with the result some turned out to be useless or 'positively dangerous surgically'. The Canadians had declined to make any commitments on the grounds they would require all the medical support they could muster. As to the Europeans, experience suggested this could be a hazardous route with a distinct health warning that with Germans, Austrians, Czechs and Poles, 'few of them had good command of English and the majority's ignorance of the language and their accent caused resentment among their patients'. Reference to their medical ethics also came in for comment and the fact these equally 'often caused resentment among British practitioners'. Altogether, the outcome could not have been clearer in confirming 'no significant reinforcement of our own medical manpower can therefore be expected from overseas and planning must proceed on this basis'.[53]

Unfortunately, the position regarding the provision of surgical support for the hospital plan deteriorated ever further. At a meeting held on 12 September 1950 between the working party and senior medical representatives of the Armed Forces, the military confirmed their requirements would reduce the general surgeon numbers available for civil defence from the figure then standing at 2,395 to only 2,066. Sifting through for grains of comfort the planners observed that there were 'thought to be' some 8,626 'specialists' and noted in the case of anaesthetists and other medical practitioners the situation did not seem to cause concern. Any relief soon vanished with the further discovery that only 455 radiologists could be called on, representing a shortfall of 43, along with a serious deficit of house officers which would have to be supplemented by general practitioners and final year students.[54]

The nature of the calculations and the anxious attempts made to balance the debits and credits through the minutiae of functional detail were pointing to the impossibility of stemming the tide of mass destruction with rigid medical hierarchies and providing a holistic medical service. Just a few months later, the tipping point came when the position really turned into a resourcing nightmare emphasised by a more specific statement on what an attack by atomic bombs meant. During March 1951, the Civil Defence Joint Planning Staff prepared an atomic bombing pattern of 20 selected targets and instructed this new appraisal required immediate incorporation into operational plans. (Appendix 1) Although an attempt to impose more certainty on the planning environment, it amounted to confirming the unmanageable situation building up month by month. The top-secret paper admitted that the assessment only represented a sample pattern for a full-scale atomic attack aimed at centres of population combined with ports and warned the number of bombs could only be regarded as 'arbitrary' and the aiming points described as 'some among many'.[55]

Notwithstanding the potentially apocalyptic scenario presented, the Ministry of Health continued to send out messages that implied a comprehensive medical service would still be on offer. Taken together with their confession about the lack of professional resources to cover the predicated disaster made to the Defence Transition Committee, which was coordinating Britain's Cold War plans, this decidedly consigned their confidence to the realms of self-delusion. Even the number of beds originally prescribe for a Phase I war had become unachievable according to the somewhat incredible revelation:

> Although the primary aim continues to be to provide a minimum continuing service in specialist hospitals and, as soon as possible after the outbreak of war, to provide 450,000 beds in England and Wales and 55,000 in Scotland in general hospitals for the treatment of normal sickness and service and civilian casualties, investigation into the numbers of medical staff likely to be available within the next few years has shown that these 505,000 beds, about 370,000 could be adequately staffed at any one time. The usefulness of the available staff, however, could be considerably increased by the employment of mobile medical and surgical teams. It is unlikely that heavy attacks will fall simultaneously in every

> area and the 134,000 unstaffed but equipped beds would form a margin which could be brought into use by the deployment of staff from areas not under attack to assist those dealing with the influx of casualties from heavily attacked areas. Proposals for composition and use of mobile teams have been drawn up.[56]

Proposals for mobile surgical teams, only 'pencilled in' until then, were quickly finalised to deal with the problem of inadequate cover. Regional Hospital Boards received further instructions during November 1952 to establish a system of mobile surgical, mobile resuscitation and mobile medical teams with the intention these would go across the country to support other hospitals, if required. Expansive promises confirmed that in addition to giving assistance in surgical work the units would deal with patients afflicted by radiation sickness, infectious diseases and gas poisoning. Transport instructions were set out accordingly:

> For transport of mobile teams, medical staff should be encouraged to use their own private cars as much as possible; mileage allowances at the prevailing rates would be payable. If private cars were not available, Hospital Group Officers should arrange for First Aid Service vehicles to be used, or failing that, should ask the local authority to provide sitting case ambulance cars, if possible. Clearly, the vehicles provided by the First Aid Service or Ambulance Service for this purpose should be diverted from their proper role for as short a time as possible, and would have to return to their depots immediately after conveying it back to its own hospital.[57]

Procedural advice of this kind does illustrate how the atomic problem was succumbing to a process of 'normalisation', an approach prevalent on a much wider scale. Actually, it mirrored the way the Civil Defence Joint Planning Staff itself saw the situation. According to their view of the new world of mass destruction 'the nature' of the civil defence task was not the problem, but rather its size in relation to the resources required. The kind of mind-set that prevailed is evident in a pamphlet which the CDJPS started to draft (but never finished) for issuing to the public so they could form street parties and prepare to deal with the aftermath of an atomic attack, in much the same way communities had arranged mutual support during the Second World War. The process of defusing 'the bomb' came in the following reassurance:

> There are some exaggerated ideas about what an atom bomb can do. The radioactivity caused by an atomic explosion would not make a town uninhabitable for years or even weeks. It would usually be quite safe to enter the damaged area after only a few hours from the time of the explosion. One or two bombs, of the type dropped on the Japanese city of Nagasaki, would not destroy the whole of Greater London. To do this would require a very large number. Bigger bombs have been constructed. But even if there were a bomb 100 times as powerful as the Nagasaki type, it would not cause anything like as a 100 times the amount of damage. – The atom bomb is a terrible weapon which can do a great deal of destruction. But if we learn the truth about both its power and its limitations, we shall find that there is much that we could do even if we were attacked by atom bombs in a future war.[58]

Behind the statement lay the essential philosophy the Ministry of Health had themselves started to prescribe to medically rationalise coping with the destructive capacity of nuclear weapons and circumvent the problem of abandonment. Embracing that approach, Regional Hospital Boards received further directives to complete other parts of the hospital plan that projected some kind of business as usual. A particularly sensitive issue related to wartime radiotherapy arrangements. Casualties were to have priority, with any spare capacity used thereafter for other purposes. Cancer patients were unlikely to receive any treatment other than nursing. Circulars laid out all kinds of possibilities relating to saving equipment, transferring it, along with sharing facilities between hospitals. An initial audit of resources suggested most regions had enough hospitals outside target areas equipped for radiotherapy to provide a wartime standard. In its most basic form the strategy envisaged that where there were no hospitals outside key areas with appropriate facilities already, then one or two suitable establishments needed to be selected with a view to moving in some smaller equipment. Even so the Ministry forbade any building work in preparation, other than the provision of a power supply that would attract a civil defence grant. Additionally, radium and radioactive isotopes held by hospitals in key areas were to be stored in boreholes, as in the last war, with hospitals to make the appropriate arrangements.[59]

As impressive as the instructions were in their comprehensiveness, they possessed the usual pattern of contradictions that cloaked the scheme with a high degree of misplaced hope. In theory, the plan aimed to establish radio diagnostic services in cushion hospitals to undertake the detection of foreign bodies, fractures, head and chest injuries, as well as blast effects. Acute hospitals sited at base areas further back were to run a full diagnostic service described as 'comparable with that provided in a general hospital under normal conditions', though only one radiologist was likely to be available. The estimated disruption time of electricity supplies forecast a failure lasting 48 hours after an attack and with that prognosis the instructions stretched the functional optimism even further. Hospitals, the Ministry of Health suggested, would need to rely on mobile units with generators and to turn that into a workable proposition confidently predicted the demand for such equipment would not be required simultaneously, so the best use of it had to be made at the time.[60] Underpinning that precept, radiologists were, therefore, to receive training across several types of unit in order they would not be confronted by the unfamiliar in the conditions forecast.[61] Altogether, this kind of layering created a vision of unfathomable positivity not only applied to the radiology side, but which also pervaded every aspect of the hospital plan to secure its resilience. In that way each perceived gap in care was covered, which in turn subordinated hopelessness and allowed mass compassion to remain as an aspirational ethical value.

Normal Service

The kind of codes of practice described were imposing an institutionalised normality on the abnormality of atomic war and in the process maintained the integrity of Carling's high-level medical care plan. This in turn set the tone for the standards throughout the casualty chain. Each casualty, especially the seriously injured, needed assurance of prompt and competent medical attention similar to the standards of the last war. Symbolic structures, therefore, were necessary to apply with consistency to provide that degree of ideological support. Inevitably, this meant overcoming many obstacles, including a reluctance to change established procedures or the inherent jealousies still festering inside medical empires. Key to keeping focus on mass compassion were the changes made to the arrangements in respect of the first aid services, a matter referred to previously. The National Health Service was to take over the responsibility in this area from the local authorities, who in World War II had set up first aid posts in schools and similar types of buildings in their ownership. Whilst giving comfort to local communities, the arrangement left many doctors and nurses awaiting their orders only to result in them being unemployed if the attack did not affect their sector. Ensuring waste on that scale never occurred again, static first aid services were to restrict their activities within general hospitals remaining after the evacuation procedures were completed and work in close conjunction with the casualty department, until required operationally. Rules laid down that one static facility for every 50,000 of the population should be provided for this purpose, principally on the periphery of target areas with 800 planned for England and Wales, the message being that scarce resources would not only be conserved, but applied principally to serious casualties.[62]

New ways of securing quick attention to the casualties outside the hospital also needed consideration. Bringing the hospital services to the injured through medical formations called Mobile First Aid Units appeared as a significant player in the nuclear organisation. Their introduction showed a classic example of small changes made during the Second World War subsequently being adapted to meet the new conditions of mass destruction. Before 1940, local authorities did have the option of supplementing their static first aid posts with a mobile facility, but not much happened in this direction until December 1941, after the major attacks on British cities had taken place. Only then did the Ministry of Health start to question the rigidity of the static post as the best means of using medical resources. More emphasis towards the provision of what were termed Light Mobile First Aid Units was then encouraged. These were to consist of a doctor, a trained nurse with a couple of auxiliaries who would go with simple portable equipment to incidents, possibly using the doctor's own car.[63] As the Blitz subsided, however, the concept did not develop much further. The Cold War really accelerated the need for mobility. In the new plan, Scotland received the support of 300 MFAUs[64] and 2,000 earmarked for England and Wales, figures not based on any estimate of the likely number of casualties, but considered the maximum number that were realistically affordable for that purpose. Establishment numbers now included one doctor, a trained nurse and nine nursing auxiliaries of the National Hospital Service Reserve. Transportation included a van to carry equipment, a station wagon or two light cars for personnel and a motor cycle for reconnaissance and communications. These units were to be centred on suitable general hospitals outside the hospital evacuation area staffed mainly through general practitioners in the locality to provide support with the allocations made shown in Table 1 reflecting the intensity of attack expected in each civil defence region.[65]

Table 1: Mobile First Aid Unit Support to Civil Defence Regions.

	Civil Defence Region	MFAU No.
1.	Northern	179
2.	E and W Riding	163
3.	North Midlands	121
4.	Eastern	66
5.	London	471
6.	Southern	97
7.	South Western	99
8.	Wales	109
9.	Midland	201
10.	North Western	303
11.	South Eastern	168

Source: NRS, HH 51/332. Civil Defence Training School, Taymouth Castle.

Although trained and staffed by local hospitals, the MFAUs came under the tactical control of Regional Commissioners, government representatives who would fight the battle for survival housed in their own bunkers. Deployment meant establishing MFAU posts wherever large aggregations of casualties appeared. Their prime purpose on mobilisation involved getting as close to casualty ring as possible and deal with what were termed 'walking casualties', the intention being to prevent hospitals being flooded and blocking facilities for the more seriously injured. Instructions characteristically promoted a string of positive medical outcomes that the unit would offer primary treatment, after which the casualty could then proceed to his own home and report to a general practitioner if further treatment or observation became necessary. Despite the fact that MFAUs might have to deal with some stretcher cases, the fundamental principle endured that those suffering serious injuries would be taken to loading points, lifted into ambulances and then transported to hospital.[66]

The revolutionary move against having static first aid posts dotted around a town was not greeted everywhere with enthusiasm and resulted in campaigns mounted against the new concept with considerable posturing. The worst case on record involved Dunbartonshire County Council which received support from their two Members of Parliament. A comment by the Health Department in Edinburgh summed up the position following a meeting that pointed to the situation developing from the personal prejudices of a senior official:

> It was quite apparent that the Council's attitude derived from strong personal views held by the Convenor. In the area in which he lives-Old Kilpatrick-static units had been very useful during the last war. He was clearly very reluctant to recognise that the conditions of a future war might be so different that a completely altered policy would be necessary.[67]

This reaction demonstrates just how far faith in the operational systems used during the last war still resonated around the whole culture of the nuclear Home Front. Without doubt Whitehall continued to be exceptionally sensitive about changing any comforting iconography unless absolutely necessary.

When looking at the iconic symbols that were to play their part in creating medical comfort zones, the ambulance represented one of the most inspirational to project the quick response to casualty needs. Invariably, it became the focus of much anxiety to maintain its clarity. The peacetime ambulance service was to be expanded by using the Ambulance Section of the Civil Defence Corps. The working party noted this principle had been adopted as the operational system of choice in deference to local councils who had staked their claim to take on the responsibility, in addition to keeping the fire service and the police under their control.[68] To cover their peacetime commitments, the *National Health Service Act, 1946* had given the County Councils and County Boroughs the option of delivering ambulance services direct by buying in ambulances and sitting cars as well as employing drivers and attendants, or indirectly through the voluntary organisations. Nonetheless, the position of even the peacetime ambulance organisation in 1948 was, to say the least, discouragingly grim. In England and Wales there were some 3,300 ambulances and of this total about 90% had more than ten years' service, or over 100,000 miles on the clock, which meant almost the entire fleet had gone past its normal life.[69] Carling's working party recognised the danger the dilapidated condition of the ambulance fleet posed and stressed the urgent need to build up the service to 4,000 modern vehicles within three years. A further recommendation suggested the purchase 1,000 commercial type lorries on behalf of local authorities to provide training vehicles for their volunteers in driving, conversion and loading on the basis these would represent the kind of vehicle obtained through the pre-attack requisitioning procedures.[70]

Scotland's organisation of the ambulance service differed in its management structure. During peacetime the Secretary of State for Health administered the service who delegated that authority directly to the five Scottish Regional Hospital Boards. In theory the Scottish hospitals, therefore, had ownership of ambulance service rather than local authorities. In practice, the greater portion of the service was, however, provided under agency arrangements by the St Andrew's Ambulance Association and the Scottish Branch of the British Red Cross Society. But, the differing pattern of management did not mean the vehicles themselves were in any better shape. The strength of the whole service in April 1949 amounted to 550 vehicles of which 60% were reckoned to be completely worn-out and mechanically unreliable, with an immediate need to provide the peacetime service with up to 600 modern vehicles.[71]

Apart from the urgent requirement to modernise the ambulance fleet across the country, Carling wanted much more done that would have involved extending the mantra of preparedness into aspects of everyday life. Proposals included manufacturers of commercial vehicles generally being encouraged to incorporate a standard form of chassis so it could be easily adapted to take the special racking fitments for stretchers and allow easy installation in the event of war.[72] Similarly peacetime ambulances, the working party suggested, ought to have a war related flexibility built in to allow their conversion to either vehicles for sitting cases or increasing their capacity from two to four stretchers. Above everything, however, emphasis was placed on the fact that modernisation of the existing fleet should be accepted as a matter of the utmost urgency, without any kind of financial constraint imposed by the Government's plans for national recovery.[73] As strange as that plea may have seemed, given the background described, many proposals were being rigorously judged against that benchmark of economic rehabilitation. An example that stands out is the impact of this policy on the type of stretchers that could be provided. It had been noted that the Americans used an aluminium frame which made them a lot lighter and less cumbersome. Even so, any ideas of converting the heavy wooden ones used by the British civil defence services were overruled on account of aluminium being regarded as 'an expensive dollar metal' and quite unaffordable in the climate of post-war austerity.[74]

Operationally, the position of the ambulance proved no less challenging to maintain its symbolic value. With the possibility all vehicles might require removal from target areas to protect them from atomic blast, much anxious debate followed. Before an attack, ambulances were required for evacuating hospital patients, as well as supporting casualty transit hospitals, duties that required a presence within the target area. Then, in the post-attack situation, they had to be available quickly to pick up casualties, in addition to being prepared to provide mutual aid to other areas. Adding a further complication, the possible disposition of depots far out in target areas then conflicted with the principle of rapid access to where casualties were likely to arise in peace. As a result, in that argument the siting of garages far away and even being put underground did not gain support both on the grounds of cost and potential conflict with peacetime priorities.[75]

Trying to deal with this bundle of competing priorities proved too much and in 1950 local authorities received a request to give consideration to their ambulance requirements by reference to the last war and the bomb conveniently forgotten. Even when revisions appeared the following year, the plan merely formalised the quandary by dispersing ambulances between local and main stations, with some on the periphery and some kept more central, all of which essentially reflected an unsolvable situation. The bagatelle of thoughts going in all directions as to where ambulances should be parked in peace and war reflected the weight of symbolism the vehicle represented, a matter clearly marked out in the ambulance training manual published in 1950:

> The speedy removal of air-raid casualties from the scene of damage to hospitals and places where they can receive skilled attention, is important not only from the humanitarian point of view but also because it plays a vital part in maintaining the morale of the public, which is essential to the successful conduct of the war. It should be remembered that the presence of ambulances at the scene of any catastrophe is regarded by the public as the outward and visible sign that help is present. This applies in both peace and war.[76]

Honourable as it might have been, the statement of intent amounted to a value becoming impossible to achieve. Early in 1951, Scotland advised the Ministry of Health of a serious 'gap' it considered existed in the casualty plan because of the segmentation of responsibilities between the first aid services of the hospitals and the rescue and ambulance services run by the local authorities. The specific task of the established rescue section of the Civil Defence Corps was restricted to giving first aid to casualties they had extricated out of the debris and, as for ambulance teams, they could not leave their vehicles. Neither did the MFAU concept run by the hospitals offer an answer. They were limited to operating at the very periphery of destroyed areas and similarly could not leave their established posts. Scotland contended this highly-compartmentalised system did not provide for the walking wounded receiving immediate attention before reaching a first aid unit, nor did it cater for the collection and giving succour to the wounded lying out in the open.[77]

Resolving the problem of the 'the gap' inconveniently raised a crucial test to prove exactly how the organisation could respond to the altering patterns of destruction which were occurring much faster than expected. An exercise called the 'London Tactical Study' confirmed the Scottish view the atom bomb had altered the tactical arrangements of the casualty chain. Ambulance journeys to cushion hospitals might be long and impeded by debris, leaving thousands of casualties unattended. 'The gap' raised the sceptre of abandonment and turned into the first threat encountered to the ideology of mass compassion.[78] Despite the fact that the situation signalled a need for urgent attention, the exercise to bridge it quickly turned out an abject failure. Domain jealousies now came into the reckoning. The possibility of casualty loading points, administered by the Medical Officers of Health and in effect becoming Mobile First Aid Unit points to cover the anticipated interruption in treatment raised a major obstacle. MFUAs were the responsibility of the Regional Hospital Boards and the possibility of the Medical Officers of Health either taking over their control or setting up another organisation altogether seriously grated with the autonomy already granted to the hospital organisation.

Only after endless debates as to who does what did the vital breakthrough occur in July 1954 and the official announcement was made: 'It is recognised that after a heavy attack large areas may be inaccessible to wheeled vehicles and bearers will be needed for the difficult and protracted task of carrying stretcher cases to ambulance loading points'. Proclaiming the painfully obvious necessarily hid the political wrangling, as did the solution. The Ambulance Section became the Ambulance and Casualty Collection Section and its detailed function finally prescribed in September 1955. The operational instructions set out a new deployment policy whereby casualty collecting personnel would 'mop up' the injured caught in the erstwhile 'gap'. They were to work in parties of seven, including a driver and a leader with a van capable of carrying the team, along with its supply of 32 stretchers, 64 slings and 64 blankets. A fleet of 4,500 vehicles suggested for use in England and Wales would go as far as road conditions allowed and casualties collected beyond the debris line and carried back to an ambulance loading point. Nor did the functional confidence end there. The model instructions suggested stretcher bearers might be assembled using members of the public or factory workers who would be organised into stretcher parties by the casualty collection personnel on the basis of four or six per stretcher depending on debris conditions.[79] These idealised structures thus ensured the casualty's position remained ideologically protected by guaranteeing hospitalisation and attendant professional care. Instructions dutifully emphasised the point further by stating casualty collection units could undertake some first aid, but any more advanced attention singularly discouraged on the grounds this would unnecessarily cause delays in the casualty reaching hospital. Appropriate to the somewhat perfunctory nature of the first aid proposed, the contents of first aid haversacks was confined to triangular and roller bandages, dressings, 3 cards of safety pins and a pair of scissors.[80] After years of agonising over 'the gap' every interest had received its due recognition, and if nothing else, maintained the sense of organisational cohesion.

The affair particularly revealed the underlying tensions within the medical domain. Operational efficiency might have been possible to attain for its own sake, but also risked bringing down the whole system like a house of cards. Moreover, for the purposes of the facade, domain jealousies actually worked in two important ways. It gave control to those who wished to preserve their authority and that eagerness could benefit the 'normalisation' process. Some of those tensions arose because of concerns that if certain protocols received approval for civil defence purposes they could eventually affect peacetime practice. Very much representing that kind of difficulty is the battle that erupted about which medical sector was to be responsible for maternity arrangements. Historically the position could not have been trickier as to whether it should fall to hospitals that were expanding their midwifery services or the Local Health Authorities who still ran a district domiciliary midwifery service. Initially, decisions favoured the latter because councils were also billeting authorities and able to offer a complete package of antenatal and postnatal accommodation arrangements in addition to maternity beds, at least if they were helped out by hospitals. The argument went that the arrangement could offer a seamless solution and facilitate the transfer of expectant mothers between maternity wards and hostels to avoid bed blocking, thus allowing hospitals to concentrate on the casualty problem.

So problematic did the issue of 'institutional confinement' become, it led to the Chief Medical Officer having to adjudicate because RHBs feared the introduction of such arrangements would eventually affect the NHS and threaten the development of obstetrics within hospitals. The final decision respected those concerns, but diplomacy still prevailed and although the hospitals were to be the main provider of maternity services in war, local authorities retained their responsibility for hostels and billeting.[81] A highly-complex paper plan to maintain an air of normality and institutional cohesion therefore resulted. Central to the whole plan hospitals outside the target areas were designated providers of maternity units of between 30 to 60 beds located as close to their established facilities as possible for normal confinements, but space reserved within the hospital itself for births likely to have complications.[82] Cast into such an institutional formwork, these maternity arrangements never changed.

Operational narratives were incredibly sensitive instruments in the politics of self-interest. They defaulted to organisational excellence and a contrived order which protected the integrity of hospital managements and through that their domain power. Very much working to that philosophy, the Senior Administrative Medical Officer remained at the heart of the hospital control framework and appropriate hierarchies established within the RHB area under his tutelage. For example, the massive potential pressure point on the frontline hospitals was recognised in 1952 and operational controls between cushion and base locations redefined. Reflecting the fact that casualties would pour into the hospitals at the front, guidance notes laid down Group Officers of cushion hospitals should have no more than two or three hospitals under their management and no more than 1,000 beds. At base hospitals, where the tempo of work might be slower, a Group Officer could have up to 2,000 beds under his jurisdiction. Their job description entailed the general operational working of the hospitals in his group, including the organisation of teams and rotas of staff, plus the allocation and economic use of beds crucial to the plan. Control over admissions, transfers and discharge of patients received particular emphasis. In reality, the list appeared to run into the realms of impossibility that included keeping his Senior Administrative Medical Officer advised of the bed situation, keeping the Secretaries of Boards up to date, maintaining contact with civil defence controls and arranging the reception of all inter-hospital transport. On top of those demands, the first aid service had to be organised, trained and deployed and in a moment of supreme optimism the instructions suggested, 'when not fully occupied by his operational duties he can take part in the clinical work of his hospitals'.[83]

Besides providing a virtual sense of empowerment to undertake the impossible, the specification of the kind quoted also reflected the exceptional planning focus on the hospital aspects of the atomic plan. Records of how this all affected hospitals directly have not survived well as most ended up being discarded when the hydrogen bomb arrived, making the national picture of progress necessarily sketchy. Fortunately, an example does exist for the Westminster Group of hospitals in London illustrating the kind of activity replicated across the country. Most of their hospitals were destined for transfer out to Park Prewett near Basingstoke, Hampshire, where the foundation of a thousand-bed acute hospital was due to take place in what had been an isolation unit and subsequently adapted to take mental patients under the *Lunacy and Mental Treatment Act*. As it happened, the choice of location did not come as unfamiliar territory. The Group had used it for one of the zone establishments during the last war to transfer Westminster's chronic patients and make room for air raid casualties in London. Members of the Westminster Hospital and Medical School staff paid two visits there during 1953 to consider the proposed arrangements. Their reports reflected the challenge of adapting a tired building with electrics and plumbing dating back to the First World War. Operating facilities were minimal, but a survey noted that to provide for the needs of a large acute unit, two large communal bathrooms were converted for this purpose during the Second World War and similar arrangements would probably have to follow in preparing for World War III.[84]

On the more positive side, Park Prewett came with its own farming estate and herds of cattle yielding 56,730 gallons of milk a year, a poultry farm supplying over a quarter of a million eggs plus an orchard and land turned to vegetables, all of which made the hospital a model of self-sufficiency. The facilities also received approval for the transfer of the medical school although rather on the lines that the premises would reflect the student position, the Dean caustically expressing his belief:

> It would probably be necessary to provide teaching facilities at the hospital in the country for not more than about 100 clinical students. The student population falls in time of war, and it is not advisable to try and increase the student numbers. The men and women coming forward for medicine in time of war are not usually of very high calibre as students.[85]

Back at Westminster Hospital in central London, the war plan required the incorporation of a casualty transit centre with 30 to 40 beds on the back of some hopeful assumptions. An explosion of a Hiroshima-size bomb anticipated over Trafalgar Square would, the theory suggested, seriously damage the structure above ground, but the hospital being at the limit of the range meant the steel framework of the building might hold with the basement giving considerable protection against the blast and gamma radiation. The heat flash problem could, the thinking went, be possible to mitigate by the removal of all inflammable items in line with windows or other openings. Then the core proposal involved transferring the unit to the basement area where a series of small rooms extended under the roadway. The layout appeared ideal for the possible separation of beds between men, women and children, with equipment provided by transferring the contents of a 32-bed surgical ward on the fourth floor. The only exception related to the first aid post, which was to function at ground floor level for as long as possible before taken below. Every aspect of converting the basement area into to a self-contained casualty transit centre, along with staff sleeping quarters, was included. For example, in the exercise the syringe laboratory became a preparation room for catering, whilst the cooking facilities themselves ended up in the sterile pharmaceutical products room. Additionally, the project incorporated the provision of emergency lighting and water along with all manner of risk assessments undertaken that included the possibility of flooding caused by ruptured water tanks and in the final event the entire hospital building being reduced to rubble leaving the occupants buried alive.[86]

Multiplying this kind of activity across the country could not have disabused the public of any major collapse in confidence on the part of the NHS to meet its wartime obligations. In reality, the medical plans and their optimistic overlays were falling quickly into the quicksand of hopeless endeavour caused by the advances in mass destruction then masked behind ambiguous phrases such as 'aerial warfare' and 'air attacks'. Undoubtedly, much of the positive thinking was down to the planning environment itself craving order and stability in the face of the unknown. By 1952, the hospital plan had combined into an incredible depiction of pre-ordained reactions. The achievement of imposing patterns of order on disorder had much to do with the way two events suddenly fused into a chase towards building 'the nuclear health service'. The first related to Carling's working party thinking laterally by not being tricked by the phasing mirage and incorporating the atomic ring of destruction as the base line for planning right from the start. The second situation came about because of the Korean War, the first armed conflict of the Cold War, which provided an impetus to an enormous amount of planning being undertaken. Any prevarication by hospital authorities, that the strains of setting up the NHS might have otherwise produced, could simply not become part of the equation.

Whitehall had been extraordinarily lucky that the medical venture continued to have all the right hallmarks of the caring and moral state as it moved with unexpected haste into the atomic arena. Instead of the hospital and casualty plan collapsing into some indeterminate level of weak medical care a new, dedicated Phase III structure might have otherwise brought, the Phase I promise of extensive care never changed. Three important principles kept that illusion intact. Firstly, mass-abandonment did not formally enter the hospital and casualty plan at any point and the resourcing shortcomings were glossed over with thick layers of functional optimism. Secondly, the system continued to project a commitment in its constituent parts to ensure it did not collapse under the weight of numbers and environmental difficulties. Lastly, the management of organisational friction also made a critical contribution with compromises made to ensure that self-interest politics did not cause a breakdown generated from within. An extraordinary allegory of medical hope therefore remained in place and proved the illusion of mass compassion was possible to project through the prism of the new National Health Service.

Chapter 2

COLD COMFORT WAR

The blessing given by *The Times* to the medical plan in 1951 held great significance, because it acknowledged the ethical framework that appeared to give support to as many casualties as possible. The medical aspects subcommittee had not set out, nor actually intended, to engage with constructing a deception, but the venture succumbed to patterns of change and these simply engulfed the enterprise. Charged with an awesome responsibility for delivering a system of mass compassion to the nation, failure in the production of a plan did not come as an option. Yet, from a position of sincerity, the proposals moved inexorably towards developing into a mythology and eventually adopted for their political value to deterrence policy. Looking at the way the Ministry of Health grew into that process is a matter for consideration to identify the critical stages of how government policy crossed that line between sincerity and subterfuge.

False Hopes

Managing 'sincerity symbolism' was by no means easy in the choices about the distribution of scarce capital resources to produce the best political impact. As mentioned in the previous chapter, the medical working party had stressed that an absolute priority, which they felt cut across any arguments over national recovery, related to the urgent replacement of civilian ambulances that were dilapidated through age and 'burnt out' by war operations. Accepted as part of the establishment of the NHS, their view prevailed and funding secured for the fleet to be modernised urgently. The position, on the other hand, regarding the provision of training vehicles for the civil defence volunteers could not have been more different. During 1949, the Ministry of Supply essentially put a damper on the idea in terms that left little hope:

> It will be very difficult for us to arrange priority for the delivery of these vehicles if their supply is left to take place through the normal trade channels. The position is that there is no priority in the delivery of commercial vehicles, distribution being left to the industry on the understanding that they

> will give preference wherever possible to the requirements of industries of national importance. We have consistently refused to grant priority for any special class of requirement and it would be embarrassing for us to do so even for so important a requirement of civil defence – and we could not make special arrangements quietly for such a large number of vehicles as apparently you would require.[1]

A Ministry of Health bid for up to 800 new training vehicles had been put on the table at an estimated production cost of almost half a million pounds. Confronted with ample evidence the country simply could not afford much in the way of supporting a decent training system for wartime purposes, the ministry surrendered without a fight. Instead, it settled on local civil defence units having to adapt any old vehicles they could lay their hands on.[2]

More difficult to hide behind the economic argument was the blood transfusion issue. Not only did blood signal survival, it represented an area where both the peacetime and wartime sides of the NHS would derive mutual benefit. Until the latter half of 1940, no comprehensive system of blood transfusion existed outside London, the service having relied on a mixture of arrangements including support by voluntary aid societies, private schemes, medical schools and municipal authorities. From there a more common and countrywide scheme resulted to provide standardised arrangements capable of being slotted into the Emergency Medical Services.[3] Ironically, the Cold War then became a catalyst for a further stage of modernisation in respect of country's blood supply network, a factor seen in the progress achieved during the first seven years. (Table 2)

A highly influential theory pertinent to that expansion of the Blood Transfusion Service came via an estimate used on radiological defence courses given at the Royal Naval Medical School, Alverstoke, Hampshire. This postulated a single atomic bomb of the Hiroshima type dropped on a typical British industrial town would produce 15,000 radiation casualties with many standing a good chance of recovery if hospitalised quickly. There was an awareness of the formidable logistical consequences. Calculations suggested the demand created by such an explosion could amount to 210,000 pints of blood and 420,000 pints of plasma for radiation casualties alone, even before dealing with the injured. Technically, other considerations also affected the blood supply situation. Transfusions were possible by using whole blood, liquid plasma or dried plasma reconstituted. However, the first two products did not travel well or keep for any length of time, whilst dried plasma remained unaffected by travel with an estimated shelf life of at least 5 years. Sourcing that more resilient plasma format still depended on the comparatively limited facilities available, then housed at a government establishment at the Lister Institute at Chelsea in London and at a plant in Elstree, Hertfordshire managed by the Medical Research Council on behalf of the Ministry of Health.[4]

Table 2: Blood Donor and Donation numbers 1949 – 1956.

Year	Blood donors	Blood donations
1949	396,167	456,973
1950	428,394	523,387
1951	465,137	593,818
1952	487,660	647,009
1953	515,632	659,674
1954	540,389	700,202
1955	591,204	759,571
1956	639,319	803,522

Source: Ministry of Health Report for the Year 1956.

If any further doubts existed about the National Health Service attempting to maintain a relatively sophisticated medical service in atomic war the message came in a clear signal sent in the second circular issued by the Ministry of Health to boost the capacity of the Blood Transfusion Service. Even without the atomic dimension, the immediate blood situation had reached a critical point. At the end of 1949, the donor panel stood at about 396,000 people producing 456,000 bottles of blood and 50,000 bottles of dried blood plasma. In addition to supporting hospitals, the Blood Transfusion Service supplied the Armed Services with their peacetime requirements for dried plasma and also a number of Colonial territories, Northern Ireland and the Channel Islands. All these places had found it uneconomic to run their own drying facilities, but the additional demand added to the problem with the need to produce an extra 24,000 bottles a year on the mainland. Whilst the amount of blood collected covered the commitments of the Blood Transfusion Service in peace, the provision of dried plasma could no longer rely on the existing facilities. Stocks of dried Canadian and American plasma accumulated during the last war were used as a stop-gap measure to supplement supplies, but these were fast running out and some of doubtful quality.[5]

Set against this unsatisfactory situation, planning started where the unachievable seemed achievable through the development of a new product called Dextran, a partial synthetic substitute. Albeit still in the experimental stage, great store was set on its possibility to reduce the demand for plasma by one-third to a half. This had the potential to dramatically change the arithmetic in respect of the atomic bomb. For example, if ten were used, estimates suggested that the product would reduce the requirement for plasma to 1,300,000 bottles instead of double that amount. Reliance on Dextran, coupled with the expansion of drying plant and a corresponding expansion of taking blood through the donor system suggested the supply problem could, therefore, be solved.[6] Encouraged by a positive outlook, the Blood Transfusion Service planned to expand the capacity of its systems to cover peacetime commitments in full and then build up the levels to meet an atomic war. The project involved a two staged approach with the immediate expansion of the existing blood plasma drying plant at Elstree to proceed with the highest priority with the intention of increasing supplies to 90,000 bottles per annum. Then for the longer term, plans for another drying plant were proposed with a view to adding a further 100,000 bottles of dried plasma per annum, except that estimates suggested it might take five years to achieve that output.[7]

Many other problems also needed addressing in the race to achieve the capacity of blood supply envisaged. The working party optimistically suggested in 1948 that both blood donors and technicians might be found in the Civil Defence Corps as a way of adding to their activities and an attraction for recruits.[8] In fact, the idea reflected not just an idealistic view of people's willingness to support the national cause, but also the immense difficulties the blood collection organisation faced in obtaining fresh supplies quickly. Recruitment of donors had already become the subject of a small publicity campaign, but the maximum possible intake regional blood centres could cope with at the time amounted to little more than a trickle when judged by atomic needs. To stand any chance of improvement, the planners were in no doubt the unsatisfactory image some centres exhibited had to be tackled urgently. Firstly, they recognised donors would not return if conditions were overcrowded and uncomfortable. Secondly, many regional centres involved in collecting blood supplies were not in good shape physically: the Birmingham premises described as 'insanitary and inadequate'. Even where decent facilities did exist, their wartime use was often prejudiced because of poor siting within target areas. Basically, the entire system suffered from being a jumble of differing situations which did little for the cohesion of the organisation and its overall efficiency either in peace or war. An urgent need to improve matters resulted in a commitment to a package of improvements with an instruction issued requiring Regional Hospital

Boards to prepare preliminary plans to duplicate elsewhere any Regional Transfusion Centre situated within a vulnerable area. A programme of earmarking suitable premises therefore began in order to establish additional bleeding centres and blood banks, all focussed on base hospitals.[9]

Enthusiastic as the plans might have been initially, by 1952 little progress followed and the reality dawned that the kind of duplication of Regional Blood Transfusion Centres suggested could not provide answers to the wartime problem of supply; an entirely new network appeared as the solution rather than tinkering around with the old. One of the most ambitious proposals of the atomic era took shape as a result with a new directive issued for twelve sites or suitable buildings to be found which could each provide between 15,000 and 20,000 square feet on a single floor. Guidelines about the size of a typical centre in these locations were drawn up which also gave targets about the annual intake of blood expected from each region and the additional assumption appended the centre should be large enough to deliver a third more in an emergency. Working at a normal capacity the expectations for regional contributions were raised to an ambitious level of a donor panel, equivalent to 2% of the population.[10]

The proposed physical expansion also came with the recognition success could not be achieved without attracting additional medical staff to the Blood Transfusion Service itself. As a career opportunity the work did not come into the attractive category, even admitted to be 'somewhat of a blind alley'. In striving to make improvements the unified Blood Transfusion Service began its formation that we benefit from today with a common management, staffing and grading structure introduced 'to avoid discontent and to preserve the homogeneity of the service'. Retaining staff at regional centres turned into an important objective with each unit assigned a medical, technical, and administrative personnel complement so it could take part in medical work other than just the collection and distribution of blood or carrying out routine tests. Finally, liaison with a medical school or teaching hospital in the region was also required to provide a more auspicious medical environment.[11]

Essential as the blood transfusion remained to underscore the intention of the state to provide the fullest care, the problem of the hospital bed also needed resolution. After discarding some radical ideas such as using old naval vessels due for scrap as hospital ships and mooring them in Northern Ireland close to hospital facilities, the final strategy suggested the accommodation package should come together in three ways. This included 100,000 beds in existing hospitals outside the target areas being established by crowding and sending patients home; 200,000 beds procured by new construction or utilising American hutted ex-hospitals and finally 150,000 beds created through the use of tents either in the form of annexes to hospitals or combined into standalone hospital units.[12] Setting out this simplistic and ordered outline of treatment space was one thing. The financial and practical reality of achieving the programme on the scale proposed in a post war Britain rebuilding its shattered infrastructure, whilst at the same time introducing the welfare state and developing weapons of mass destruction, was quite another.

Making matters worse, the hospital plan soon fell victim to the political vortex of world events. With the fall of China to a Communist regime in 1949 and the onset of the Korean War in 1950, concerns over the domino effect were met by a policy of rapid rearmament. Skilfully pushed through by the Labour Chancellor of the Exchequer, Hugh Gaitskell, a military budget of £3,600 million agreed in 1950 then increased to £4,700 million in January 1951.[13] Momentarily, it also seemed a serious attempt would be made to bombproof Britain at the same time as the military initiatives. The argument went that if improvements to civil defence preparations did not materialise in tandem, then the strengthening of the armed forces would be to no avail as civilian morale would decline and nullify the deterrent effect. To bombproof the entire country, even if it were possible, involved sums so vast that if the Soviets were not to destroy everything, then some prioritisation required working out so the country did not do the job for them. The Government's Defence Committee had requested a balance sheet be prepared to make some sense of the problem covering not only shelter and early warning systems, but also the functioning of ports, public utilities and communication systems and to protect such vital infrastructure by either duplication or strengthening. The project came with a certain pragmatism that a start had to be made somewhere without the cost seriously interfering with the country's economy and social policies, so the sums had to reflect a four year schedule of expenditure towards a finality in 1957.[14]

Project estimates were slotted into a four-year programme of expenditure under three categories that placed a wide interpretation on the term civil defence and not just on what had previously been 'air raid precautions'. So this included many items possessing a military value such as communication networks, war rooms, and warning systems essential to the control systems of the Royal Air Force.[15] Category I included schemes considered vital to the civil defence of the country impossible to improvise at short notice. Category II involved projects of a more secondary importance that ought to be completed, or at best brought to a reasonable point of completion. The last section, Category III, related to a nebulous set of imperatives for which no policy yet existed. Estimates for the exercise were to be based on assuming full employment, existing price levels, the extant value of sterling and 'did not purport to be accurate in detail' but intended to show the general levels of expenditure required. Constructed on this completely rickety financial appraisal, the estimated costs of CAT I projects amounted to £136,998,000; CAT II £248,663,000, and CAT III £550,432,000. The three categories added up to an eye-watering total of £936,093,000.[16] Whilst representing an unbelievable financial mountain, the whole effort still had a built-in air of dejection with the afterthought appended that, even if the whole of CAT I expenditure were invested, 'the country's civil defence measures would not, by the end of that period be anything like adequate'.[17]

Admitted to have been prepared 'in some haste' and 'broad guesses', the Ministry of Health put in a total bid of £227.5 million. A significant portion of that, amounting to £97.5 million, was to provide for expanding or building new hospitals specifically to meet civil defence needs. Under normal circumstances, the Treasury reaction to the submission would probably have been unequivocally negative. However, because one of the duties imposed on the National Health Service included the provision of medical support for military casualties who could not be treated in military hospitals, somewhat begrudgingly the Treasury allocated a figure of £10 million under CAT I expenditure towards underwriting the civil defence beds and blood transfusion projects. This provided for the building of hutted annexes to hospitals in evacuation areas, hutted hospital complexes, and hutted accommodation for expanding the Blood Transfusion Service all based on a timescale between 1951 and 1954 for completion.[19]

For the hospital annexes, six variants of the Emergency Medical Service huts used during the Second World War were considered and two chosen as standard designs for the programme, one to provide 40 beds and the other 36, including 4 cubicles. Alternatively, hospitals received the option to put the unit towards expanding the accommodation available for residential nursing staff with a capacity to provide single rooms for 25 nurses. Instead of the old coal or wood burning stoves, which had been the bane of the wartime hutted unit for their smoke and dirt, plans incorporated central heating as the modern equivalent. Other features to reduce the austerity look of the last war, included bedhead lighting and even provision for wireless cabling so radios could be installed later using hospital amenity funds. Generally, the specification for equipment to fit out the units was described as requiring a level based on a 'minimum peacetime standard, but in some respects 'rather better' than it would have been if it were only intended for use in war'.[20]

The massive budget was split with £9,000,000 allocated towards constructing approximately 600 ward huts, producing around 22,800 ward beds. For the Blood Transfusion Service, calculations suggested £1,000,000 should be allowed for building the twelve duplicate centres and a new drying plant. On receiving Treasury approval, with another

£2,500,000 added for fitting-out costs, Regional Hospital Boards in England and Wales received notification of their allocation during December 1950 and asked to nominate hospitals in their areas for expansion.[21] The Treasury stipulated huts must be located to provide a peacetime use that did mean the practical demands of actually finding the right location for the extension did add certain difficulties, not to mention delays. Adequate back up using the existing services of a hospital, as well as securing linkages to operating theatres, kitchens and X-ray departments were just some of the complexities involved. Notwithstanding those practical problems, the project received a favourable response since it often provided much needed space during the first phase of establishing the NHS. Also the capital cost did not fall on hospital budgets and came out of the civil defence vote as did the maintenance, until the huts were put into use.[22]

Then, suddenly, in the Cold War diary of events, December 1950 became notable for a government decision to accelerate defence preparations and strengthen the active forces as quickly as possible in the light of the Korean situation. This meant readjustments to the civil defence projects in CAT I with a revised completion date set at December 1952, down from four years to two. All other civil defence preparations needed to be kept to the original timetable with any deficiencies accepted as inevitable.[23] In real terms, the tactical spurt in the rearmament programme meant the narrower area of civilian defence had been demoted to a category of lesser importance. The move represented a watershed in the planning doctrine that military-related measures should take priority over the safety and welfare of civilians, a policy shift that meant nearly all the eggs were to end up in the nuclear basket as the main force for peace.

The idea the nuclear Home Front was likely to become ossified into a virtual irrelevance did not impress the father of post-war civil defence, Home Secretary, Chuter Ede and he protested vigorously about the dangers this posed. His move, however, lost any immediate impact as Labour had descended into ideological disarray and in the death throes of its second term of office.[24] What did make Ede's protest notable is his insistence that if no major improvement were made to the situation, then the Cabinet would need to accept collective ownership of rationing civil defence expenditure as a formal policy rather than just allowing the position to drift endlessly. Ede won his point and the shared recognition he wanted received formal ratification on 29 January 1951, evidenced by a short, yet important minute which recorded 'the deficiencies in Civil Defence should be accepted'.[25] Unquestionably, this revealed the fundamental hypocrisy of the civil defence services being propagandised 'The Fourth Arm of Defence'.

Because the National Health Service had a duty to provide the Services with medical support, the freeze was lifted which gave cushion hospitals priority for the first batch of wooden huts to be erected in their grounds. Even so, the project did come with a stern warning that approval to the building programme did not mean the entire hospital bed shortage for civil defence purposes would be met in this way. Despite that proviso, the down payment made by the Ministry of Health could not have been more impressive given the many restrictions which capital projects were being subjected to in austerity Britain.[26] The profligacy even caused the Ministry of Health to raise anxieties that highlighted the difficult conditions being faced. Attempting to keep the peace by bolstering morale in the direction of the deterrent was fine, but as the Ministry indicated, the effect on civil projects such as securing the future of the National Health Service itself could become counterproductive by undermining public confidence in a different way. The Ministry nevertheless received an assurance their civil defence expenditure was still possible to accommodate without disturbance to civil programmes. Any concerns they might have harboured were rebuffed on the grounds: 'the absence of civil defence preparations might have an even more serious effect on public morale'.[27]

If the Ministry of Health considered the hutted accommodation a reckless statement of intent, another came in the form of a purchasing binge on an unprecedented scale to further underwrite the attention promised to the atomic casualty. Originally, the programme for establishing the hospital and first aid services involved equipping 150,000 new general hospital beds in England and Wales, plus the addition of 10% to cover the needs of Scotland. The rationale behind the purchasing policy was that priority of acquiring strategic equipment should focus on areas where production difficulties or shortages of materials meant a high risk of supplies being unobtainable through requisitioning, diverting or increasing production. Against that reckoning, the Ministry of Health and the Department of Health for Scotland received an allocation of £36 million to cover civil defence requirements.[28]

Eventually the Ministry's foreboding about the financial largesse the programme represented turned out to be fully justified. From the national economy perspective, the effects of the armament agenda and its ancillary projects were enormous. Whole swathes of British industry including aircraft production, motor, radio and radar manufacturing were supporting the defence sector. The consequential loss of exporting capacity, coupled with a deteriorating labour and materials situation due to rebuilding the post war civic structure, provided the circumstances for a calamitous situation to build up. In the end, it reflected in the construction of the hospital huts themselves. Attempts to manage the building process in terms of cost and timing came to nothing; the whole project falling foul to the rabid inflation mercilessly engulfing the entire economy. As a result, the estimated project costs rose by nearly half as much in just a few months. In truth, the battle to control costs could not be won. Inflationary tendencies in the post-war rebuilding of Britain were affecting coal, freight charges, building commodities and labour charges, all of which impacted hugely on construction projects.[29] Worries also arose over the supply position of materials such as piping and boilers, then subject to an 18 month delay.[30] Competition for steel fuelled the shortages, including the building of a hanger for British Airways at London Airport and the help of the Ministry of Works sought to gain priority in regard to civil defence work.[31]

In reality, the pressures, which the Government itself were experiencing, mirrored the dire economic situation out in everyday life. Its own economic survey published in March 1951 described the conditions as 'harsh and unpleasant' with blame put on military spending, but at the same time resolutely stating the programmes needed to be pushed ahead without delay as the price of peace. Absorbed by a self-convincing rhetoric, the document pleaded, 'it places on us all the duty of accepting with patience the shortages and high prices that world rearmament entails, and of doing everything that we can, as producers and consumers, to eliminate waste and inefficiency'.[32] The appeal, however, fell on stony ground and the electorate mired in shortages and uncertainty did not see the situation in those same terms. During October 1951 Labour lost the election to the Conservatives. With a new political battle to save the country from within, whilst still protecting it against the external threat of communism, something had to give and became rather a question how those two issues were to be politically reconciled which would in turn influence the future direction of the wartime hospital and casualty plans.

Deceptive Appearances

After taking over the reins of power in October 1951, the Conservatives began slowing down the military programme. Civil defence clearly did not come on to the agenda for special attention. The economic policy review for the Cabinet made by the Chancellor of the Exchequer issued on 17 May, 1952 defined the nature of the problem and inevitably impacted on the way the 'nuclear health service' could be regarded. In one sense, the National Health Service might have been a core contributor towards building up, as the Chancellor put it 'a strong, free and prosperous country,' but it had also become part of the problem. Britain was now heaving under the weight of commitments to provide better health services, schools, house building, and slum clearance. At the same time the country had embarked on a colossal rearmament programme which, of course, included the manufacture of atomic bombs.[33] Conservative Chancellor of the Exchequer Richard Austen (Rab) Butler warned the defence budget risked destroying the country's balance of payments, his concerns reflecting the intricate politics involved. Undoubtedly, the task of dealing with the situation was proving politically challenging in view of the implications for some of the elements that underpinned the welfare state. For example, in areas such as the removal of food subsidies cuts risked increasing the cost of living index and consequently opposed by the Ministry of Labour in its quest to hold back wage demands. The welfare state undoubtedly weighed heavily on the Chancellor's mind with the National Insurance fund as he put it, 'running into a dangerous state of indebtedness owing to the number of old people'. In order to counter this position, even ways of inducing the elderly to stay in work longer came on the political list of matters being examined.[34]

As a result of trying to cut the economic knot of rearming, improving living standards, fulfilling overseas commitments and defending sterling, the impact on 'the nuclear health service' arrived with a dramatic and sudden blow to its expansionist ideals. Both the hospital hut programme and extension of the Blood Transfusion Service suffered. Rescheduling, delays in commencing work, delays in obtaining materials and roaring inflation meant only a fraction of the grand plan had actually been put into effect. Once almost embarrassed by the money thrown in their direction, the Ministry of Health found it necessary to save projects in mid-stream and cautioned stopping construction would risk deterioration of the fabric and heavy claims by contractors.[35] The alarm was also raised about the modernisation of the blood service inexorably bound up with preparing for World War Three, and now put at risk:

> One criticism that may be made is that we should have had to incur part of this expenditure on the blood transfusion service anyhow and therefore it is not a proper commitment for the Civil Defence Expenditure Programme. The answer to this is that this in essence is a programme of expenditure for war purposes though it brings us a concurrent benefit in peace; if we were considering only our peacetime needs we should be proposing something different and less expensive, because we should have expanded the service more slowly and to a smaller extent. For defence purposes we have been compelled to build a large drying plant (and later on

> a second drying plant) in addition to 12 new transfusion centres to deal with the greatly increased intake of blood needed to provide an emergency reserve of plasma. Had this emergency reserve not been needed we could have managed with one smaller drying plant and with little or no increase in the number of transfusion centres.[36]

The Treasury did concede to the completion of certain projects, but overall the picture looked singularly unpromising. In 1950, a four-year construction programme promised much.[37] Economic reality, however, intervened. Only the first stage of the hutted hospital plan reached completion and provided fifty-four ward units, space enough for a meagre 2,100 beds in England and Wales and 456 in Scotland.[38] One consolation for Scotland was that part of their grant had been spent in a different way which plugged some major gaps in their civil hospital plans on the back of the atomic blueprint. Their allocation included a sum of £400,000 to rebuild the Alexandria Hospital, Vale of Leven, especially to provide support for the evacuation of Glasgow hospitals. In addition, the Princess Margaret Rose Hospital Edinburgh benefitted from extensions and a blood transfusion unit and laboratory provided at Law.[39]

The abrupt halt to the hutted accommodation project put into sharp focus the hospital bed situation. Worryingly, it showed little signs of improvement and held obstinately at an estimated shortfall of some 200,000 beds. As a last resort, Regional Hospital Boards had to inspect and earmark sites for tented hospitals to reduce the deficit to the tune of 85,000 beds (including 10,000 in Scotland and Northern Ireland). However, any initial exuberance over tented hospitals providing the solution to the bed problem soon began to be plagued by doubts. On further reflection, the planners acknowledged whilst tented hospitals were satisfactory for the Armed Forces, who had a large number of male staff and patients, the canvas option for civilian use was 'far less suitable for use as civilian hospitals with a high proportion of female staff and patients of both sexes'. Nonetheless, there appeared no alternative and the policy needed to continue with the Ministry of Health said to be examining the mixed ward issue.[40]

Another discouraging subject to join the lengthening list of premises problems stemmed from hopes that the Ministry would have a free hand over acquiring the ex-Service camps and hutted hospital accommodation built by the Americans for use in the last war. Unfortunately for the Ministry of Health, this potential supply also contracted unexpectedly. The War Office refused to relinquish its interest in these assets, leaving the Health Departments with only enough huts under their own control to bring down the bed deficit by a paltry 6,000 beds.[41] If a way out existed, it lay with the Ministry of Health being allowed to earmark school premises so these could be secured by requisitioning. A countrywide process had been set up for this purpose through an Accommodation Clearance Register maintained by the Ministry of Works. The procedure was limited to buildings in possession of government departments, local authorities and certain public bodies. However, a scramble by many ministry departments to reserve buildings for their own wartime needs meant the exercise ended in considerable uncertainties as to who should get preference.

In fact, the Whitehall rush to earmark school premises reached quite histrionic proportions, which reflected badly on government planning machinery. About 700 primary and secondary schools were earmarked across the country and along with the Ministry of Health, the prime competitor for space turned out to be the War Office, particularly for mobilisation centres and to a lesser extent the Ministry of Works and the Admiralty. The totals represented some quarter of a million school places and included over 30,000 boarding pupils. Other requests involved seven special schools for handicapped children, twenty institutions of further education and thirty-three training colleges, mostly for women teachers. In the case of the Ministry of Health, their bid involved 204 schools, with a potential loss of 75,100 places.[42] Far from being assured of securing these properties, however, the Ministry were still left to complain that the system, based on a 'first come first served' arrangement, often prevented them obtaining the most useful type of property for the care of casualties.[43]

At a meeting of the Defence Transition Committee, now in its fifth year of weaving together the country's military plans, Frederick Armer, Deputy Secretary at the Ministry of Health made a plea that 'the nuclear health service' faced 'an alarming shortage of beds' which might have to be made good by tentage, even against medical advice. Armer stressed that all he asked for was a way to reserve buildings for planning purposes which involved no actual work being carried out. Nonetheless, the Cabinet Secretary Norman Brook as chairman of the DTC imposed his mark on the proceedings to ensure the facade was not extended any further and accused his colleague of unnecessary empire building.[44] Consequently no action to sort out the hospital premises fiasco appeared. Instead, it left the Ministry of Health high and dry, with a potentially embarrassing problem on their hands.

That sense of chaos also surrounded the civil defence purchasing strategy. Although a working party had produced what appeared to them a coherent plan, any good intentions of abiding by its principles disappeared when much of the funding began to be syphoned off to protect all kinds of political problem areas, particularly textile manufacture. At the start of the

Korean War a bout of abnormal buying across the world was followed by a slump in prices as no further orders were placed. France and Australia imposed import restrictions and the textile industry toppled into recession, hitting the industry hard, women workers especially affected. In the UK the worst-hit regions were Lancashire, Cheshire, the West Riding and South Scotland. With falling cloth prices, a spiral of uncertainties aggravated the position further. Clothing factories deferred purchases of cloth and consumers stopped spending rather than risk paying for cloth at the old rates.[45] Attempting to protect the home textile market from the downturn in demand, the Government went on a buying spree to fill every nook and cranny of possible need for cloth. This included purchases for the army, the Home Guard (recalled during the Korean War), the civil defence services and even blackout material appeared on the list.

Prime Minister, Sir Winston Churchill, had also sent a personal minute to his Home Secretary expressing the political imperative to spend, spend, spend:

> It is absolutely necessary that special efforts should be made to bring unemployment in Northern Ireland down from its very high level of over ten per cent at the present time, or three times the rate in Great Britain. The production of pre-fabricated housing interiors seems one hopeful step, but every method should be considered. I am relying on you to fight this battle and bring the matter to Cabinet when you want support. Not only is this our black spot, but it is a black spot in the most prominent position, i.e. a bull's – eye. There is no reason why Northern Ireland, with its loyalty to the Union, should be the most penalised of all.[46]

The command was actioned in number of ways. The Home Office wrote to the Minister of Health demanding a new production plant for penicillin be established in Ulster, explaining: 'This unemployment is not only economically disastrous, but politically dangerous and the strategic importance of Northern Ireland makes it essential that Her Majesty's Government should avoid antagonising the population by apparent indifference to their problems in peace'.[47] Probably the most dramatic move came with massive orders of certain textiles which were arranged under the *Acceleration of Textile Orders* issued as part of the defence programme to alleviate the recession in the cloth industry described. Translated into consumables, a mountain of 600,000 sheets and pillow slips, together with flax duck to the value of £1.095 million for the manufacture of canvas, surfaced as one of the greatest 'white elephants' ever to be created as a result of civil defence policy.[48] With money being thrown at the textile industry vested interests also came out of the woodwork to secure a slice of action. Rayon manufacturers, for example, claimed the cotton industry had been favoured unfairly which then led to long procurement delays whilst tests were undertaken to manufacture sheets and pillows using a rayon/cotton mixture.[49]

By way of complete contrast, the Treasury applied a strict code of practice in respect to other sectors to avoid unnecessary expenditure, and directed stockpiling could only be undertaken for items which might be difficult to procure during the hypothetical warning period of six months before war breaking out.[50] Adopting this as a benchmark, it was considered that drugs in common use, such as antibiotics, could be made available at short notice. The exception to the rule related to opium. During 1939 a policy of buying in the product had been introduced to process into morphine and an initial supply of 44 tons purchased. As the war progressed, further imports were made of Turkish opium, amounting to 230 tons. The estimate of normal consumption in the UK was calculated at some 55 tons, part of the processed supply being exported, particularly to the Commonwealth. By 1949, the stocks in the UK were very much below normal and stood at 14 tons held in reserve by the Government and 40 tons by the trade. Considered a vital commodity, with a heavy demand by other countries, an increase to 100 tons as a strategic stock was in the circumstances considered essential to procure on the grounds of being critical to the needs of peace and war.[51]

A functional thread of confidence also appeared right the way through the purchasing strategy. The list included 10,250 sterilisers of various kind, 250 operating tables, 6,500 instrument tables, 1,600 patient and theatre trolleys, 9,500 tubular ward screen frames, along with 225,000 detachable covers and 235 theatre lamps. Embodying an eclectic collection of items they, and much more besides, possessed an aspirational value some kind of peacetime normality was still possible. Sometimes obsolescence resulted in the application of contradictory policies. For example, 3,330 oxygen cylinder carriers were ordered on the one hand, but on the other, more brutal decisions were taken which made their usefulness somewhat doubtful.[52] In the case of oxygen, just one medical supplier existed in the British Oxygen Company. Out of their 27 factories only 21 manufactured oxygen for medical purposes and most of these were vulnerable to attack.[53] As a safeguard, an idea floated to invest in French machinery and secure some form of local supply, which could be more strategically distributed, received a less than enthusiastic response by the Home Office. They curtailed the matter abruptly with their view that if an attack occurred then 'medical treatment will become a good deal more primitive that at present and oxygen may be one of the things we shall have to do without. Indeed oxygen may be more important for the oxy-acetylene cutters which will be needed to remove steel girders from important roads or railways'.[54]

With some inevitability, the kind of disjointed and expedient purchasing policy began to be felt, and worse still, risked becoming public during civil defence exercises. The resulting deficiencies hit the area of first aid badly. A working party had designed a special first aid pack for use by Mobile First Aid Units, but the Ministry of Health held out no hope whatsoever as to its introduction in view of the stringent financial controls being imposed.[55] It was just one element amongst many where the fault lines were appearing. During just two years, the procurement exercise in all its forms had become a series of failures to hang the critical symbols of operational capability on Carling's hospital and casualty framework. No modern training ambulances existed, much of the blood transfusion plan had been discarded, the premises strategy was in a state of disarray and in the case of support equipment, most of it simply reflected a shambolic rush towards meeting other political objectives.

Secret Confessions

Entangled by a myriad of complications with no extrication seemingly possible, civil defence appeared to have no future. Taking a historical viewpoint it is the political machinations about the shaky structure that finally demonstrate the support the organisation could still muster through its perceived value to deterrence policy. In a statement marked 'Top Secret' the Minister of Defence made it quite clear the Cabinet could not have it both ways, particularly as the development of nuclear weapons had changed more rapidly than had been forecast two years earlier. He put his point forcefully: 'Severe cuts cannot be made without industry, the Armed Forces, and before long our Allies realising that our rearmament programme is being emasculated and is taking second place to housing, consumer goods, and social services, which are remaining virtually unaffected'.[56] Caught by the inevitable financial squeeze that followed civil defence received no favours. Commenting about the Home Secretary's attempt to restore the fortunes for civilian protection, a note by an unidentified civil servant summed up the position: 'Civil Defence must for the time being eat of the crumbs which fall from the general rearmament table'.[57] Prime Minister Churchill himself had few qualms about being brutally frank regarding future funding, a fact seen in a move to disabuse his Secretary of State of any ambitions to undertake a comprehensive civil defence programme:

> While he appreciated the Home Secretary's anxiety about his responsibilities for civil defence, he doubted whether it would be justifiable to devote to civil defence large sums of money which could be more profitably used in active defence measures, which would be a more effective deterrent to war or if the worst came, more valuable in the early stages of a war.[58]

Notwithstanding those negative sentiments, Churchill still recognised the propaganda advantages of the civil defence organisation to underwrite political capital. The advice he gave to his ministers, in effect, became the ideological doctrine adopted for the remaining years of its life, succinctly put in the following way: 'Although it would be wise to do enough to create an impression of activity in civil defence, care must be taken to avoid spending large sums of money on measures which would pay no dividend'.[59] In other words, a very deliberate and focussed public deception was to be pursued based on cost and perceptual effectiveness. If a name for this policy had not yet emerged, it soon acquired one that surfaced in quite an unexpected way. A Parliamentary Select Committee on civil defence spending concluded civil defence in the UK was a 'facade', and the Civil Defence Corps, the backbone of the organisation singled out as 'an organisation in name only', its peacetime function having 'no central executive peacetime direction or control'. Neither did the way the textile industry had been favoured escape attention, the Select Committee even uncovering a spend of £646,000 on coloured blankets with Treasury collusion and made without any estimates demanded. Extravagance on this scale had been further compounded by the discovery of nearly £80,000 allocated to buying in Women's Land Army underclothes 'to save it going on to the ordinary market'.[60] Overall, the civil defence programme according to the Select Committee added up to a financial disaster of both overestimation and under-spending.[61] The most serious jibe referred to the entire organisation being no more than a facade which implied it lacked operational validity and preparations were too far removed from possible mobilisation. Sparing no quarter in the embarrassment stakes, the committee waded in with the overall comment that the objective of government was 'not to prepare for an immediate war or even for an early probable war, but only to prepare to prepare for war'.[62]

What the Select Committee's report did elicit was a secret insight into the deepest thoughts of Ministers over the civil defence problem. Documentary evidence of their political fears is revealed in a note the Cabinet Secretary, Norman Brook, who had also served the Attlee administration, prepared for his new political master. The briefing to Churchill on the Select Committee's scathing criticism stripped policy back to an uncomfortable truth expressed in the following way:

> So far as concerns policy this report by the Select Committee on Estimates is misconceived. The purpose of the Government's defence policy is, not to prepare for a war regarded as inevitable, but to take all practicable measures to prevent war. The major part of our defence effort has therefore been directed to strengthening the Armed Forces; and it is reasonable and logical that civil defence should have been allowed to lag behind. This was the policy of the previous Government. The Select Committee have used the word 'facade' as a criticism; but in fact neither this Government nor the last have ever intended to do more than build a facade of civil defence.[63]

A handwritten comment by Churchill, addressed to the Home Secretary alluded to the costs of civil defence, but his few words also propelled the belief system into the Cold War as one of its most audacious psychological weapons. This confirmed: 'You should see this I think it is too much anyway for what is after all only a facade'.[64] By concurring with the name, Churchill effectively baptised the itinerant child of deception which would proceed to grow in its intensity until 1968. In respect of making a public announcement, such candidness clearly did not come into the equation. A discernible, collective paranoia engulfed ministers as to the public response and considerable agitation expressed about the Select Committee going outside their terms of reference by criticising civil defence policy. To explain the Government's position, the publication of a White Paper came in for consideration, a way forward that the Home Secretary favoured as opposed to a departmental response to Parliament. On the other hand, Iain Macleod, Minister of Health, one of the most able ministers in the Conservative Government, expressed concerns that reveal the kind of political tightrope the facade had become. He warned civil defence should neither alarm nor concern the public and the question of additional expenditure had to be kept out of the debate, all the issues laid out in the following minute:

> The Minister of Health, while agreeing that a strong reply was necessary, expressed the view that we should be careful to avoid alarming the general

public. To issue a strongly worded White Paper on Civil Defence policy as a counter to the criticisms of the Select Committee would be bound to raise public hopes that fresh developments in Civil Defence preparations were imminent and that more money would be spent in the immediate future. Unless, therefore, prior agreement had been reached with the Treasury that public demand for increased expenditure could in fact be met, there would be a risk of causing widespread disappointment and disillusionment. The Press criticism of Civil Defence preparations arising from the publication of the Select Committee's Report, may have been given undue prominence because of the temporary absence of other political news at that time, and it would be wrong to assume that the general public were greatly disturbed by the report. To reply now in the form of a White Paper would only encourage the Press to take it up again, and in this event they would be bound to pick out the weaker points of the reply, so that our last state would only be worse than the first. It was clear that on the whole the general climate would be against increased expenditure. For these reasons, he would prefer that the reply should take some form other than a White Paper.[65]

Iain Macleod's recommendation that it was essential to dumb-down the problem as constitutionally as possible prevailed. Following that course, the issue was dealt with through a robust response made to Parliament by the Home Secretary Sir David Maxwell Fyfe. The text also circulated amongst all the civil defence organisations because it defended their integrity by arguing the civil defence case as being consistent with known government policy. Both Labour and Conservative administrations were said to have followed the same guiding principle, 'that is directed to the prevention of war and not to the preparations for war considered to be imminent, or even inevitable'. Military force as a deterrence factor had, it was stressed, the first claim on resources, the purpose of civil defence planning being 'to build up a nucleus of an organisation with a view to its subsequent expansion if necessary'.[66]

The official line to counter the allegations that civil defence was nothing more than a facade may have been fine for public consumption, but inside Whitehall a new appreciation privately came to the same conclusion through a more terrifying process. Because of a strategic review in March 1953, a Home Defence Committee was established, the seriousness of the situation reflected by its membership. Chaired by Sir Norman Brook, the Cabinet Secretary, its members included the Chiefs of Staff, the Permanent Secretaries of the Home Office, Ministry of Fuel and Power, Ministry of Transport and a senior representative from the Treasury. Approved by the Prime Minister, its terms of reference were to ensure consistency in war planning between the military and civil agencies in the defence of the United Kingdom in a future war and to report to the Defence Committee.[67] Amongst the tasks a study of the effect by an attack with 200 Nagasaki/Hiroshima-type atomic bombs on the United Kingdom was to be undertaken. The term 'facade' did not appear, but the exercise predicated on the basis: 'it might well be found what was required was not a mere intensification of our present arrangements but an entirely fresh approach, as it was already clear that we should never be able to afford in peacetime all the physical measures needed to fully mitigate the effects of air attack on such a scale'. The underlying military assumption suggested the Soviets would not concentrate all their weaponry on single targets, but aim at areas containing elements of the greatest number of target systems including communications, food distribution centres, manufacturing, power, oil supplies, and port facilities. Based on that supposition, the bombing distribution for the purposes of the study assumed 132 atomic bombs assigned to civilian target areas (35 falling on London), 40 bombs allotted for attacks on atomic air bases and the remaining 28 held in reserve to replace bombs not reaching their targets. As a result, 1,378,000 people were estimated killed and 785,000 seriously injured across the United Kingdom.[68]

The Ministry of Health looked at their plans for dealing with 700,000 casualties in England and Wales classified as 'seriously injured', plus the requirement of the Services for a possible 88,000 beds for their wounded, quite apart from the civilian and Service sick. Taken as a whole, the Department's conclusions contained in the report *The Initial Phase of a War* did not make for good reading. Assuming 180,000 people required urgent attention within 24 hours to deal with abdominal, chest, head, joint and severe limb injuries the medical facilities were found wanting on an unprecedented scale.[69] Making a secret confession, the Ministry acknowledged massive shortages in all areas including blood supplies, dressings, drugs and anaesthetic materials. Furthermore, because of the intensity of the attack, the flexibility of the hospital plan flouted in public could not, came the admission, actually offer first aid through mobile teams. No patient transfers were possible to areas free from attack due to ambulance coaches being destroyed or unable to operate across the resultant fields of debris. 450,000 beds had been the aim, but a further confession confirmed only some 250,000 could be established, though even this figure was cloaked by doubts and the likelihood expressed that some 50,000 of these would be inside tents. In the compendium of failures one particle of hope suggested because so few beds would be provided, 'it is unlikely that there would be difficulty in providing an adequate staff of nurses and medical auxiliaries'. Faced by this horrifying risk assessment the Ministry was caught by an uncustomary air of dejection and the Department confirmed, 'the hospital service would be quite unable to cope adequately with the large number of casualties which are assumed to have occurred in an attack of the degree propounded'.[70]

Only a few weeks after the pomp and ceremony of the Queen's Coronation, the nation's most senior military men and civil servants also added their concerns about the effect of such an attack on morale. They collectively warned that the British stiff upper lip encapsulated in the last war as 'taking it' could no longer be relied on.[71] Such an astonishingly bleak picture might have suggested the point had been reached where any kind of survival regime could have nothing further to offer. On the other hand, if as Churchill believed, the facade could play a part in deterrence policy and its ideological components such as 'the nuclear health service' turned towards protecting the wartime spirit of defiance, all was not lost. The connotation of 'facade' had been publicly heralded as a matter of incompetence representing a massive failure in coordinated planning which had been allowed to drift aimlessly at great expense to the public purse. In that regard, Whitehall was actually spared being cast in the less-honourable position of outright deceiver. Moreover, the advice given by the Minister of Health to his colleagues that the public should not be alarmed by greater expenditure on civil defence now conveniently fitted in with the economics of indulging in both welfare for the masses and weapons of mass destruction. The facade had somehow become a comfort blanket too good to discard.

Chapter 3

SURGICAL SPIRITS

On the face of it, the new National Health Service and its common systems seemed an ideal organisation to pull in all kinds of directions and produce a logical way of dealing with the weapons of mass destruction. As atomic revisionists, Carling's people were a world away from the kind of difficulties faced by the medical planners preparing for the Second World War. Before the NHS, they had to contend with bringing together all the diverse buildings, equipment and professional services in the equally differing patterns of healthcare systems that existed. They included the private practice sectors, voluntary and municipal hospitals, in addition to all the associated support provided by local authority and public health officialdom. Eventually, these assorted elements became fused into a national structure called the Emergency Medical Services, but still left many elements of care outside. Certainly, by comparison to that era, the reordering of the physical assets of the National Health Service was possible through the legal necessity of hospital administrators acting as agents of the Minister of Health. However, for all the commonality provided by the new physical framework, the situation as far as surgeons, hospital doctors and general practitioners differed considerably. At first, the Ministry of Health saw the problem in terms of requiring a new contract of mobilisation and deployment to run in parallel with peacetime terms and conditions of service. For certain, by adopting this view the issue could not have presented a more challenging task since the setting up of the National Health Service.

Hood's Prescription

Gaining the support of the medical profession by means of such new contracts became regarded by the medical aspects subcommittee as a fundamental principle of dealing with the atomic bomb, a matter always referred to officially as, 'the control of medical manpower in war'.[1] Control in the context of planning for nuclear war meant 'absolute' control in a military sense requiring obedience to centralised orders and discipline. Many problems of the atomic battlefield appeared surmountable by subjugating the medical profession to that ideology. These included the preservation of medical resources before an attack; securing a mobile service possible to move to areas of greatest demand and finally to maintain a balance between the military and civilian needs when it came to the division of the scarce medical resource. But then transferring those objectives into practical terms meant deconstructing the National Health Service after its construction and some of the most acrimonious power struggles imaginable. As an exercise it very much presented fertile ground for old wounds to reappear, particularly as to who had the right to control doctors and whether they should be controlled at all.

Historically, the problem of 'controlling' the medical profession had its roots in the Second World War. A major issue included the painful process of drip-feeding medical resources from the civilian side to the military that eventually left civilians with a medical system close to collapse. When hostilities began in 1939, the pool of medical practitioners in Great Britain and Northern Ireland numbered about 45,300, of which 1,400 held regular commissions.[2] At first, volunteers were called for. It was not until April 1940 the Ministry of Labour and National Service declared the *National (Armed Forces) Act 1939* would be applied to medical practitioners so they could be conscripted in their professional capacity. All medical men, whole time or part time, were to be called to the colours, though limited to those under the age of 41.[3] The impact of conscription hit the junior medical staffs in the Emergency Medical Service hospitals hard and only strong representations made by the hospital authorities kept 'key' individuals working for the civilian side.[4]

As 1940 ended, 7,500 practitioners had received their call-up into military service, which left 36,400 practitioners on the civil list, some 5,000 of those being over 70 years of age.[5] This precipitous reduction, even without further calls on the civilian medical services, had an immediate effect. Not just the numbers caused complications, but the quota system itself used to harvest conscripts by age proved equally troublesome. Choosing medical men of 41 and younger meant some communities suffered more simply because of the age structure of general practitioners in their area. Other problems occurred when some newly qualified doctors, who failed to obtain house posts in the well established hospitals fought shy of appointments in the EMS system, especially where these units were outposts in rural districts. Instead, they bided their time as locums working in general practice until receiving their call up papers. At these hospitals great shortages of medical personnel developed which in turn precipitated the temporary transfer of staff from large towns, particularly to deal with the casualties repatriated from overseas.[6]

Confronted by a crisis of confidence, the Government had to respond immediately. A small but powerful committee under the chairmanship of Sir (William) Arthur Robinson (who had just retired from his post as Permanent Secretary to the Ministry of Supply) was appointed and returned its verdict the following month. The Robinson Committee's most important recommendation called for a central organisation to be established which could settle questions of priority in the division of medical resources between civilian and military needs. Fiercely resisted at first by the Minister and the Secretary of State for War, they eventually relented, but not without protecting their position by insisting men with practical experience of military medical service should be included in the decision making process.[7]

Designed to take a more measured approach to conscription, powers were vested in a new body called The Priority Committee which started its work during June 1941 with Geoffrey Shakespeare, Member of Parliament and Parliamentary Under-Secretary for the Dominions, at its head. An immediate package of measures resulted. The Ministry of Health cut back the medical establishment of hospitals and brought in another 300 alien practitioners, in addition to the Americans and Canadians already allowed to practice. By June 1941, this permitted the release of 126 British doctors for military service.[8] To even out the depletion of medical resources, especially where a higher incidence of younger doctors had their practices, the Ministry of Labour and National Security increased the call up age for medical practitioners by five years.[9] For the first time, the Ministry also introduced the conscription of women doctors who were unmarried and born on or after 18 December 1910.[10] Finally, the more efficient use of resources came through various changes, amongst the most important being those to the civilian Emergency Medical Service that allowed for the redirection and transfer of whole-time medical staff between hospitals during times of urgent need. On their part, the Army and Air Force were required to deliver economies by pooling resources where possible. For example, instead of anti-aircraft and barrage balloon commands each retaining their own medical facilities, a sharing arrangement on an area basis had to take place.[11]

Well-intended as they were, the revisions did little to improve matters. The fact remained the Services needed more and more doctors as the war turned increasingly to attrition rather than defence. The call up arrangements operated on the basis that the Service Departments would notify the Priority Committee of their needs, with discussions following about the numbers that were possible to spare. Once approved, the conscription process itself operated through the machinery of the Central Medical War Committee. For general practitioners, the quota system kicked in and imposed downwards onto the Local Medical War Committees. In 1941 the calculation for the exercise involved an assessment based on the number of doctors becoming surplus to an area after making an allowance for one general practitioner per 3,000 patients for an urban population, one per 2,400 patients living in rural regions and one per 2,700 patients in mixed areas. Despite that neat theoretical division, by the end of 1942 more than half of the total population of England and Wales were in an area where the allocation had risen to more than 3,000 patients to each general practitioner and at times the doctor patient ratio even climbed to 4,500, far above the recommended levels.[12]

Decanting medical practitioners in this way eventually reached breaking point. As the Chief Medical Officer remarked in his report on the medical conditions during the war, 'the normal inflow of new practitioners was completely diverted to the Services, even those found unfit for the fighting services being almost all absorbed by the hospitals, while death, retirement and breakdown continually depleted the ranks of the seniors'.[13] Attempts to find new ways of satisfying the ceaseless call for medical quotas by the military inevitably caused immense problems in healthcare more generally. All kinds of expedients emerged during 1942 to mitigate the problems. Qualification times for doctors under training were compressed and the clinical part of the medical curriculum reduced from three years to thirty months.[14] Mental hospitals and other institutions, which really could ill afford to give up their medical cover, were raided for additional medical manpower.[15] Even a scheme to extract the diversity of local authority medical appointments appeared and Public Health Officers became the target of Ministry of Health Circular 2881. Issued in May 1943, this captured a hitherto mercurial band of medical professionals and placed them into one class called 'public health medical staffs of local authorities,' a move allowing the sector to be milked more easily.[16] The results were some of the most disturbing and by 1944 clinical cover for maternity services, child welfare and the school medical service sometimes dropped to unconscionable levels. Although the shortage crisis of medical manpower in various civil hospitals was the subject of a review during February 1945, the only comfort extended to a tacit acknowledgement of the importance of the different specialist fields such as the laboratory services, radiological services and the tuberculosis service, but no increases in resources actually materialised to alleviate their plight.[17]

There were other problems for civilians. Whilst the Emergency Medical Services appeared to provide a common system of care and were often cited as a precursor of the NHS, the prime purpose of the organisation had been to provide medical facilities for the civilian and Service casualties due to enemy action. Gradually the categories were relaxed, but despite that the system remained a highly regimented and bureaucratically-controlled regime when it came to admissions policy. Categories included the police sick, police casualties, civil defence workers wounded whilst on duty, and unaccompanied evacuated children.[18] Towards the end of the war many other classes of war workers were added, for whom the best treatment was available to allow them to return to their important duties. At the other end of the humanitarian scale, however, distinct problems arose, with women and children making up a large part of a growing waiting list for medical attention. In Birmingham alone, a review undertaken in 1942 showed the Children's Hospital turned away at least four or five medical cases daily. The Queen Elizabeth Hospital in the same city reported the number of women seeking gynaecological treatment had reached unprecedented levels and lamented that even with the accommodation and staff available 'it would take years to work off'.[19]

Devising a plan to provide mass compassion for the atomic era, therefore, required a radical overhaul because on the record of the last war it also raised the spectre of mass neglect. With this kind of experience behind their thinking, the Ministry of Health decided its key objective must be to take 'effective control' of the entire medical services of the country. During the last war, it had been necessary to 'gain' control due to the disparate collection of medical resources available before the National Health Service came into being. With the establishment of the NHS, the Ministry of Health did have control over many medical services, but contracts, committees and careers bound these up into a difficult resource to unravel. All the various elements had a complex relationship with each other and 'effective' control really meant deconstructing the entire system and reconstituting in ways that would create more flexibility if the risk of the Cold War turning hot was to be covered.[20]

For general practitioners especially, a new doctrine based on such flexibility along with subservience to new codes of practice represented uncharted waters bringing a shadowy uncertainty. If they were not called up, their future remained unclear with the possibility of having to support local hospitals acting as auxiliary surgeons, supporting Mobile First Aid Units at the scene of devastation or becoming part of a new domiciliary service able to cover home visits or community care. Especially worrying loomed the great anathema of placement under the control of the local authority civil defence systems and even worse direction by local health authority Medical Officers of Health. This in many respects represented the allegory of centralised state care they had fiercely resisted before the National Health Service had been finalised. In particular, it meant submitting to local authorities who had gained enormous concessions both directly and indirectly by way of the *Civil Defence Act 1948*. Using this legislation, local politicians could enhance their local prestige with nuclear salvation used as an extension of civic duty, all of which represented dangerous territory with a history. Government had found the perfect self-interest group in the local authority willing to re-enact the past glories of the Home Front. For general practitioners working within a system that had acquired such influence therefore meant a trip into unfamiliar territory and a position completely alien to their desire to keep full control over their destiny. Not surprisingly, the journey to turn the concept of medical manpower control into an operational reality began to assume dreadful proportions as Carling's vision of a unified medical force took on a shape and form designed not by a civilian, but a military doctor, Sir Alexander Hood.

Based on the principle the medical system must be capable of mobilisation within minutes of atomic bombs falling anywhere in the United Kingdom, Hood proposed to put every doctor and surgeon into a special medical unit. According to the medical general's predilection for militarisation this meant 'It should have a disciplinary code and ranks to ensure in all circumstances an automatic chain of command and proper relationship with the Fighting Services. The uniform might well be battledress with a distinguishing flash'.[21] Officially, the organisational model used the excuse of efficiency for its introduction stating: 'The chief virtues of a unified medical corps would be to avoid competition, and uneconomical use. It was considered all doctors irrespective of age should be brought into it, although it was realised that the policy of compulsory direction of men above military aged might be criticised'.[22] A major advantage seen in the unification proposal was, so the theory went, that it would allow doctors earmarked for overseas postings to continue working in Britain and avoid wasting their services whilst waiting for their official appointments to be realised. That was not all. Another issue creating an impetus for more control emanated from a belief, particularly strongly held by the chairman of the medical aspects working party, that many of their medical colleagues had evaded their wartime responsibilities during the first two years of the war. Consequently, it was a matter put high on the list for addressing to assure equality of sacrifice operated without fear or favour.[23]

Key to meeting these objectives, the working party felt the way forward required the preparation of a register of doctors by age and physical fitness capable of use on a geographical basis. Information of that kind would then permit a sieve process to operate allowing the identification of doctors under 45 for training as potential members of a National Medical Corps. Secondly, doctors over military age labelled as 'fit and mobile' were to serve in the corps as the most 'portable' resource, whilst doctors identified 'fit for local service only' would remain within designated locations. At the very heart of the plan came the principle of a unified command that required it to be highly centralised and as powerful as possible. Fleshing out this operational objective meant the NMC would be organised on a regional basis under a Whitehall supremo, the Director General National Medical Corps, with each region having its Deputy

Director General.[24] The allocation of doctors to commands would fall to the Director General, with the planning of area services in the regions undertaken by his deputies in consultation with Principal Medical Officers of Health in the public health service and Senior Administrative Medical Officers in the hospital service. Whilst an internal assessment of the proposal by civil servants at the Ministry of Health did not argue with the committee's view the direction processes conducted by the Ministry of Labour had been 'an embarrassment in the last war' a good degree of scepticism about Hood's quasi 'militarisation' plan did exist. An internal report warned: 'Any conception of a medical corps implying (if that was even intended) continuous discipline and regimentation, not merely liability to be directed, would probably be unpopular with the profession as too bureaucratic even as applied to the National Health Service'.[25]

Undaunted by the prospect of a bad reaction, the medical aspects team were gripped by a determination to go through with the concept. As a first step an outline document with the administrative formality of calling it the 'Skeleton Plan' made its appearance. Recognising the difficulties of unifying the entire medical profession under a regimented scheme going far beyond anything attempted during World War Two, the proposal provided an appropriate inducement. The conscription or 'employment' section involved similar arrangements established by the end of the last war covering two main areas of responsibility. This involved the introduction of a National Medical Committee as a strategic point of reference with ten eminent medical practitioners appointed on the lines of the old Medical Priority Committee. Its remit included giving advice to Ministers on the use of medical manpower and the allocation of doctors between the three fighting services and the civilian medical services. For dealing with the actual recruitment side, two subcommittees of the National Medical Committee were proposed, one to cover England and Wales and the other Scotland with the intention they should manage a web of Local War Committees equating to the wartime organisation responsible for offering guidance on the enlistment of individual doctors.[26]

A distinctive change did arise in the pigeonholes medical practitioners would find themselves in for the purpose of recruitment procedures, a move designed to ensure the appropriate professional bodies could become more involved in the process. The three sectors consisted of firstly, general practitioners, secondly, hospital consultants, specialists and university teaching staffs, while public health officers came under the third functional division. Professional interests, therefore, appeared adequately covered with the package even giving assurances conscription was possible to challenge on hardship grounds. This side of the Skeleton Plan, therefore, seemed to represent nothing more than a benign organisation giving the medical profession the same degree of self-governance it had enjoyed during the Second World War.[27]

By contrast, the second half of the plan, referred to as the 'operational' side contained arrangements that could not have been more different to the comfort zone of the old wartime protocols. Even though the general view prevailed these might be 'too bureaucratic', they were adopted and codified without compromise as originally outlined and effectively put into blunt reality the most drastic philosophy ever proposed for the medical establishment of Great Britain. Everything came back to the critical factor of 'effective' control. In the first place, the recruitment process no longer was to depend on a proclamation of war, but conducted during peace to achieve a constant state of readiness. Secondly, and this related to the deconstruction side, conscription would not only be applied to those of military age, but to the entire medical profession below the age of 65.[28] Once agreed for medical practitioners, a similar operational arrangement would come into force in respect of dentists, ophthalmologists and pharmacists. Breathtakingly bold, the scheme in reality placed the entire medical profession under permanent notice of martial law.

Though the strategy could not have been clearer, the politics of introducing it were both complex and contentious, especially because three very powerful interest groups needed to give their blessing to the scheme. They were the Services, the medical profession and the Ministry of Labour and to stand any kind of chance of succeeding, the game plan the Ministry of Health prepared anticipated all the problems they might encounter in dealing with these sectors. Devious to the last, their mandarins proposed to apply a progressive form of peer pressure with the Armed Services targeted as the most receptive, followed by the medical profession and then endowed with that powerful consensus the Ministry of Labour would feel sufficiently pressurised to surrender all their powers of direction and vest these in the Minister of Health direct.

In many ways, the Services had no real interest how the medical profession might look, so long as their own medical position remained largely unaffected. Reflecting that situation, it took only a few weeks for the Ministry of Health to gain this crucial support. A reasonable inference might be drawn this quick success merely represented an outcome based on furnishing the military with an easy solution to their manpower needs in war. The consummate irony of such a swift agreement was, however, much more to do with their fears over the future of military medicine in peace. For the military medical services plans to use the medical professions more economically under a semi militarised National Health Service posed a subtle danger with the potential to harm, if not destroy, their wartime prerogative of treating the military casualty exclusively in military hospitals. Post-war economic pressures meant cuts and constraints were always on the political agenda, especially under the dour Sir Stafford Cripps, the Chancellor of the Exchequer and architect of the country's post war austerity programme. Wearing his military hat, General Sir Alexander Hood had himself expressed concerns in stating categorically: 'He felt that we were in serious danger from the National Health Service'.[29] To counteract the danger and secure economies on their own terms, Service Ministers established the Medical Services Co-ordinating Committee as a means of reassuring the Treasury of their good housekeeping. Chaired by John Newling, an Under-Secretary at the Ministry of Defence, (who would in due course consider the Skeleton Plan), its terms of reference were to ensure the 'maximum co-ordination and the elimination of duplication, and by such means, the greatest possible economy of medical personnel and material consistent with maintaining efficiency and readiness for war'.[30]

There is little doubt the emergence of the National Health Service had begun to cause problems for the military medical services in terms of justifying the complete range of medical cover they provided in the UK not only for soldiers, but also for their families. The NHS with its good geographical spread of relatively consistent resources offered an alternative capable of delivering better economies of use, particularly where the military were thin on the ground, rather than establishing separate Service facilities. Even more perturbing to their medical independence, the national coverage of the NHS could be used to good effect in atomic war planning rather than expanding military hospitals which anyway were mostly in militarized zones and likely Soviet targets. Added to those threats came a more pressing and urgent problem. Membership of the National Health Service offered better career prospects to medical practitioners compared to the pay and conditions available in the Royal Army Medical Corps. It gave a real choice between a stable career within the expanding NHS or the alternative of having to practice in a military machine run on cheap conscription to defend an increasingly hostile rump of empire. Naturally, the preference for civilian medicine prevailed, which seriously depleted the establishment figures of the military healthcare system. Also, having to endure further suffering in the Chancellor's pay freeze, it did nothing to help the dire situation with the result that the whole system was heading towards total collapse.

All kinds of ideas whirled around in desperate hope that from somewhere an answer to the recruitment problem of the Services could be found without breaching the Chancellor's pay policy. Minister of Health, Aneurin Bevan, started 'hares running' with the idea National Health Service specialists might be granted leave to join the Forces on condition their pension rights were preserved. Of course, this did not offer a workable solution. Transferring specialists from the civil to the military spheres involved complex, if not intractable difficulties such as the loss of seniority in the NHS and subsequent reinstatement. Outright blackmail joined the list of possible solutions. A proposition even proposed that Registrars who were to become surplus due to the restructuring process within the hospital sector could receive preference when they reapplied for NHS posts if they had volunteered for military service. The whiff of coercion eventually reached the House of Lords. Webb-Johnson, surgeon to Queen Mary, advocated to his peers that all full-time appointments in the NHS should carry an outright obligation to serve in the armed forces.[31] Detecting an opportunity, the Director General of the Army Medical Services spelt out with less political correctness how that process might work, particularly affecting those who had never served in the Forces:

> There appears to be no attraction to N.H.S. specialists to volunteer to serve. A specialist who is 'dug in' in the N.H.S. will not want to leave his job voluntarily and go abroad for a period of 18 months unless there is some inducement. The only inducement which might be offered would be again if service in the armed forces would be regarded favourably by the Ministry of Health when assessing more senior appointments, and such a candidate would be given preference provided his professional capabilities are satisfactory. If this suggestion is not accepted then the only way of obtaining such specialists is on the basis advocated by Lord Webb-Johnson, namely that full time appointments might carry with them the necessity of a period in the armed forces. Selection would preferably be from those who for some reason or other have never served in uniform during the war.[32]

Far from seeing all these fears and problems that beset the military medical establishment as a disadvantage, the Ministry of Health embraced the situation and steered it towards agreement over the National Medical Corps. Primarily the tactic involved giving comfort that whilst more fusion of civil and military medical facilities was necessary, certain elements of Service medical support were possible to preserve. For example, the Ministry of Health agreed the expansion of existing military hospitals could take place where strategically possible, but put a stop on the construction of new facilities. The Ministry of Health also fully recognised the concerns of the Services about the loss of morale their people might suffer if left too long under civilian care and confirmed transfers to a Service-based establishment would be permissible when patients were fit for light duties. Extending the principle, the Services were also to organise such rehabilitation and convalescent centres they might need to bring those in recovery under military discipline as soon as possible. Finally, important promises about military administration confirmed the status of the uniformed medical officer remaining at the heart of preserving the health of the soldier and the maintenance of fighting efficiency.[33]

In particular, the basis of the expansive medical illusion was defined by the 'underlying principle' that whilst the medical profession would be pooled, ostensibly to cover both the needs of civilians and the military, the national interest demanded priority would be given to Service casualties to ensure the continued effectiveness of the fighting services. The Ministry of Defence received this fundamental reassurance by way of a secret understanding, a matter covered in a most oblique statement of intent in the Skeleton Plan:

> The underlying principle is that in a future war the best and fullest use in the national interest must be made of all available doctors and hospital facilities. Both were severely strained in the last war; in a future war the Health Departments' assumption, is that they may well be quite inadequate to deal with all casualties in this country.
>
> The Services could not be given overriding priority for all their actual and potential needs at the expense of the civilian population. Equally, however, it did not follow that the best use of medical resources in the national interest was to pool them all and to treat everyone, civilian and service alike, equally. On the contrary, the Forces must, in war, have the necessary priorities to enable them to function at fullest possible efficiency. The Health Departments accepted this.[34]

Based on these pledges, the Newling Committee ratified the Skeleton Plan on 11 August 1949, illustrated as a flow chart in Appendix 2. With such powerful backing, it effectively dragged in the approval of the Ministry of Defence, the Ministry of War, together with their respective Ministers, all of which provided an alliance of exceptional value to the

Ministry of Health. For both parties it embodied the ideal compromise where the significant looked insignificant and crucially seemed to provide the catalyst in putting doctors and surgeons into a para-military organisation.[35]

Turf Wars

Unluckily for the Ministry of Health, things were not entirely as straightforward as they had hoped. Talks with the Services regarding the mobilisation of doctors, dentists and surgeons had been kept secret as a part of a clearly defined strategy.[36] In parallel with those discussions the Ministry of Health also started to engage with the medical profession through their professional institutions. The tactical direction chosen involved these organisations appointing representatives to attend a meeting at the Ministry so the proposals could be put to them 'in confidence'.[37] Enticing the grandees of medicine with just the right degree of information to generate curiosity rather than controversy is evident in the Ministry's deliberate choice of approach which suggested: 'It would be a mistake to give the organisations a detailed description of our proposals in advance as we think they would tend to harden against it but it seems necessary to give them some idea of the main points to be discussed, which can be expanded verbally at a meeting and followed up with a detailed memorandum at a later stage'.[38]

For that reason, the Ministry's invite gave nothing away about the totalitarian club the medical profession was to join. Couched in agreeable terms and given under the signature of Miss Enid Russell-Smith, the Under-Secretary to be responsible for much of the negotiation, it anaesthetised the atomic dimension with a polite summons: 'the Ministry would like to discuss with representatives of the medical profession the steps which ought to be taken to control medical manpower in war'. Requesting advice on policy for the allocation of doctors and the medical representation proposed were all carrots of possible influence the Ministry negotiators knew would entice their potential adversaries to attend in a receptive frame of mind.[39] Many of those involved bore the scars of negotiations over the NHS with personal and professional animosities included in the mix time had never healed. Two in particular stand out. Dr Charles Hill, Secretary of the BMA since 1944, had mounted a final and intensive campaign against the NHS. Known famously as 'the radio doctor' for his broadcasts during the war, he also nurtured political ambitions and eventually became a Member of Parliament in 1950 for Luton as a Conservative and National Liberal. Lord Moran, the President of the Royal College of Physicians and Churchill's personal doctor, on the other hand, had helped Bevan both psychologically to deal with the BMA and practically to support him with the nationalisation of the hospitals by bringing in the consultants. An unbridgeable gulf existed between the two men. Moran had written privately to the editor of *The Times*, describing Hill as 'a demagogue' and whose 'mind is without depth or balance – not a wise man'.[40] Moreover, Lord Moran, marinated in professional status to ensure his institution held the highest ground, had little time for general practitioners and even less time for women medical students. In 1924, like many administrators, he had as Dean of St Mary's Hospital Medical School, ended the admission of women allowed during the First World War. True to form, a file note left at the Ministry of Health indicated: 'Lord Moran telephoned on 6 October about the meeting on Monday next, to discuss Medical Manpower in Wartime. He said that he was not anxious to sit round a table for two or three hours to discuss what should be done with General Practitioners and that the most important matter for consideration was the allocation of Consultants and Specialists'.[41]

Unquestionably, the gathering of this eminent group presented the Ministry of Health with a challenge requiring utmost diplomacy. The date of the meeting depended upon the availability of Sir Alexander Hood before his departure to take on a new post as Governor of Bermuda. Working to that schedule, on 10 October 1949, medical professors and knights of the realm packed into the conference room of the Ministry of Health in Whitehall. They represented the Royal College of Surgeons, the Royal College of Physicians, the Royal College of Obstetricians and Gynaecologists, the Royal College of Surgeons, Edinburgh, the Royal Faculty of Physicians and Surgeons Glasgow, The Society of Medical Officers of Health and the British Medical Association. All these were the professional bodies destined to serve on the proposed National Medical Advisory Committee. With only one other woman present amongst twenty-eight men, Miss Russell-Smith (Later Dame Russell-Smith) embarked on a serious charm offensive. Russell-Smith, as a senior civil servant, had been very much involved in the establishment of the National Health Service itself so would have known much about those she faced and the way to deal with their foibles. She did not disclose the existence of the Skeleton Plan, the one agreed by the Services, but suggested to those gathered their views were important to hear before the finalisation of any documentation. Creating a further sense of ownership, the meeting was sworn to secrecy, with the command that under no circumstances could there be any kind of publicity or press announcement.[42]

Internal Ministry of Health notes setting out their understanding of the meeting suggest step two turned out to be just as successful as the first that had secured the agreement of the Services. The firm belief prevailed the response given by the organisations had at least been positive, evidenced by a comment: 'It appeared at the conference that the representatives present were prepared to accept a scheme on the lines sketched out in the document, though it is, of course, always possible that they may have second thoughts when they see it in black and white'.[43] Even the thorny question of the National Medical Corps seemed to survive its first outing, with Dr Charles Hill giving tacit approval on condition that the scheme did not involve any kind of compulsion. How far this nod of approval reflected the degree to which the Ministry of Health had left out the less savoury parts of the plan is not possible to identify, but overall the result appeared to Ministry officials to be a promising start.

When the official response of the British Medical Association arrived on the 29 December 1949 nothing seemed to suggest it represented anything other than a collective wish to move the Skeleton Plan towards a swift conclusion. The Association suggested they saw 'no good reason for dissolving a machinery, that of the Central Medical War Committee and the Medical Priority Committee, which has worked with efficiency for the past ten years'. They went on to make constructive comments on the proposals, typically focussing on the committee structures and appeal processes. Then, the Ministry of Health must have felt they had hit the political jackpot. Having considered the direction procedures, Sir Henry Soutar, Dr Peter Macdonald, Major-General Sir Percy Tomlinson and Dr Charles Hill on behalf of the British Medical Association collectively confirmed: 'No comment is made on the central theme of a National Medical Corps under the control of a Director-General with statutory powers of direction' and 'The Director-General should be a medical man.'[44]

Taken altogether, the reactions seemed to signal the prospect of a satisfactory outcome and in a memorandum the Ministry jubilantly proclaimed, 'There seems to be hardly anything between us'.[45] The response of the Medical Women's Federation amounted to a blank canvas, saying they had considered the Skeleton Plan 'paragraph by paragraph' and approved the proposal in its entirety. No doubt flattered by being given a voice in the debate they added: 'The Medical Women's Federation is glad to be included in the professional bodies to be consulted and will be prepared at all times to contribute to the best of its ability'.[46] By mid-February 1950, the Ministry of Health recorded an impressive tally of approvals in principle from the BMA and the Society of Medical Officers of Health. The Royal College of Surgeons considered women doctors should not be subject to more direction than other women of the same age, a point ironically in conflict with the blanket approval of the Women's Medical Federation. Other than that, their remaining proposals were so confused it was felt it would be necessary to explain the scheme again. The Royal College of Obstetricians and Gynaecologists gave their general agreement, subject to the Services agreeing the scheme. The file note indicated, 'they have already done so on the Newling Committee, but the profession have not been told about this', an exceptional revelation about the careful, not to say clandestine, way the Ministry were establishing their position.[47]

With everything pointing to an agreement over the formation of a National Medical Corps being reached it seemed incongruous anything further could stand in the way, particularly as the situation in Korea threatened to turn into global war. Yet the seemingly-inexorable movement towards a successful outcome met the immovable, intransigent and exceptionally irate form in the Ministry of Labour. Instead of cooperation in the national interest, a sideshow of self-interest politics erupted with volcanic force. Getting the Skeleton Plan agreed involved treading on the bureaucratic territory of another Ministry in a major way. The proposed National Medical Corps represented a cataclysmic change in the policy relating to conscription and the direction of labour, still the responsibility of the Ministry of Labour and National Service (giving its full title). Ensuring their absence from crucial meetings and withholding background papers had secured enough time to obtain the agreement of the Armed Forces and muster a formidable alliance to put the opposition under immense peer pressure. The course of action taken is very apparent in the correspondence between the Ministries before the final showdown. It contained an air of nervous jollity, but shows the veil of secrecy which the Ministry of Health had drawn over the matter.

Sensing they had become victims of a conspiracy, Gilbert Nash, Under-Secretary at the Ministry of Labour and National Service, had requested sight of some of the papers he knew were circulating. Even so, he was advised by his opposite number Sydney Wilkinson at the Ministry of Health: 'I think it would be better if you could possess your soul in patience a little longer until the Newling Committee have disposed of the matter unless, as I said before you feel you should see our proposals earlier'.[48] Eventual discovery of the contents of the Skeleton Plan by the Ministry of Labour raised a sense of complete disbelief, a fact amply shown up by a covering note to Sir Harold Wiles, Deputy Secretary that squarely laid the subterfuge at the door of Enid Russell-Smith's department:

> Sir Harold Wiles. I think you should see these papers. I am extremely disturbed at the developments they indicate. I am very sorry to see that we did not insist on having a copy of the document in its initial stages. It is quite clear in the letters from Mr Wilkinson that he was most anxious that we should not see the document, anticipating

that we would not agree with the Ministry of Health's proposals.[49]

The indignation expressed by Ministry of Labour and National Service reflects the extent to which they felt cheated. Not only did they consider the proposal trespassed on their domain, which included the mobilisation of manpower resources for the whole country, it also interfered in other spheres of medical arrangements including factory doctors that came under their jurisdiction. On 9 December 1949, they informed Russell-Smith there were fundamental points of policy on which they could not agree and advised her: 'You cannot proceed with your discussions with other bodies on the assumption that your proposals are acceptable to the Government as a whole'. Any hope of a reasonable settlement dissolved with the statement 'there is not much common ground between us and we must dissociate ourselves from the memorandum you have issued'.[50] Those few words then started a turf war as to who should have the power to control medical profession. Protecting their legacy, the Ministry of Labour argued doctors had to be under the same kind of control as the rest of the population and saw 'the gravest objection' to compulsory enrolment in a corps of all members of a particular profession without any regard to what was happening to the rest of the population.[51]

One last attempt by the Ministry of Health to pressurise the Ministry of Labour into submission by suggesting a *fait accompli* in respect of the Skeleton Plan seriously backfired. Relations deteriorated still further when the Ministry of Health ignored the request to stop and continued talks with medical representatives until found out again after the Ministry of Labour discovered the position through other channels.[52] From the files at The National Archives, it is possible to deduce the civil servants dealing with the Skeleton Plan at the Ministry of Health hoped that the Cabinet would finally arbitrate on the issue.[53] They had every reason to be confident about things going their way. The Services were in favour of the Skeleton Plan to the extent the Director General of Medical Services Royal Navy had expressed some surprise that the plan, originally promised to become operational by the end of 1949, had not yet materialised. It was also felt the Minister of Defence would support the Ministry of Health's position at a Cabinet meeting.[54] Whilst everything seemed to be progressing in the right direction, unfortunately for the Ministry of Health this momentum suddenly stopped because of a General Election.

When hostilities eventually resumed, the antennae of Cabinet Secretary Sir Norman Brook picked up on the dispute at a completely unrelated meeting with the Ministry of Health. He immediately wrote to Sir Godfrey Ince, the Permanent Under-Secretary of the Ministry of Labour saying, 'I gathered that there was a difference of view between your

Department and the Ministry of Health' and suggested before the question was referred to Ministers there ought to be preliminary discussions between officials to least clarify the issues at stake.[55] In fact, Brook's intervention ended the Ministry of Health's plan to create the bandwagon with medical and military backing. His summons to the Cabinet Office of Ince, and Newling on 4 April 1950 exhibited both his personal standing as well as self-assurance in being able to keep good order. At least part of what transpired appears in a minute prepared by a Ministry of Health official. In short, it amounted to an expression of deep-rooted mistrust of the medical profession by the Ministry of Labour and they felt they were the department to control medical resources. Ince referred to the dubious call up arrangements conducted by doctors during the last war and added victimisation to the list of offences in suggesting they were too frightened to use the appeals procedure for hardship because of possible persecution by their fellow doctors if they did take that route. Things did not get any better. Sir Godfrey Ince saw no problems in his department, the Ministry of Labour, dispatching a large number of doctors to a specific area and deal with an atomic attack. Indeed, his wrath took in the whole machinery and he questioned whether the Presidents of the Royal Colleges as members of the Medical Priority Committee and the proposed National Medical Manpower Committee should advise the Government on questions of medical manpower at all. The whole tirade came wrapped in an overall condemnation: 'He reiterated that he could in no circumstances agree to doctors dealing with doctors and said that this was the only profession that had these arrangements which should cease. Reference was made to dentists, pharmacists, dispensers and opticians who had special schemes but he and the Chairman agreed that these were all the same breed'.[56]

Brook's remark as 'the Chairman' may have appeared as nothing more than jovial banter but for the record of his subsequent rationalisation of the position that the minutes reported:

> Ministers were not 'war minded' at present and he was reluctant to put a paper to the Cabinet at this stage. Although sundry 'guesses' have been made about the initial stages of any future war, the enemy might decide not to use the atom bomb. The forecasts of casualties in the early stages of World War II had been somewhat inaccurate.[57]

These were extraordinary statements made by the most senior civil servant who had intimate knowledge about the Government's atomic bomb programme and the Cabinet's increasing defence consciousness following the Berlin Crisis. The meeting had taken place before the real jolt of the start of Korean War some weeks later, but there were other preoccupations. These included the possible costs to the NHS, which were already spinning out of control, not to mention the unknown risks of trying to impose a national service liability in peace on the entire medical profession. All these things were not exactly political winners for a Labour government that had gone to the country on 23 February 1950 and returned with a majority of just five seats. Any attempt to mobilise the entire medical profession into a para-military force could have simply tipped the entire calamitous situation over the edge.

Because of Brook's involvement, the Ministry of Labour was empowered to develop a new strategy through the auspices of a revised Skeleton Plan for consideration by the medical profession about their future control in war. Firstly, the Ministry of Labour made sure the bid for total power over medical resources by the Health Departments did not go further. It sent a clear message the responsibility for medical manpower would not rest with the Minister of Health or the Secretary of State for Scotland, but on a committee of the Cabinet and that in implementing policy the Health Departments would act only in consultation with other Ministers concerned.[58] During the process of demolishing the Ministry of Health's bid for supreme authority over all things medical, the proposal to establish the corps came in for an extraordinarily astute move. Sir Harold Wiles sent out a questionnaire to the Ministry of Health asking them to justify, with hard evidence, the decision to recommend the formation of a National Medical Corps and requested details of its proposed structure and ranks, as well as the pay and conditions proposed. Looking at the briefing notes Under-Secretary Wilkinson prepared for his colleagues to formulate a response, the fact that emerges is just how vague the basis for the mobilisation plan really had been all along, a position underlined by the admission that absolutely nothing was available conceptually about the way the NMC proposal would work in practice:

> If we are going strongly to advocate a corps we must say and be able to describe in much greater detail than we have done so far how we would organise and dispose it. So far we have fobbed off questions of uniforms, ranks, etc., by saying that we had not yet worked out the matter so closely, but we cannot hope to take this line successfully very much longer.[59]

Once the seed of self-doubt took root it merely grew, the consequences becoming all too clear at an internal planning meeting that took place at the Ministry of Health in Whitehall on 11 September 1950. Chaired by Sydney Wilkinson, the main backers of the plan, Sir Ernest Rock Carling, Sir Claude Frankau were in attendance as well as Miss Russell-Smith, along with a representative from the Department of Health for Scotland and other, more junior, civil servants. Their combined thoughts added up to the fact nobody could actually defend the strategy to any great extent, if at all. A key belief evasion had taken place during the war was shattered when one of the junior civil servants suggested the problems had been largely due to the vagaries of the quota system itself and it was this that caused many more recruitable doctors to be left in one area than another because of age structures. Eventually the meeting finally accepted the conspiracy theories were unfounded and that if there were problems the war itself had magnified these out of all proportion. A minute of that decision provided an appropriate epitaph to the whole affair in admitting 'that earlier insistence on a National Medical Corps had perhaps gone too far'.[60]

Although the central plank of the National Medical Corps disappeared because of the self-inflicted mortal wound, it still left the mechanics of how the medical profession should be mobilised and deployed to meet an atomic attack for further consideration. The Ministry of Labour were just as keen that the medical profession should come under a more stringent form of control. Indeed as the meeting with Brook had also drawn out, the two sides were not actually far apart in their suspicions about 'doctors dealing with doctors'. The second Skeleton Plan still reflected that to some degree with the proposed appointment of a Director-General to control the civilian medical services, principally on the basis somebody would eventually need to have overriding control. In the new order of things, his powers of direction would emanate from the Ministry of Labour and National Service and delegated as necessary.

Regarding the vexed question of conscription, the Ministry of Labour made some moves towards acknowledging greater speed was essential to mobilise doctors and surgeons in an atomic emergency. Although the ministry did not want any kind of enlistment to commence prior to the formal declaration of war, to compensate for that, it conceded to the preparation of a voluntary compilation of a register of all medical practitioners well in advance of hostilities giving information on age and mobility. Compulsory registration either shortly before or after the outbreak of war could then cover any gaps.[61] Another concession did stand out as an acknowledgement the existing Defence Regulations represented an outdated means to deal with an immediate response to an atomic attack. Constitutionally these were only possible to pass when the international situation deteriorated to the point when war seemed inevitable, by which time it would be too late. Recognising the dilemma, the Ministry of Labour suggested the Ministry of Health should proceed quickly to enrol doctors on a voluntary basis so that some at least could be organised into the mobile groups and rely on the remainder up to the age of 65 being called up to bring the organisation to its full potential. The compulsion then applied would be the same as for the civilian population generally with the added advantage of including nurses and medical auxiliaries.[62] Apart from these changes, the administrative side dealing with constitutional and committee matters remained much the same as in the original document and a new Skeleton Plan B emerged for the medical profession to consider.

Doctored Orders

With the pressures building up over Korea, an agreement in respect of the revised Skeleton Plan may well have seemed a formality when it came to gaining the approval of the medical profession, especially in its watered-down form. However, as luck would have it, the resumption of talks also coincided with some of the most acrimonious negotiations about pay and conditions in the National Health Service during the period 1949-1951. Looking back today to the founding of the NHS in 1948, one might wonder how in just twenty four months the bright dawn of the new medical era could have darkened so quickly. Two issues collided to produce a furore of seismic proportions. Firstly, the full costs of creating the National Health Service were coming home to roost. A combination of freewheeling expenditure in setting up the system, combined with a rush by the public to take advantage of the 'free' services offered, inevitably had an impact beyond imagination. So just seven months following the start of the new service, the Minister of Health had found it necessary to request a large supplementary appropriation of almost £53 million, amounting to a stunning 30% of the original budget estimate. If that was not bad enough, a year later yet another appropriation this time of £90 million, nearly 40% of the estimated running costs for 1949-50, rested with political discomfort on the Treasury table.[63]

Secondly, against a barrage of bad publicity and the Treasury determined to curtail the NHS costs to predetermined limits, Dr Solomon (Solly) Wand, Chairman of the BMA Council demanded the central remuneration fund be increased by £16.5 million from the sum actually available which amounted to £41.5 million. Pitted against an intransigent Treasury, BMA negotiators eventually threatened a strike along with a refusal to sign National Insurance certificates. During their discussions, the BMA Council noted with concern that an extension of the Defence Regulations had been declared by the Government which took them to December 1951, a move allowing the Minister of Health to assume emergency powers if general practitioners decided to come out of the National Health Service.[64] The BMA retaliated and prepared its own battle plan. A 'phantom' body called The British Medical Guild, established in 1948 to collect 'fighting funds' with the purpose of enabling trade union style actions to be undertaken, was put on full alert with a promise to provide all legal support necessary. Strike action may not have materialised, but the episode uncomfortably brought the medical profession close to statutory direction and control for the first time. Not until the issue went to a judicial adjudication by Justice Danckerts in March 1952 followed by a settlement of nearly £10 million in favour of the medical profession did some kind of normality resume, but the whole episode left a bitter taste.[65]

Behind the BMA's sensitivities also lay the painful deliberations conducted between 1943-1948 regarding the kind of structure that a national health system should adopt. These had gone through several reports including Beveridge, Maude and Willink, all milestones along a tedious and often acrimonious route that attempted unsuccessfully to appease the medical profession to bring them into a universal system of state medical care. British medicine had evolved during the pre NHS days into a commercially orientated business with many individual practices, a fact that left an instinctive aversion to anything that could threaten that element of independence and turn them into civil servants. With an extraordinarily complex history behind the setting up of the NHS, this had a profound effect on the way the BMA in particular saw the world across a negotiating table. It faced a government prepared to nationalise much of Britain's industrial and transport infrastructure, and for that matter grab the hospitals from municipal control. Everything therefore went through a microscopic process of consideration to filter out any speck likely to threaten their medical independence. It could also make dealing with the BMA deceptively congenial. Often the finest of detail or a sudden panic attack could scupper negotiations, just when they seemed on the right track, a fate that necessarily awaited the progress of Skeleton Plan B.

When the Ministry of Health sent out letters marked 'secret' during September 1950 to those organisations representing the medical profession there were no apparent signs of any insecurity about returning to the issue of wartime controls. The correspondence included a copy of the Skeleton Plan referred to as 'the revised scheme' along with an invitation to attend a meeting on the 20 October 1950 at the Ministry of Health offices in Whitehall with the optimistic aim of 'reaching final agreement'.[66] Writing on behalf of the BMA, then-Deputy Secretary Dr Angus Macrae acknowledged receipt, but took the opportunity of reminding Miss Russell-Smith worries over a war in Korea were causing 'much disquiet' in the profession. Bearing in mind the publicity given to other civil defence plans, he requested the secrecy requirement be relaxed so the Association could make some announcement about the arrangements, which the meeting proposed might conclude.[67]

Once again, the event was a grand gathering of the great and the good of the medical professional bodies and appeared to generate an enthusiasm to get the issue of medical manpower control sorted out once and for all. Under the chairmanship of Sir William Douglas, Permanent Under-Secretary of the Ministry of Health, all the right strategic decisions were made to set the framework of committees which would hold good until the final plan appeared in the *British Medical Journal*. It was the thing the medical profession, particularly the BMA, excelled at to ensure their professional interests received due protection at every level of decision making. When it came to constructing committees for conscripting the medical profession for war service, the principles adopted followed the procedures of the last war, as far as possible. A case-in-point involved the new National Manpower Committee destined to advise the Government. Constitutionally it represented only a change in name from the old Medical Priority Committee. Reassuringly, membership of this elite group of ten medical men and women was again to come through nominations of the main professional bodies and confirmed by the Minister of Health, the Minister of Labour and National Service, the Minister of Defence and the Secretary of State for Scotland following the practice started in 1941.[68]

Determined to stay with the wartime template, even the idea the national recruitment committees should be subcommittees of the National Manpower Committee met with complete resistance to ensure any kind of political linkage was removed. Instead, the old wartime hierarchies were adapted to fit into the structures of the National Health Service. Two independent groups in the form of the Central Recruitment Committees, one for England and Wales and another for Scotland were to operate in the same way as the previous Central War Medical Committee, their status assured by a wide range of representation from the medical profession. Keeping the same self-regulating powers the profession had enjoyed in the past became critical. These began at the centre and then trickled down into the Local Recruitment Committees which covered the entire profession across the entire country. For the medical profession this represented an essential safeguard to maintain their power base and protect themselves against the rapacious government controls they perceived were behind every change to established protocols. The importance of this was not lost on the Ministry of Health who saw 'no harm' in allowing the illusion of total self-governance to persist.[69] Following that path of complete control, attempts to put a representative of the Ministry of Health as chair of local committees, ostensibly to prevent victimisation, were stopped in their tracks. With one voice, the meeting asked Sir William to make it a matter of record 'the profession should be dealt with by their own colleagues'. Neither was anything to prejudice the system from within and Local Recruitment Committees were to be elected annually thus ensuring miscreants could be weeded out. Imposing such means of self-protection at all layers of influence, however great or small, came with a final demand for the wartime protocol to be reinstated involving nominations for call up being delivered to the Services directly by the profession and not through any government machinery. Though arguably a symbolic detail, it still represented an obsession over government interference hardly conducive to the task in hand.[70]

The big test over control, of course, lay in the need to achieve a consensus over the direction of the civilian medical services in wartime, particularly since the plan no longer possessed military connotations. Certainly, the omens seemed good. The meeting approved the principle that all doctors, both men and women up to 65 and not in the fighting services on the outbreak of war would be subject to direction by a Director General. Crucial to the whole concept, this now provided the means for introducing a centralised command structure.[71] With that essential element in place and the committee framework for selecting doctors agreed the whole scheme seemed to be heading in the right direction at last. Adding to the air of consensus, the meeting agreed an amended Skeleton Plan should be prepared and for this purpose a small subcommittee established immediately consisting of five medical men, including Dr Angus Macrae, Deputy Secretary of the BMA. His appointment was crucial in suggesting that any agreement reached would be subsequently 'rubber stamped' when the final proposals were submitted to the BMA's main ruling committee.[72]

When the final outline did emerge, the January 1951 revise of the Skeleton Plan represented an extraordinary collegiate effort to produce a system having little to do with atomic warfare, but more about defending the power interests of those organisations involved. Looking at this document it is possible to appreciate why the Ministry of Health had always preferred the backing of military law. Between the Ministry of Labour and the medical subcommittee's wish to ensure the medical profession were not to be victims of direction, the clause regarding their position under atomic attack had been watered down to an obsequious level of legal triteness:

> Attacks with weapons of atomic, biological and chemical warfare would, of course, put an unprecedented strain on the medical manpower available, and it would be essential that in any emergency those doctors required to deal with the

> situation should carry out promptly and without question any orders given by the Director-General or his authorised officers. Leave to appeal against a direction (before it had been complied with) would operate. The Director General would be guided on the question of the medical needs of an area by the Central Recruitment Committee, who would in turn be advised by local committees.[73]

Tying the actions of the Director General of Medical Services into the committee system and allowing an ambiguous form of leave to appeal against his orders entirely sums up the way the BMA saw the question of control. Proof of that somewhat irksome pudding came when the plan reached the full BMA Council. The main antagonist appeared to be the venerable Dr Solomon Wand, who clearly had no intention to regard the plan as anything more than another potential threat to his organisation. The minute of the debate, which records his objection and the reaction of his colleagues, reveals the enormous tension between the organisational interests of the BMA and playing its part in any humanitarian emergency:

> Dr Wand expressed concern at the arrangements in the skeleton plan under which, immediately on the outbreak of war, the entire profession could be placed under the control of a Director-general of Civilian Medical Services. He foresaw the possibility of direction to such an extent that it might be impossible to return to independent practice after the emergency had passed. The Committee expressed general agreement with this view, but it was considered that no objection should be raised to the preparation of plans for the full mobility of the profession in an extremely grave emergency such as might be expected to occur, for example, in atomic warfare.[74]

For all the affirmation about continued cooperation, Wand had cast a long shadow over the plan, particularly by sowing the one seed of organisational doubt about the potential threat the arrangements might have to the future independence of the profession. His concerns came like a bolt out of the blue for the Ministry of Health. The annotations made on their paperwork clearly show they believed the BMA had accepted the principles of the Skeleton Plan through the auspices of the subcommittee. What it really showed is just how the BMA were past masters at playing the committee system. Infuriatingly, the BMA Council made up its mind a relationship had to exist between the nature of the war and the degree of control the medical profession could allow government to exercise. Passing on their concerns to the Ministry of Health, just eight days before the meeting planned to be the final hurdle, they provided their view as to how the control issue had to be handled:

> In the first place, the Council believes that doctors will give better service voluntarily than under the discipline of a semi-military machine, and it considers it to be of the first importance that control of the medical profession in time of war should be introduced only to the extent that circumstances render necessary. While it may be essential to make plans in advance for the full mobility of the profession in grave emergencies, such as might be expected to occur, for example, in atomic warfare, the Council is anxious to be assured that the powers of direction proposed will not be used in conditions of warfare such as have been experienced in the past and that, save in circumstances of extreme emergency, doctors will not be recruited, whether for military or civilian work away from home, except with the approval of the Central Recruitment Committees.[75]

True to form, the BMA had regressed into one of its most awkward defensive shells by 'nit-picking' everything they considered had a threatening tone which reflected the fact the British Medical Association had met its nemesis. Whilst on the recruitment side it deemed its interests adequately protected by means of the committee structures, the direction and control issue created for them a dangerous power vacuum. This put commands in place of committees and in the mind of the BMA left the medical profession vulnerable to government interference. Set into its most obsessional frame of mind the Association felt the wording of the Skeleton Plan was 'tactless and unfortunate' and jumped on the words 'direction' and 'control' which in its view needed to be replaced by the more acceptable term 'recruitment'.[76]

Applying tactics of this kind really started the endgame by pushing the Ministry of Health into a complete state of exasperation. Whereas the principle behind the Skeleton Plan had been total flexibility within seconds of atomic bombs falling, the BMA idea imposed a new dimension as to how the circumstances of a deteriorating situation would dictate the recruitment process and whether its labyrinth of committees could be dispensed with. Demonstrated by a debriefing note, the Ministry of Health clearly regarded the BMA's stance as the final straw, concluding: 'We can say that no doctor will be recruited for military service otherwise than with the approval of the Central Recruitment Committees, but we clearly cannot say that no doctor will be recruited for civilian work without their approval: we must have some scope for quick action in an emergency'.[77] With the urgent need to bring the administrative procedures for conscription to a close, the further question about operational control seemed to offer only months of further wrangling, and even then, little guarantee anything would ever be resolved given the BMA's total allergy to compromise over the issue.

Making matters worse, the concerns over government interference harboured by the BMA grew even deeper. It then caused the relationship between them and the Ministry of Health to deteriorate to its lowest level just at a time when some kind of mutual give-and-take was called for. Because of the endless arguments over the mobilisation plan the 'screening' of doctors for war service had climbed further and further up the Government's agenda as the Korean crisis deepened. This involved the process of sifting through those demobbed after the war, but still with a liability for military service in the event of a national emergency. By far the largest reservist category was the 'Z class' and the Government's Defence Committee provisionally agreed that over 600,000 in this category should be considered for possible recall to military service. Because of the large numbers, many doctors were involved and the BMA offered to undertake the screening of these to ensure their call up did not adversely affect the National Health Service. However, instead of generating unity and consensus, this suggested approach actually created a level of distrust and disunity between the medical profession and the Ministries of Health and Labour which led to an incredible game of mutual stubbornness being played out at a critical moment in the nation's history.[78]

Between them the Ministry of Health and the Ministry of Labour agreed they would not surrender to the BMA on their interim measures until the complete package had been agreed especially the issue of control and direction. In a belligerent mood, both Ministries decided to accept the political risks of a delay in order to achieve their objective. The Ministry of Health signalled that sense of determination when the Department itself secretly began screening consultants and specialists working in the NHS. Principal Medical Officers of the Ministry of Health undertook the clandestine exercise in consultation with Senior Administrative Medical Officers of the Regional Hospital Boards. Of course, keeping such an operation under wraps proved impossible and when discovered, the BMA reported being 'astonished and alarmed by the action of the Ministry of Health and is protesting vigorously against this move behind the back of the profession'.[79] By then the degree of internal wrangling stretched the patience of Major-General Bainbridge, Director of Manpower Planning at the War Office. He felt obliged to send out a warning to the Ministry of Labour and National Service on the 7 February 1951 that should mobilisation occur before any so-called proper procedures were in place the Services would simply take those doctors they required for military service regardless of the dislocation this might cause in the National Health Service.[80]

Obviously anxious not to lose their legacy of administrative control in the event of the Services taking unilateral action, Dr Macrae, acting in his new role as the Secretary of the BMA, threatened Miss Enid Russell-Smith with a statement in the *British Medical Journal* exposing her failure to deliver timely advice to practitioners about their call-up status. Such was the mood of hostility that suggestions even emerged about hauling Miss Russell-Smith before the Services Committee of the BMA to voice its concerns and if that did not work, then the BMA would have to approach the Government directly and get an interim process of screening started at once.[81] Accepting it had run out of alternatives, and unwilling to sacrifice the reputation of a senior civil servant to its cause, the Ministry of Health caved in. Dr Macrae won a simple, but effective interim arrangement, which at least protected the BMA investment so far built up.

Put in its simplest terms, the Central War Committee, still in place since the last war but due to be replaced, was to send out nominations of reserve doctors to Local Medical Committees and these in turn would consider the effect on local medical services. Crucial in that manoeuvre was the fact the Local Medical Committees already existed as part of the National Health Service to represent the interests of local practitioners. These were to form subcommittees for screening, a tactical stroke of genius, which effectively anchored the process into the medical heartland of the BMA and allowed them to prove their capability of handling conscription without outside interference.[82] The Local Medical Committees received some 800 names for possible recall as the BMA had demanded and asked 'to recommend whether or not doctors could be spared from practice in an emergency without serious dislocation of the civilian medical service'. Each doctor also had an opportunity of representing his case personally if he considered grounds existed for an appeal in that respect. In the absence of other arrangements, the Ministry of Health also undertook the screening of reservist doctors working in hospitals or the public health sector.[83]

These moves secured the high ground for the BMA in their continuing battle over the Skeleton Plan. With the panic over screening ended, they could then pick off at will any further challenges to their position and did so with a consummate ruthlessness.[84] The net result was a foregone conclusion. When Miss Russell-Smith chaired the last great meeting of the profession on 28 March 1951 the minutes confirm it degenerating into a grand crescendo of obsession with committees, their final numbers and appointment procedures established. As to direction and control, she waved the white flag by announcing the issue had not been put on the agenda and closed the matter accordingly:

> As regards that part of the skeleton plan that dealt with the operational control of the medical services in war-time, the Chairman suggested that it would be premature to come to definite conclusions at the present time. Plans were still being worked out, and it was the intention to consult the medical profession from time to time as definite proposals were crystallised.[85]

The official surrender document came when the BMA published details of the committee plan in the *British Medical Journal* of 2 February 1952. The introduction amounted to a masterful piece of political diversion, given that after a year of negotiations the achievement amounted to just a newer version of the old wartime committee system. The BMA Council confirmed it had given 'some consideration' to the new scheme that laid down the composition of the new central and local recruitment committees. It was perfectly clear in the structure as to why they had agreed. Looking at the construction of the two Central Recruitment Committees, the most important outcome related to the English and Welsh structure consisting as it did of 45 representatives, of which 27 were either members of the BMA or associated with it. Without doubt, that position must have given the BMA considerable comfort about its influence being in no way reduced.[86] Doctors had ensured their position of control had not been usurped and the NHS would not be enveloped by some backdoor plan of total medical control. Those who were to be controlled were effectively in control.

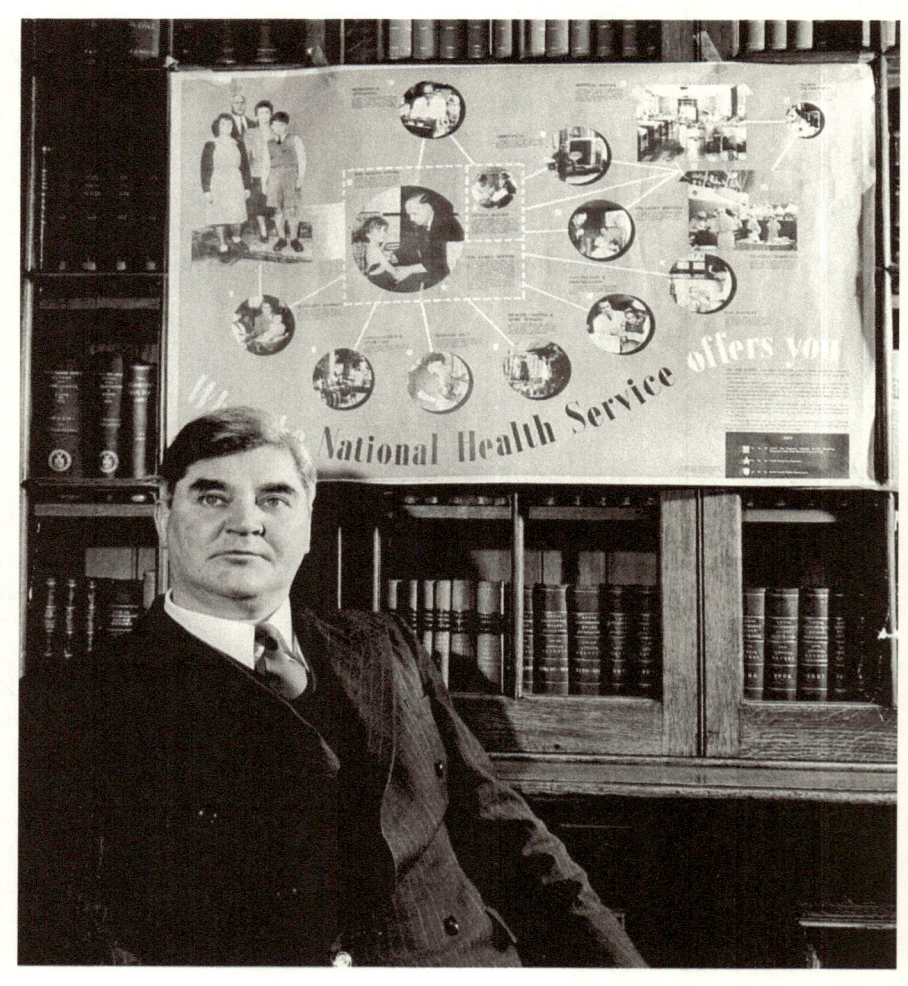

1. Aneurin Bevan, the political father of the NHS in 1949. Behind him is a poster used to promote the new era of state medical care.

THE NEW
NATIONAL HEALTH SERVICE

*

Your new National Health Service begins on 5th July. What is it? How do you get it?

It will provide you with all medical, dental, and nursing care. Everyone—rich or poor, man, woman or child—can use it or any part of it. There are no charges, except for a few special items. There are no insurance qualifications. But it is not a "charity". You are all paying for it, mainly as taxpayers, and it will relieve your money worries in time of illness.

2. The official notification about the start of the NHS distributed throughout Great Britain during 1948.

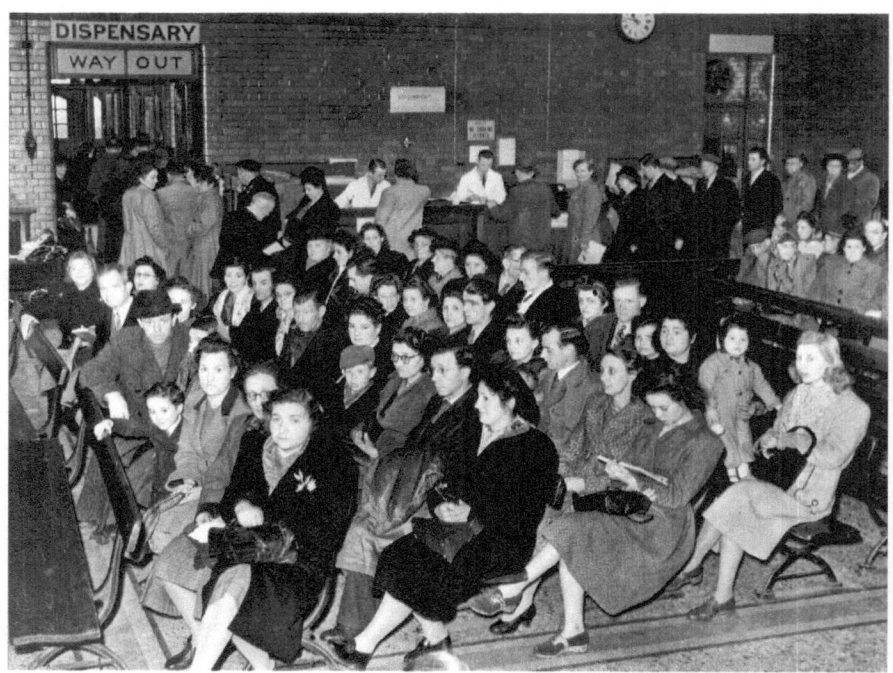

3. An East London hospital in April 1949 with outpatients making appointments and in the waiting area. Demand for treatment was completely underestimated and the rush to take advantage of the new NHS arrangements caused stress in the medical profession over the terms and conditions of service originally agreed.

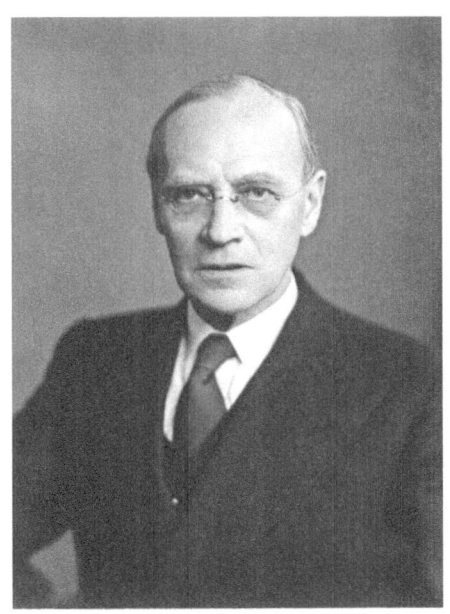

4. Sir Ernest Rock Carling.

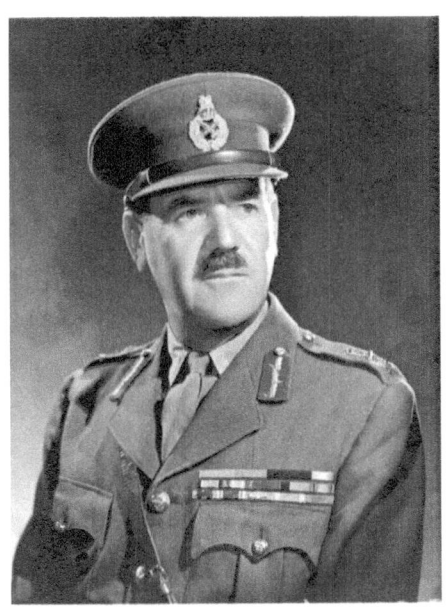

5. Sir Alexander Hood.

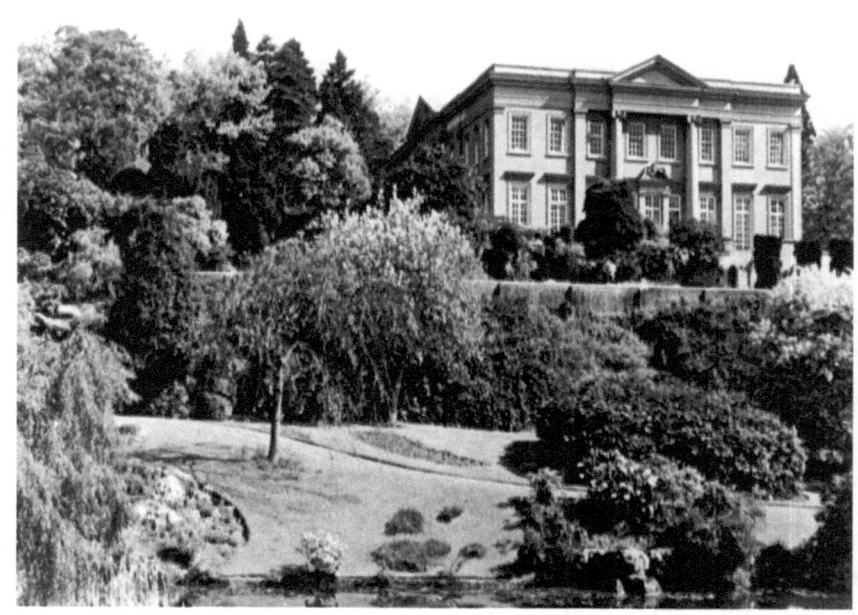

6. & 7. The Civil Defence Staff College, Sunningdale Park, Ascot with a lecture in progress about the atom bomb.

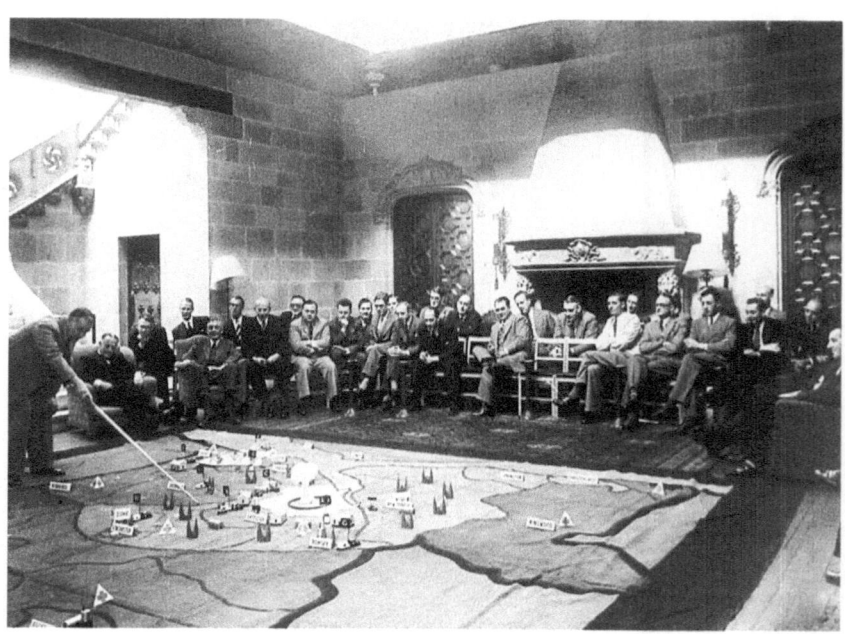

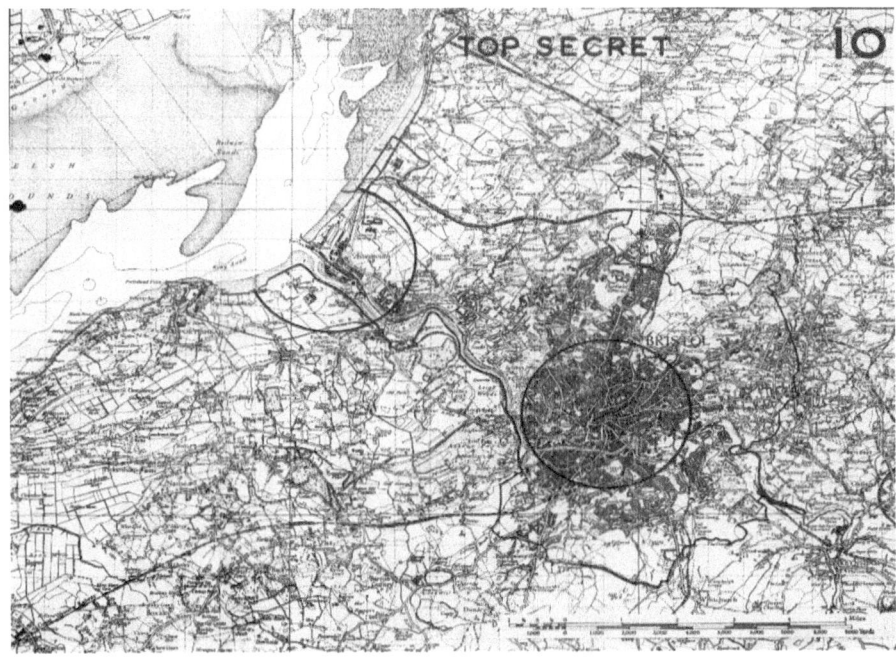

8. Target map showing the two damage rings of a Hiroshima-size bomb on the port and civilian centre of Bristol.

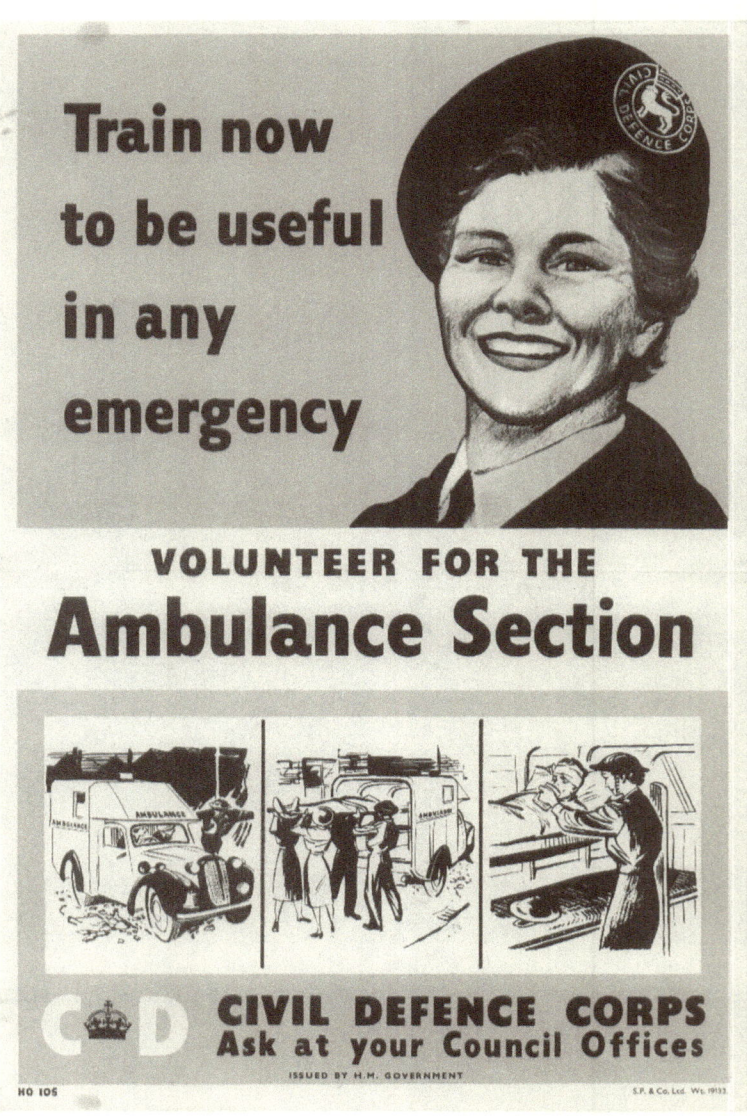

9. 1950s poster. The recruitment of ambulance crews projected the ideal that casualties would receive the best medical attention possible.

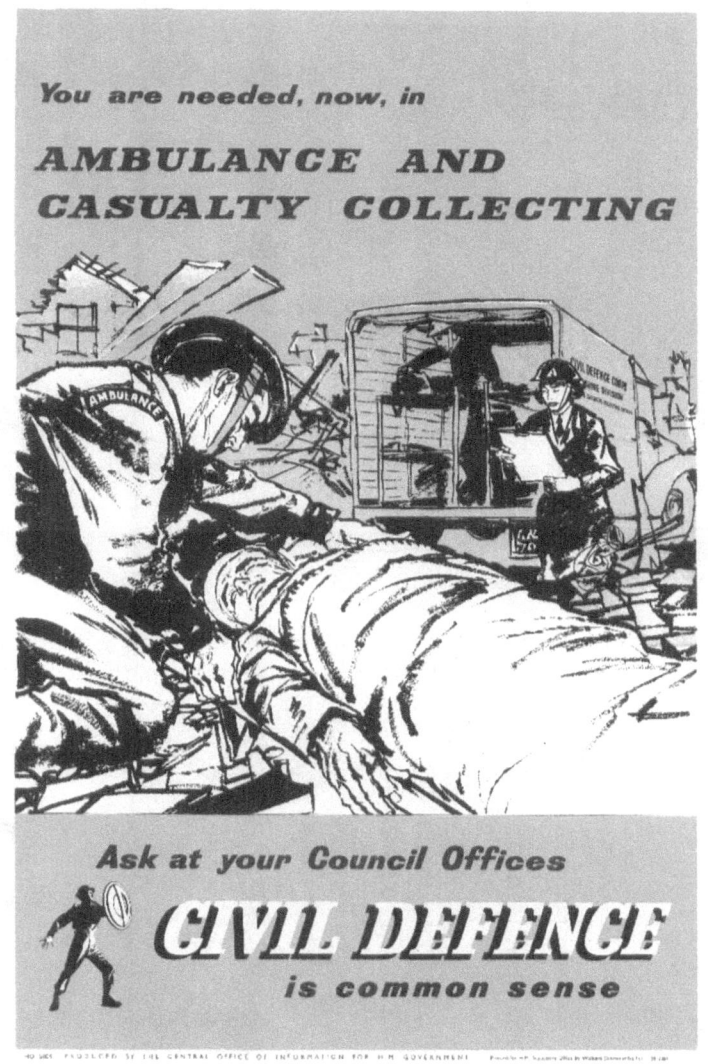

10. The image of swift and comprehensive attention to the nuclear casualty was reinforced by adding Casualty Collection to the Ambulance Section.

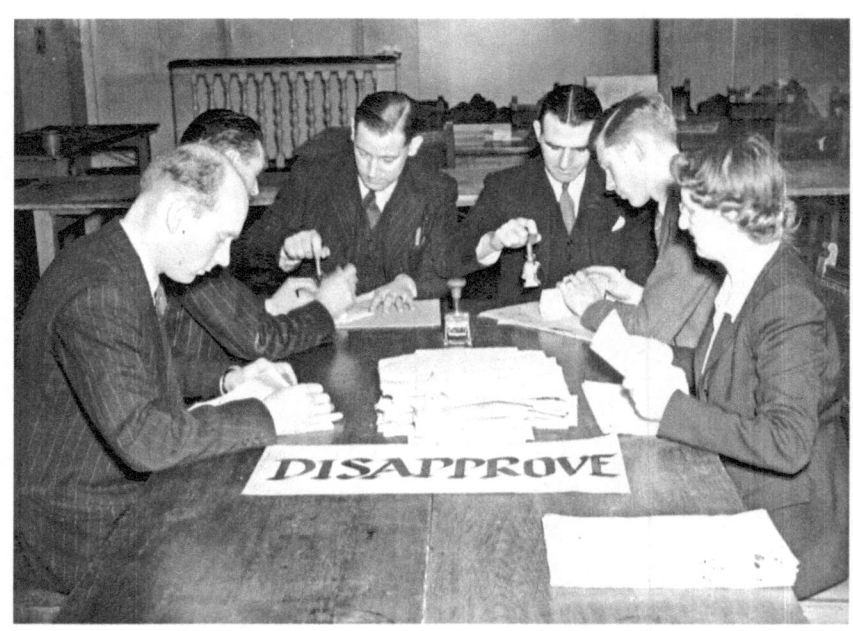

11. The anti-NHS table during the counting of votes in April 1948 at BMA House, reflecting the deep divisions about the scheme.

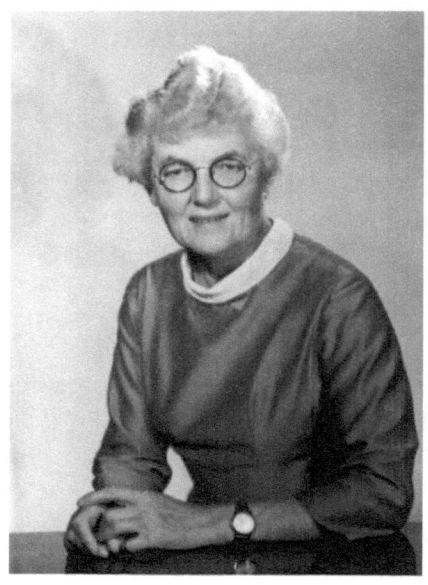

12. Dame Enid Russell-Smith

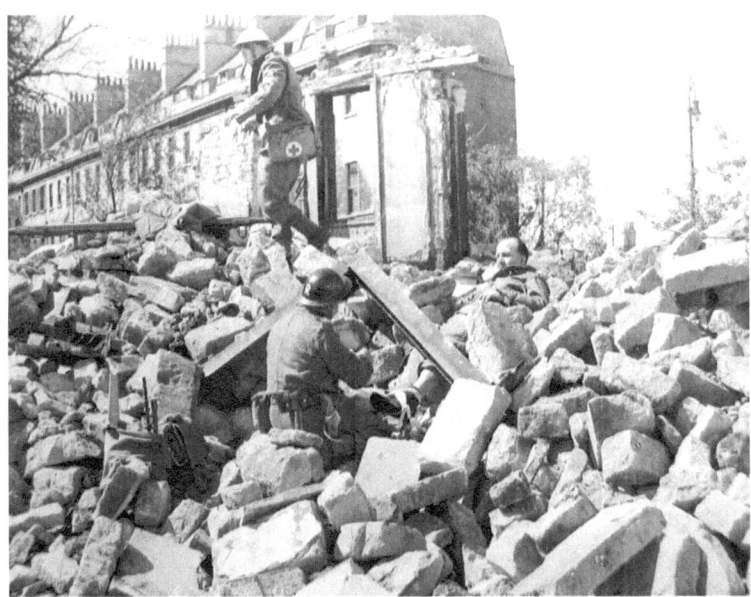

13. & 14. Bomb sites and special rescue training grounds all provided reassuring signs of supporting the nuclear casualty.

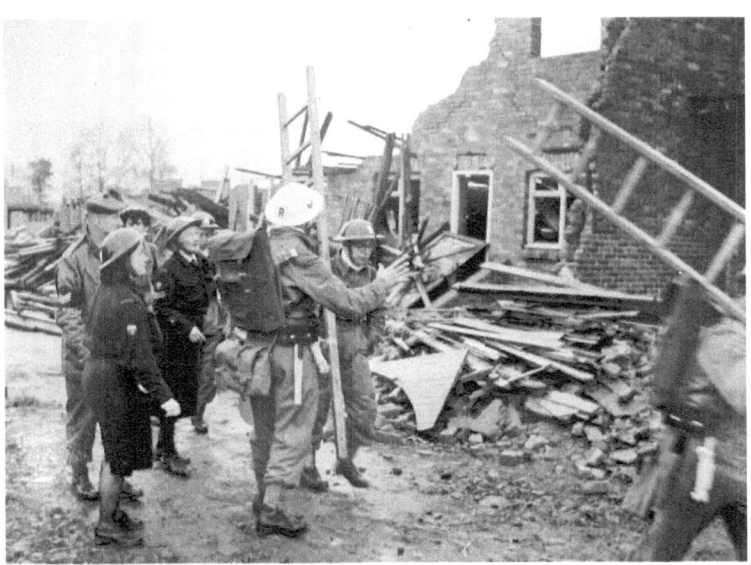

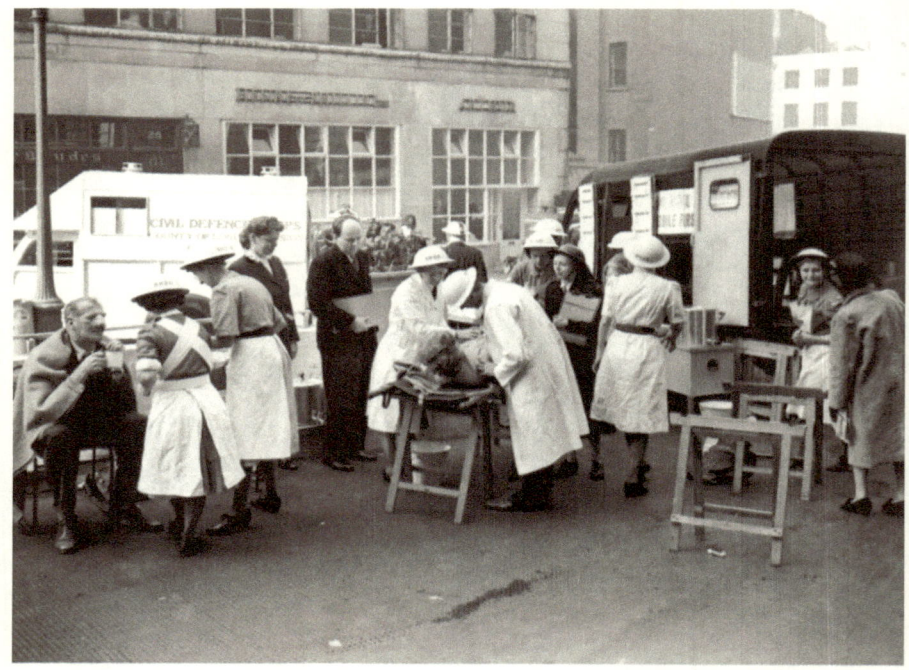

15. A Mobile First Aid Unit exercise presented to Iain Macleod, Minister of Health and Miss Pat Hornsby Smith, Parliamentary Secretary outside the Ministry's London Headquarters during October 1952.

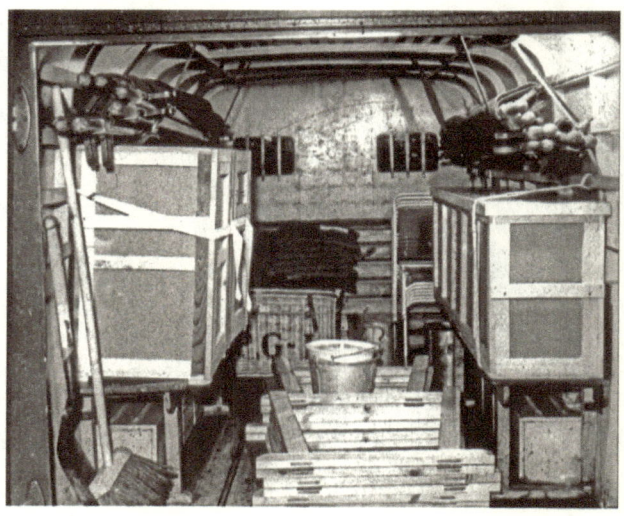

16. Home Office best practice photo of a MFAU van fully packed and ready for frontline support.

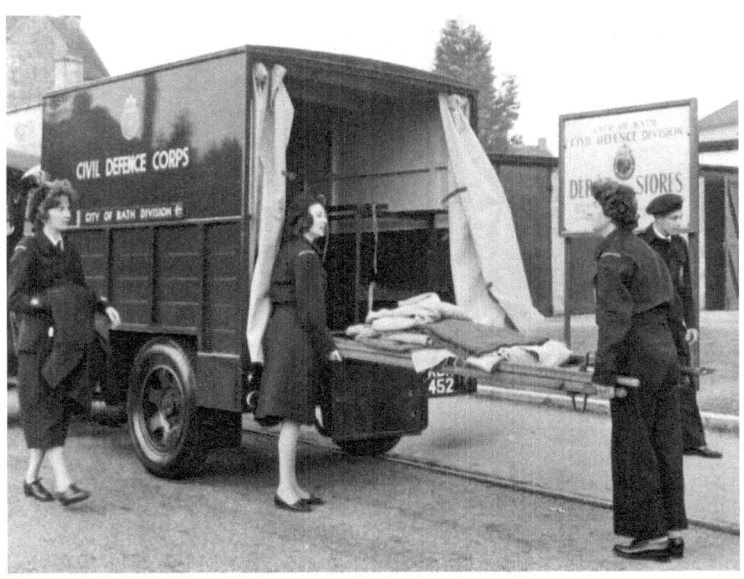

17. & 18. Examples of preparing and loading civil defence ambulances fitted with a special racking system to hold four stretchers.

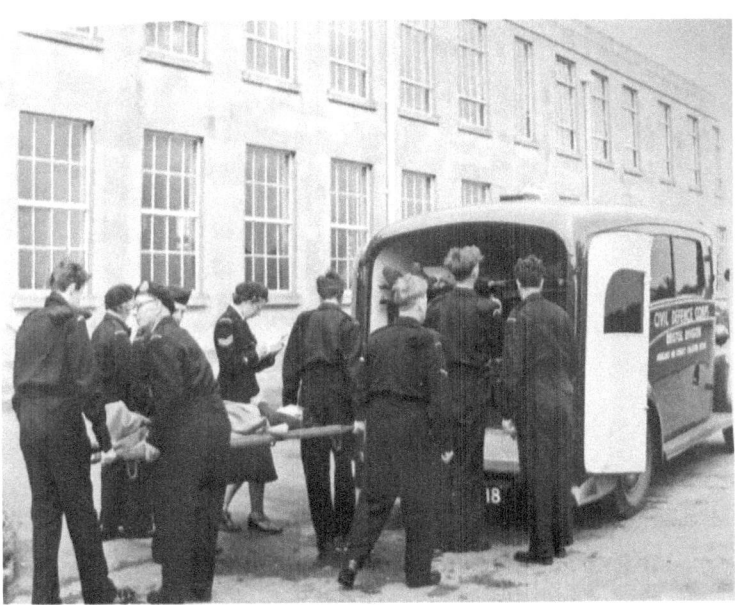

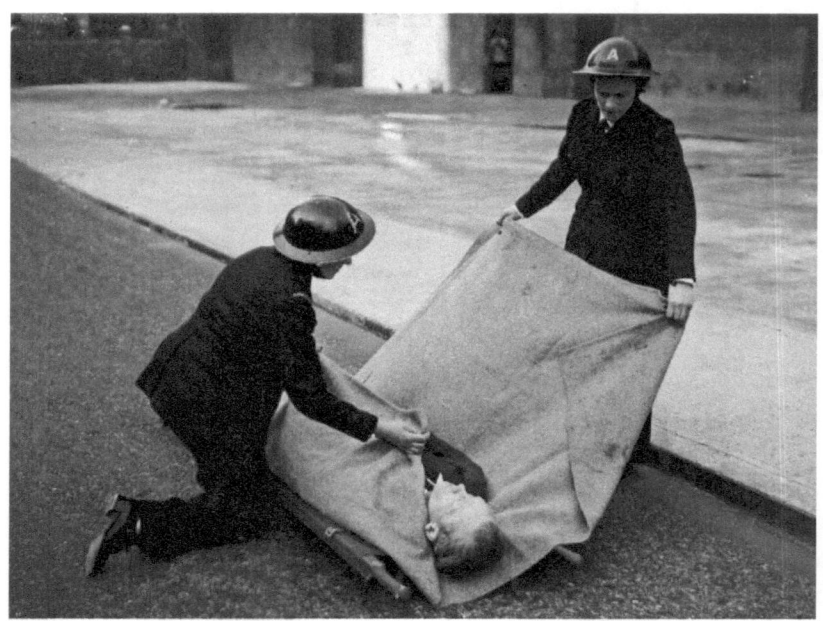

19. & 20. Wrapping it up. Ambulance crew demonstrate the method of dealing with an atomic casualty during the early 1950s.

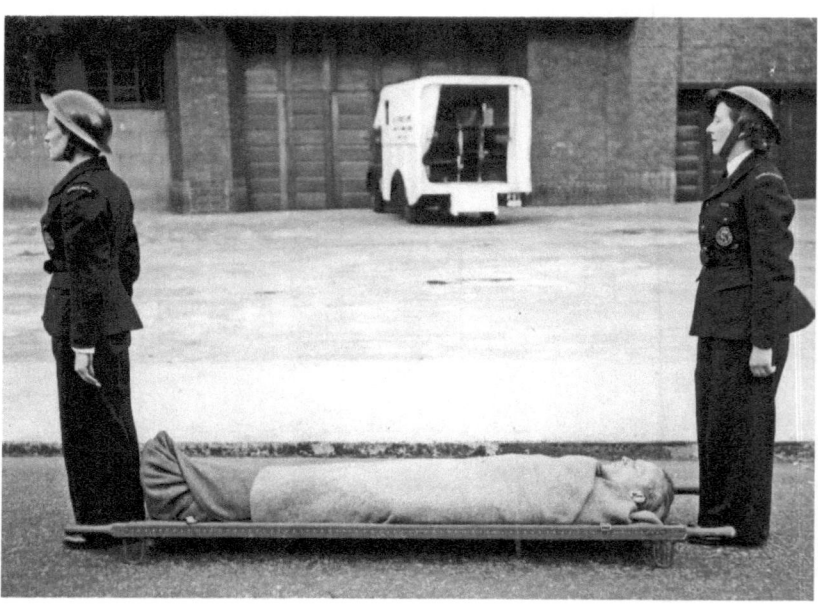

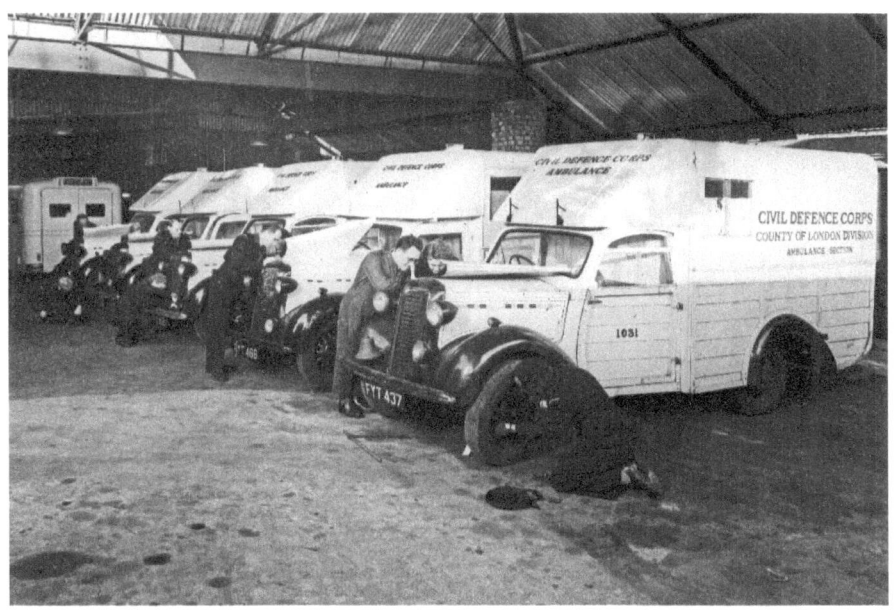

21. & 22. Civil Defence ambulances of the London County Council and Bath showing the collection of different vehicles that made up the section.

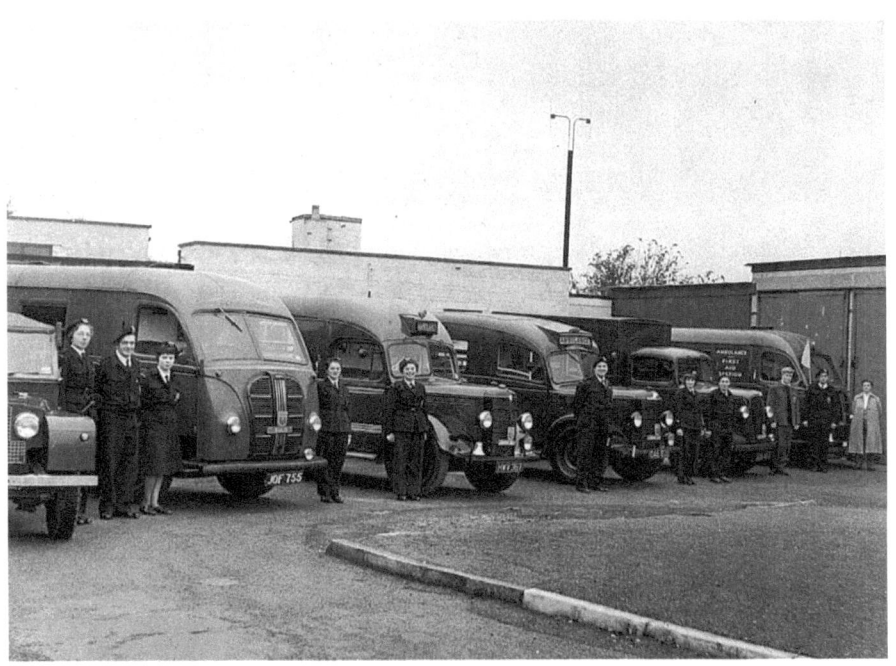

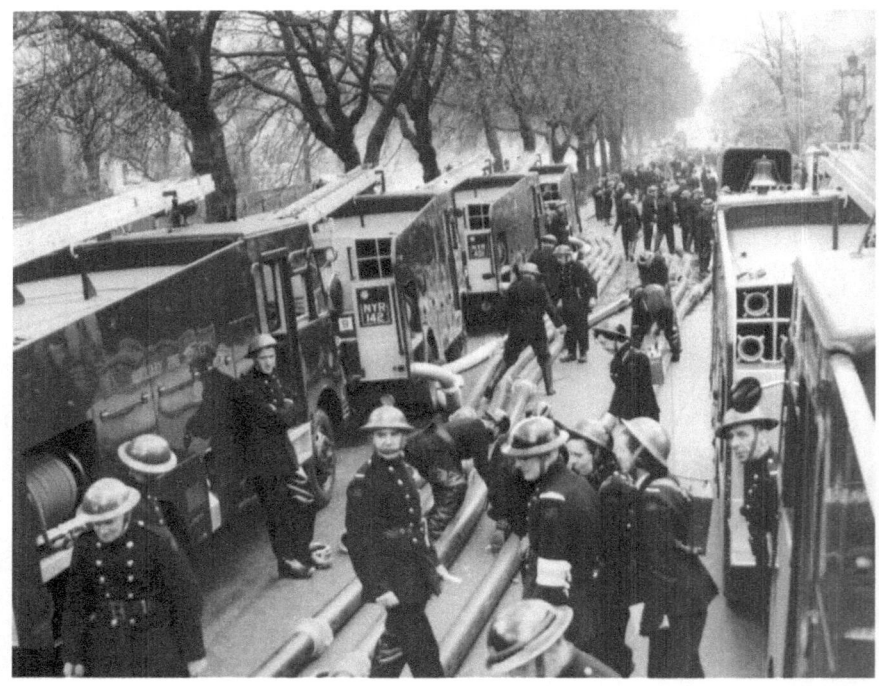

23. When it came to equipment, the medical services found that they were the poor relations of civil defence, often having to use dilapidated second-hand vehicles as ambulances or mobile unit vans. The picture showing a national training exercise by the Auxiliary Fire Service illustrates the nature of the problem very well with the attendance of powerful 'green goddess' pumps and use of a special plastic hose designed to carry massive quantities of water.

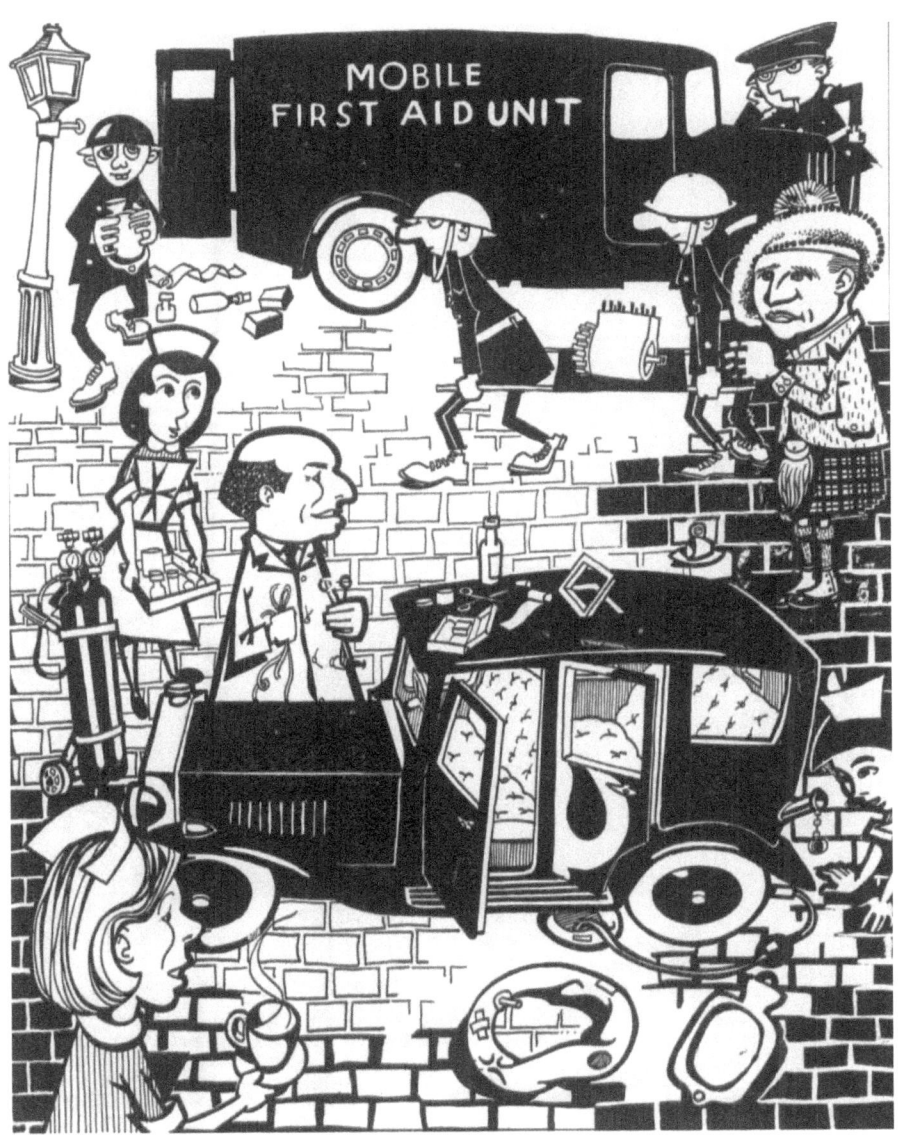

24. Cartoon from an in-house NHSR Newsletter of December 1953, titled 'Ready for any emergency' complaining about the state of vehicles in the volunteer medical services.

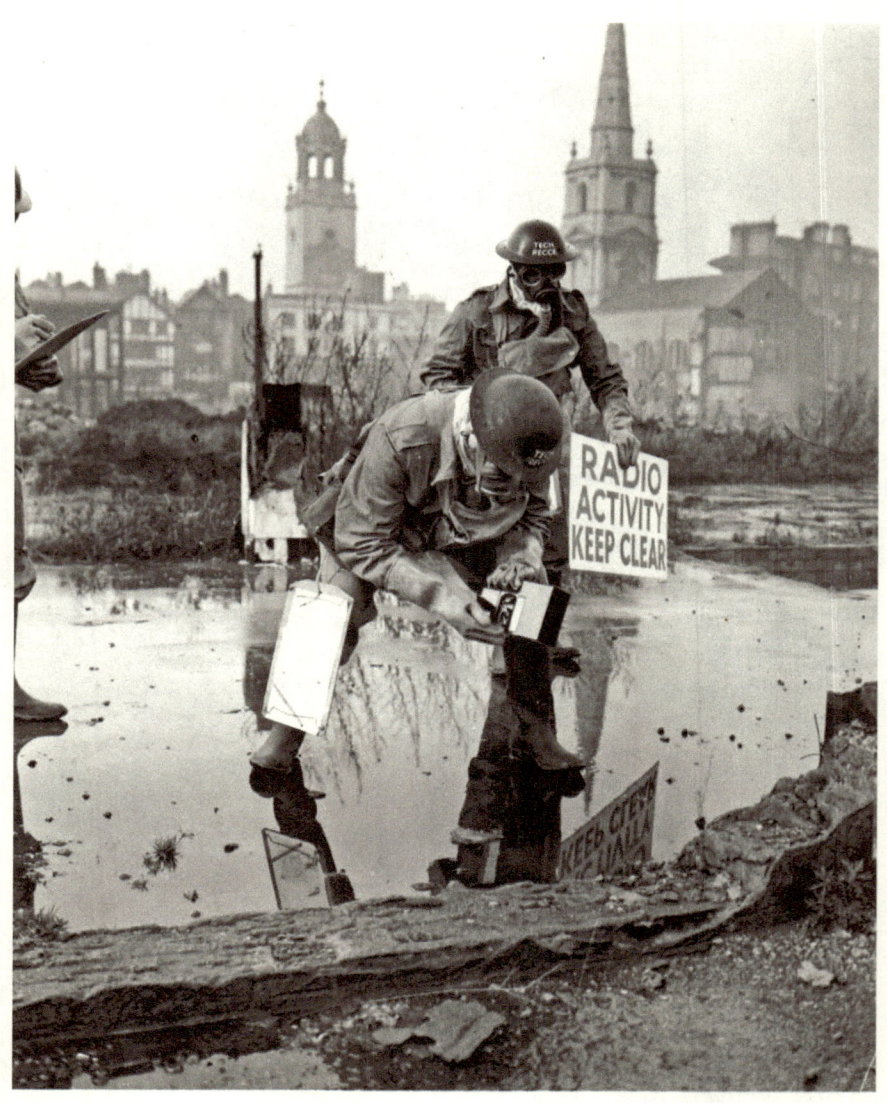

25. One of the first full atomic exercises carried out in in a bombed out area of Bristol during 1951. The stark conditions depicted against a background of radioactive contamination rarely entered the medical arena which preferred conditions under where casualties would receive the best attention.

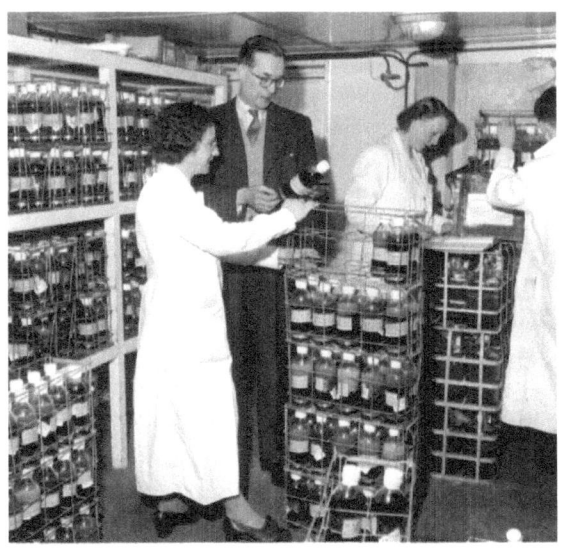

26. Bottles of blood at a London hospital, 1954.

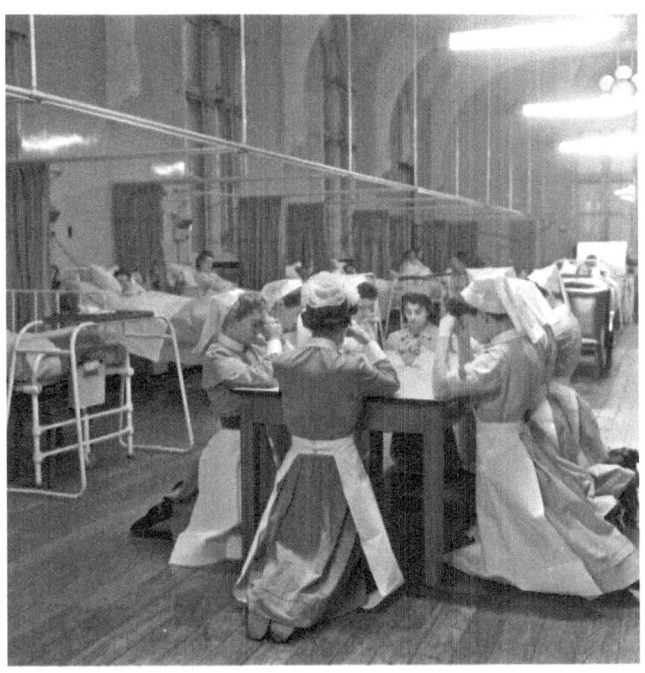

27. Nurses pray before starting their shift, 1956.

Chapter 4

FACADE FATIGUE

The failure to bring the medical profession into 'the nuclear health service' by way of a formal agreement may have equally suggested that its days as a psychological cornerstone of the civil defence facade were numbered. By an accident of Cold War history, however, the very absence of that contractual liability proved to be one of the strands which contributed to its survival. Although the institutional entity of the National Health Service appeared to be part of the facade, it did not mean that all of its constituent elements actually were involved directly. Instead, surrogacy and perception entered the equation and in many ways turned 'the nuclear health service' into a virtual reality by using volunteers and its administrative components to actuate the vital impression of total commitment by the NHS to the nuclear cause. The approach especially fitted in well with the new economic mantra of maintaining the ideology of nuclear survival in place at least cost. Unfortunately, the route also began to push the entire structure towards a political disaster zone. Buying in sincerity symbolism to amplify and link the NHS to its nuclear role became a soft target under the budget cuts that arrived with increasing vigour just when the emergence of the hydrogen bomb and its infinitely greater power required better representation. A new factor soon came into the vocabulary of deceit. The notion of counter value emerged in the form of 'illogicality' which began to corrode the integrity of the belief system and brought it to the brink of collapse at a time when Britain was being drawn ever further into an arms race developing with breathless intensity.

Bomb Shock

The great symbol of atomic defiance in the local community existed in the form of the local civil defence control centre allotted to priority target areas from where those inside would conduct the lifesaving battle within their communities. These self-contained structures proudly boasted an eighteen-inch thick concrete roof and floor along with fifteen inch thick concrete external walls. Despite the look of solidity, the programme had not been without its moments of difficulty. At first, building specifications demanded construction entirely above ground, but were later revised when the realisation struck home such a position would make the bunker less secure against an atomic blast and a semi-sunk alternative was devised.[1] Also, the allocation of bunkers was restricted to the most important target areas, including London, Thames-side, Merseyside and the Clyde. Later the scheme included other cities also considered vulnerable such as Bristol and Coventry. The project also fell victim to the capital investment restrictions and the timely provision of ventilation plant especially suffered. A progress report prepared during 1953 complained about the general inertia and although work on 79 centres had started, no less than 113 had to be abandoned because of rationing of materials, particularly steel.[2] Naturally, those structures completed under the painfully restrictive conditions described came to represent an epic achievement in overcoming economic adversity. The eventual handover of the controls provided not only the opportunity for much civic ceremony, but gave a platform for government ministers to publicly state the support they were affording local communities to defend themselves. One such occasion received special attention in the *Civil Defence* magazine when Home Secretary, Sir David Maxwell Fyfe opened a new control centre in Kensington, London, just off the high street. An article described the ceremonial inspection of the concrete monolith made in the company of the mayor. Later at the town hall, the Home Secretary used the moment to flatter local politicians in terms that underlined the priority assigned to the project for the public good:

> Their new control centre, so skilfully planned and equipped, was the latest of a number of control centres that now stood ready in different cities and towns. Many of them are adaptions of existing buildings, but most of them are, new buildings designed and constructed for the purpose. When you consider the many other pressing demands on building materials and manpower, this is a valuable accomplishment by the civil defence authorities.[3]

Inside these bunkers, Medical Officers of Health were to play a pivotal role in the medical scheme of things. Their assignment of wartime duties was defined in 1951, but only after their representative bodies protested the civil defence plans initially published by government departments did not sufficiently recognise the contribution they could bring to the atomic dimension. Rectifying the omission, many areas of responsibility were extensions of their civil functions. They were, for example, to check and control outbreaks of infectious diseases of all kinds and look out for subversive attempts to cause disease or spread its prevalence within communities. Really, the MOH post became an organisational receptacle to hold every imaginable public health crisis because of overcrowding in billets or through homelessness and the general breakdown of public amenities. The brief included aspects such as the contamination of water, food, problems with sewage, as well as the burial of the civilian war dead. In addition to those professional responsibilities, came the control function to build the vital bridge between the local authority civil defence controls and the wartime management of the hospital organisation, particularly as Regional Hospital Board areas and civil defence regions did not coincide. (The relative position illustrated by Maps 2 and 3 at the front of the book) As the official responsible in England and Wales for the ambulances and inter-hospital transport, the task of linking those elements with the hospital organisation also ended up in his court. Fortuitously, none of that kind of operational control caused friction and actively supported by hospital administrators on the basis attempts had occurred to saddle them with this responsibility, but which they resolutely felt they did not need.[4]

Nonetheless, continuing to play the political game through these symbols became increasingly difficult as the Cold War drove an arms race of Olympian dimensions. An incident then surfaced on 1 March 1954 when the US Atomic Energy Commission undertook a hydrogen bomb test above ground at the Bikini Atoll in the Marshall Islands. Its consequences appeared to consign any kind of civil defence ritualism to history. Code-named BRAVO, the veil of secrecy suddenly lifted and embarrassingly exposed the combination of a miscalculation in the science of the explosion and unforeseen changes in wind direction. The fusion of events caused radioactive fallout to cover vast distances exposing 28 Americans at a weather observation station and 236 Marshall Islanders to dangerous levels of radiation. Worse still, some eighty-five miles east of Bikini the Japanese crew of a fishing vessel called *Lucky Dragon* suffered contagion by the fallout debris whilst out at sea. By the time they reached port on 14 March, most of them exhibited symptoms of radiation sickness. A secret evaluation on the test, prepared by the AEC, provided a forbidding script to the beginning of a new age in mass destruction. The blast had produced fallout in the form of an elliptical pattern covering an area of 8,800 square miles. As the new reality, it defied any human dimension and took the American security services some ten months to consider the public relations implications. Anyhow, attempts at subverting the truth were pre-empted by an article published by Ralph Lapp, an American nuclear physicist (who had worked on the Manhattan Project to develop the atom bomb), in two American magazines before the official version emerged on 15 February 1955.[5]

The Government suddenly faced a public relations disaster as the news freewheeled unexpectedly through the usually tightly controlled networks of publicity on mass destruction. The British Press had a field day due to the fact the Government knew nothing of the test and the sheer power it represented with the mushroom cloud making especially good front page copy. For example, the *Daily Express* suggested how the mushroom shape, reaching a height of 25 miles and a width of 100 miles, would be visible from Brighton if the bomb had fallen on London.[6] The Home Secretary, Maxwell Fyfe tried to pour as much cold water on the bad news as possible. He did so in a speech to Parliament and attempted to allay fears one bomb could wipe out Britain with the suggestion that there would still be 'marginal areas where much could be done by an efficient civil defence organisation'. Fyfe also struggled to demolish the fallout threat, which had engulfed the Japanese fishermen, by noting they had recovered and adding: 'If they had all remained below deck level I am advised that in all probability symptoms would not have developed and the resulting alarm of the public would have been avoided'.[7]

Because of the profound shift in destructive power, civil defence met its decisive test of political sustainability. Certainly, the prospects of the organisation surviving seemed in doubt sooner rather than later when the predominantly left-wing Coventry Council chose to break ranks with convention and withdrew their support for the organisation to follow their own political agenda. With civil defence always regarded politically neutral, the ability of the protest to attract publicity also added another layer of discomfort insofar as the psychological weapon was being used for the first time against the Government itself. Furthermore, the move provided an intensity to the action no other place could possibly achieve. Legendary for suffering the loss of its cathedral during an intensive attack in the Blitz, which the Germans coined as 'Coventration', news of the rebellion spread across the world and received with particular interest in America. What the affair put at risk, if other authorities followed, related to the loss of the public health arm of 'the nuclear health service' and the vital involvement of the Medical Officer of Health. Unnervingly, Home Secretary Maxwell Fyfe added his prediction of an even greater calamity that sent a shudder through government about the possible damage the mutiny could to deterrence policy itself:

> There was little doubt that the decision of the Coventry City Council to abandon their civil defence work had been promoted by left wing politicians who believed that it was useless to try and protect the civil population against the effects of nuclear attack and that this justified the adoption of a neutralist attitude in our international relations. This line of reasoning might lead to a demand for

the withdrawal of the United States strategic air forces from the bases in the United Kingdom.[8]

In point of fact, the stance of Coventry that civil defence could only be regarded as 'make-believe' in the face of the new destructive capacity converged with the Government's own appreciation of the situation. At a meeting of the Official Committee on Civil Defence, held in the Cabinet Office on 11 May 1954, between the Ministries, the Home Office and senior representatives of the Armed Forces, those involved confirmed secretly that government had got it wrong on the hydrogen bomb by implying it differed from the atom bomb in degree rather than kind. Political realisation at last dawned the effects of a hydrogen bomb were actually very different, which made local authority controls useless and 'the public probably had not yet appreciated the appalling devastation which would follow hydrogen bomb attacks and did not realise that all amenities would disappear and that a sheer struggle for survival would follow'.[9]

Whilst the municipal mutineers of Coventry were forced into line by a combination of factors including the Government calling in commissioners to run the city's civil defence services, the political parties showing solidarity and the local electorate expressing its own disapproval at the General Election, in the long term the mutiny left its mark in a number of ways. In terms of upsetting 'the nuclear health service', the destruction of the local authority pillar of support would have been disastrous practically and politically. Further grist to that political mill also appeared in the *Peace News*, a pacifist newspaper. It reported that the Medical Association for the Prevention of War (founded in 1951 by a small group of distinguished doctors to provide a forum to handle the problem of nuclear ethics) had given its backing to Coventry Council in a resolution that provided a medical perspective on the issue:

> Our membership comprises only medical practitioners and students, and in consequence the Association is deeply aware of the impossibility of any country finding adequate resources-in terms of medical manpower, suitable hospital buildings, drugs, blood transfusion facilities, and so on-to deal with the terrible results of even a small series of atomic explosions of the now outdated Hiroshima type. The newest weapons so dwarf this in their potential effects that we consider the only entirely realistic piece of 'civil defence' is to make certain that these weapons shall never be employed.[10]

With this medical diagnosis joined to the Coventry blackmail note, it heightened the danger that any political action giving credence to the protest could make the hospital plan politically useless. Moreover, the difficulties showed no signs of abating as Whitehall itself eventually became fully-appraised of the potential capacity of a hydrogen bomb to wipe out the nation in a study undertaken during 1955. A report prepared on the subject 'The Defence Implications of Fall-Out from a Hydrogen Bomb' gave a hint of the human tragedy its contents would represent. Conducted under the chairmanship of William Strath (a senior official from the Treasury, who also had extensive experience in military related ministries) his team had evaluated the effects it would have on defence policy and associated problems of civil defence. No extensive nuclear capability existed in Great Britain at the time and therefore the major cities considered as the main targets of a Soviet attack. The first survey of the potential horrors of the hydrogen bomb assumed a possible strike by just ten ground bursts in the ten-megaton range, the minimum regarded to neutralise the nation. Instead of the usual optimism found in civil defence narrative, Strath painted a picture of Stygian gloom whereby not a single part of the country could be regarded as immune from the effects. In the absence of any preparations made in advance, the study warned a successful night assault on the main centres of population would kill about 12 million people and seriously injure or disable 4 million others. Casualties on such a scale were described as intolerable since it meant the loss of nearly one third of the population, including a disproportionate share of the skilled manpower on which the future of the country depended.[11]

Adding yet more gloom, another assessment suggested an estimated further 13 million people, many of them suffering radiation sickness, would be pinned down for at least a week. Stark new language added an urgency largely lost in the apparent taming of the atomic bomb. It indicated: 'The fire hazard from nuclear attack dwarfs all previous experience to insignificance'. A hand-drawn diagram attached to the report showed a radioactive plume caused by a hydrogen bomb dropped on Bristol being driven by a south-westerly wind across to Humberside. Against this calamitous picture, Strath counselled living with the bomb meant a new uncertainty for the post war generation and had to be addressed in some way, a matter stressed in the following terms:

> Finally, the attack would fall with devastating suddenness. All preparations would have to be ready in advance and brought to a high state of efficiency. It would be folly to trust to

> improvisation. The price of unpreparedness would be catastrophe. Inefficiency and indecision in the execution of plans would be hardly less costly.[12]

If the threat was to be met, Strath laid down the foundation of a new approach that meant weaving permanent vigilance into the fabric of society. This included the provision of a fallout monitoring and warning system, compulsory protection of new houses, shelters on the outskirts of target areas against fallout, some protection against blast and heat as well as extensive stockpiling of food and materials on a scale never before envisaged.[13] Sinister aspects of social control surfaced, suggesting a degree of force would be unleashed throughout Britain on a scale never experienced before. Any mythological nostalgia for the spirit of the Blitz evaporated with the recognition: 'hydrogen bombing would place a very severe strain on public morale and on the forces of law and order'. Martial law, the study predicted, had to be accounted for in plans with a regional military commander appointed who would 'if called upon exercise his common law powers to take whatever steps, however drastic'. In order to assist the transition from civil to military control, the report entered even darker areas of policy making with reference to flexible systems having to be put into place, normal judicial processes suspended and ominously 'war zone' courts set up for 'the prompt disposal of criminal cases'.[14]

Medical plans also received the Strath treatment. The report highlighted a need for new medical ethics to be applied involving a complete change in the relationship of the citizen and the state when resources were simply no longer available to support every individual. Pitilessly frank, the new reality came with medical concepts that during the last war would have been unthinkable:

> Plans to relieve the more serious casualties must at all costs avoid overtaxing the able-bodied manpower which survived the nuclear offensive and exposing a large proportion of it to the dangers of radio-activity in the course of relief operations. It would be quite unrealistic to hope to maintain anything like normal medical standards. There would also be grave problems of priority in dealing with a wide range of casualties some of whom would have no hope of recovery. We understand that the chief difficulty would be to distinguish those who, in addition to having received burns or other injuries, had also been exposed to a lethal dose of radiation and who would therefore ultimately die,

and on whom it would be wasteful to expend scarce medical resources.[15]

For the first time, those unthinkable thoughts formally challenged the idealised pictures presented by attentive medical services and instead promoted the concept of abandonment on a massive scale to conserve resources for rebuilding the state. Epidemics due to the dislocation of sanitary services would add to the death toll and required special precautions. Self-help appeared as a possible answer to those less injured with 'good food and good nursing and rest provided by family and friends', but probably untenable with the prospect of a further line in the credit column of mass death being added. So whilst the lid of Pandora's box had been lifted a little exposing the myth that social control could be relied on using local democratic processes, it was quickly closed with the order the assumptions were not to be revealed to local government under any circumstances.[16]

Strath's report, of course, meant that the casualty plan had to be redrawn which then presented a challenge on an unprecedented scale. To undertake the task, new arrangements were introduced involving departmental working groups and using *ad hoc* committees for dealing with specific issues. Carling's illustrious committee was, therefore, no longer involved. By far the most spectacular response that resulted through this planning approach came in the revised stretch factor to the NHS hospital organisation. During 1956 the National Health Service in England and Wales had 477,000 beds, two thirds of which were still in the special needs category, the majority of those allocated to the mentally disabled.[17] From this starting point, along with the Scottish beds, the new hospital plan was to be extended into a staggering total of one million beds, double the previous number and geared to the assumption the warning of war would be no more than seven days.[18] Unfortunately not one word remains on departmental files, either in Scottish or English archives, as to how this new figure came into being and the circumstances of its adoption. The audit trail of decision-making of the kind available behind the Carling atomic proposals is missing in its entirety. Whether the silence came about by accident or design is impossible to say.[19] Whatever the reason, it leaves a vacuum in the historical process that intriguingly ran parallel with much of the Suez Crisis and could have been of great value as to the assessments undertaken heightened by active military operations.

Enough evidence remains, however, to show that a titanic struggle took place in the revisions made to the atomic plan. The very first conceptual proposals set out in July 1955 immediately prepared in response to Strath have survived. These reveal how the planners, challenged by weapons hundreds of times more powerful than the atom bomb, added further elements of normalisation to the old atomic plan such as using tents on an epic scale that would be pitched by the army once the fallout patterns were identified. Even an idea to tempt more doctors during peace to support target areas materialised, with housing and equipment suggested as part of their NHS package so that 'a general practitioner-cum-home-nurse service' could be provided.[20] By the end of that first planning cycle, the Ministry of Health even had enough to roll out the old mantra: 'The object is to provide as much general accommodation as possible for war casualties, both civil and military, and at the same time to continue to provide for the essential needs of the ordinary sick and injured and for 'special' patients of whom mental patients, mental defectives and the chronic are the most important categories'.[21]

Eventually, some of the first ideas such as the canvas solution remained, whilst others were discarded. Despite those elements of normalisation, when Regional Hospital Boards received the final plan during 1957 for implementation a twist of some irony surfaces through the instructions. The wording suggests that the increase in beds may not have been the result of attempting to keep the ideology of mass compassion intact, but actually signified the beginnings of a policy of mass abandonment. There was still a distinct desire not to let go of at least some of the ethical values of the Blitz. In particular it was said: 'The role of the hospital service in the initial intensive phase of any war must be, therefore, to provide essential treatment for as many of the sick and injured as possible, even though this may mean restricting treatment to a minimum in some cases and accepting reduced standards of staffing and accommodation'. On the other hand, Regional Hospital Boards were told that the approach described was to be regarded as a new policy where the hospital bed would be used 'to do the greatest good for the greatest number', a code that only certain injuries were to be dealt with.[22] Further evidence of that position rests on the way the previously well-ordered medical system was totally collapsed. Beds were not to be set aside for the specific use of one category of patient and patient need at the time would finally determine the functional distribution of the beds throughout the country.[23]

On the face of it the regime seemed to encompass the seismic shift in medical ethics Strath had alluded and now recognised this in organisational terms. But as the next chapter explains, neglect of the seriously injured took many years to formalise with more precision than the first awkward steps made in that direction. Really, the new hospital scheme itself was nothing more than a monument to abandonment, almost self-destroyed even before any attention from Soviet bombers. Indeed the hospital situation mirrored the general retreat from the atomic arrangements. With the hydrogen bomb being no respecter of local authority boundaries the old controls were crashed and replaced by a system that scattered new ones across huge distances outside target areas. Control centres were earmarked at schools, army centres and even prisons, but with a lack of money not much in the way of physical work undertaken that simply produced an extraordinary nuclear folly on a grand scale.

The position with regard to the casualty plan was no less dramatic. Keeping hospitals outside target areas now significantly altered the all-important bottom line as to how much existing, useable hospital space remained. In the case of London, Birmingham, Manchester, and Merseyside a circle designated the *Hospital Evacuation Area* was to be drawn with a radius of 15 miles from an assumed ground zero. Elsewhere hospital evacuation distances were less severe, but still involved a radius of 5 to 10 miles, although the lower figure regarded as the very minimum and an extension preferred provided the additional beds lost were not disproportionately high. It presented a predicament admitted by the Ministry of Health that raised 'a high degree of risk of losing buildings'.[24] Taking the case of Edinburgh, for example, a radius of seven miles measured from the General Post Office and assuming a one megaton ground burst meant the loss of 36 hospitals which equated to a peacetime total of 7,500 beds having to be found elsewhere and before any expansion.[25]

Outside the evacuation areas, the battle to save casualties would occur in a sector called the *Main Hospital Area* extending 20 to 30 miles from a central point in the main built up conurbations and 10 to 20 miles in the case of others. With a greater blast power the hydrogen bomb also caused another problem as it meant target error by Soviet bombers could magnify inaccuracies considerably. To overcome that possibility, a new concept appeared through the designation of a *Standstill Area* which meant hospitals in a five mile wide ring adjacent to the *Hospital Evacuation Areas* were to be cleared of patients, but nothing more done beforehand. Should they subsequently survive these hospitals would then take the first call on the admission of casualties by cramming in as many as possible before space in the main hospital area became operational.[26] Within the outer periphery of target areas, no more than 15% of the existing general beds were to be retained as *Home Cover Hospitals* for the essential day-to-day needs as in the atomic plan.[27]

One million beds may have had a ring of the caring state in public propaganda, but the package had become so diluted internal instructions struggled with what it actually represented. In England and Wales 450,000 *Grade I* hospitals or *Acute Hospitals*, as they later became known, and 50,000 in Scotland were to offer something resembling medical attention which the Scots described as 'simple techniques and austere standards'.[28] With that degree of dilution applied to the so-called best standard, the second level of hospital care in *Auxiliary Hospitals* shared out in the same way amounted to little more than a political conscience saver. Half a million beds were to be opened on a crash basis after the attack in schools, hotels and large stores, their control and administration undertaken from a parent acute hospital where the necessary medical kit would be held in special packs until required. This part of the medical package envisaged provision of 'little more than covered floor space for casualties with the minimum of medical attention and equipment'. Putting all this together, *Auxiliary Hospitals* were, therefore, likely to provide little more than shelter for casualties waiting admission to an acute hospital or for those who had already received treatment, but not fit enough for discharge.[29]

Even the flimsy one-million bed promise appeared more precarious as the military priorities agreed in the Skeleton Plan years before began to raise new problems. At first, the Ministry of Health secured important assurances from the War Office that greater integration of Service and civilian medical facilities was possible and the following statement of intent given:

> The War Office planned to recall only those doctors needed to fill their order of battle; the remaining doctors on the reserve would be available for the National Health Service. Those recalled would be for units proceeding overseas, for the Territorial Divisions supporting Civil Defence, and there would be some required for static units in the UK engaged on mobilisation duties. All three Services had issued instructions that their static, non-operational units in the UK should play their part in local Civil Defence plans. This would ensure that the Services' local medical facilities could be co-ordinated with Civil Defence plans.[30]

A raft of other common procedures followed, particularly at the expense of the Royal Air Force that agreed to waive certain specialist medical facilities in the initial stages of a war for the exclusive treatment of burns and plastic surgery.[31] Unfortunately, the value of the co-operation promised then vanished when new tactical appreciations suggested the hydrogen bomb would create a far higher call on NHS resources by military casualties than first thought. The original plan of the Army had involved expanding military hospitals to take up to 10,000 casualties, but now many of these were located in the extended target plans. New appraisals estimated 22,000 military casualties would occur during the opening phase of a war in the UK and up to 78,000 casualties might require evacuation from Europe.[32] The Royal Navy added further concerns about their hospitals at Portsmouth, Chatham and Plymouth that were now in target zones and threatened to fall back on the National Health Service and requisition suitable buildings for their medical needs whenever or wherever that might become necessary.[33]

The NHS, therefore, seemed at risk of facing a nuclear Hobson's choice over having to support Service casualties, but preferring to maintain its public image as a provider of civilian services. On further investigation the realities of moving casualties from the continent to the UK were such that reports concluded movement would be impossible in the chaotic circumstances, which then turned the problem the other way around. In other words, if the NHS was unable to support the numbers of casualties on the mainland, then the UK medical system had to provide greater support on the continent instead, especially on German soil, where the British Army of the Rhine would take the brunt of a Soviet land invasion. Just as the whole situation seemed to be reaching an organisational impasse, the Ministry of Health expressed concern about the possible implications of the situation and it would have to ensure not too many doctors ended up in the Services to the detriment of the UK. On this note, nothing more transpired and the position left on the basis that discussions would continue.[34]

Everything about the new hydrogen bomb menace might have emphatically pointed to a hopeless situation but the Strath report nonetheless offered a remarkable lifeline to the future conceptualisation of the facade. Whilst fully recognising the desperately horrendous conditions resulting that would follow a megaton attack Strath still maintained a conventionalist outlook by approaching the hydrogen bomb as a resourcing problem. Indeed, the approach was in many ways positively encouraged by the assumption that ten hydrogen bombs would only destroy one quarter of the country's industrial production. Percentages were even applied to the likely deliverability of medical supplies, if that is, the bombs fell in the right place. The list of outcomes expressed in percentage terms included: surgical dressings and plaster 44%; surgeon's gloves 45%; syringes and needles 59%; surgical instruments 20 %; penicillin 67.5 %; insulin 26% and X-Ray apparatus 20%, although the production of X-Ray film would entirely disappear. Underpinned by this outlook, it was not beyond the bounds of possibility to sustain the publicly acceptable face of nuclear reality by reshaping the illusion of the atomic age to show the immeasurably greater power of thermonuclear weapons was still possible to manage through logical solutions.[35] In fact, the reaction to Strath had a distinct sense of déjà vu.

Stockpiling large amounts of just about everything seemed to be the answer and the inevitable committee formed to assess what had to be put on such a list, including medical supplies.

'Medical supplies' meant equipment in the widest sense and included everything required to care for both the sick and injured with a price tag of £85 million.[36] Dressings alone accounted for £14 million of that sum. A massive expansion of X-ray equipment for the rapid diagnosis of blast injuries appeared on the list in the form of mobile and portable units costing £2 million, which in turn led to doubts whether the call on the X-ray film needed to the value of another £2 million could be met from current production.[37] The steep curve this spend represented that would keep Britain intact on some kind of social thread even led the planners to the view at least £3 million would have to be handed out in subsidies so manufacturers could increase their production capacity and meet the demand the nuclear shopping basket represented.[38] If cost alone did not reflect the immensity of the proposals then the final estimated need for storage certainly did with a requirement for three million square feet suggested for the purpose.[39]

When the Prime Minister took receipt of the entire shopping list during November 1955 to provide Britain with some nuclear resilience, the paper submitted began with a sheepish preamble: 'Prime Minister, we are in difficulties over what has hitherto been called the civil defence programme'. 'The difficulties' mentioned were an understatement with huge implications. To bombproof the nation against ten hydrogen bombs amounted to £1,878 million. Of that total, the largest items were the food stockpile at £138 million, an oil stockpile costing £121 million and shelters put at £1,250 million.[40] Prepared under the direction of Home Secretary, Major Gwilym Lloyd George, the national plan for survival left nothing, but nothing to chance, even down to vast supplies of nails and tea. The British 'cuppa' thus took its vital place as the saviour of national morale:

> The Ministry is satisfied that tea is an essential item in the wartime diet if full benefit is to be obtained from the other items in the diet and people able to carry on the essential tasks on which survival of the nation depends. Arrivals from abroad would be seriously reduced after attack and commercial stocks would be largely destroyed. Experience makes it clear that for British people, tea is a necessity for survival.[41]

Along with the morale booster of tea, shelter for all had not escaped attention in the age of welfare equality. Plans included the construction of small shelter under living room floors approached by a trap door, the idea compared to an inspection pit in a garage. Undaunted, Lloyd George resolutely defended his new Home Front as psychologically essential and maintained: 'Alarming as these figures are they should not appear so to the man in the street while we are spending a sum of £1,500 million a year on defence'.[42] But the proposal arrived at a time when the facade of civil defence, linked to amassing large quantities of so called lifesaving goods, felt the effects of an economic slowdown. The first signs of trouble had already become evident in an internal Cabinet statement on 16 December 1953 with the Chancellor prefacing his note: 'I am much concerned about the prospect for civil supply expenditure next year'. In truth, the country's finances were spinning out of control, even before the hydrogen bomb had been added to list of problems. The civil supply forecast, that included the social services and agricultural subsidies, suggested a figure of £121 million over budget whilst the defence programme showed a net increase of £70 million.[43] Civil defence spending, the soft political option, suffered and pegged immediately at £60 million, ostensibly a temporary measure while the implications of the hydrogen bomb were thought out. Any hopes of a revival of fortunes were invariably blighted during the next financial round when the Treasury announced the very maximum the country could afford to spend during 1956-7 for bolstering the Home Front should not exceed £50 million pounds.[44]

Challenged by the financial illogicality, a possible public outcry due to the brake on civil defence expenditure again exercised the political resourcefulness of Cabinet Secretary Norman Brook, who in June 1954 posed a singularly important rhetorical question to the Prime Minister: 'This creates a problem – The trend of government expenditure cannot be concealed. How then are we to justify a policy of spending <u>less</u> on civil defence when the hydrogen bomb has convinced the public that the risks and dangers to the home front are <u>greater</u>'. Conveniently, the *Statement of Defence Policy 1955*, (Cmnd.124) came to the rescue and disguised the more frugal future of civil defence in the wider context of national plans under an umbrella organisation called 'Home Defence', which included the internal support of the armed forces and the paraphernalia of government control epitomised by deep and secure bunkers. Intriguingly, the question thereafter came down to whether the facade could somehow be maintained given Brook's financial Chinese puzzle had taken a definitive step to hide its essential fragility from public view.[45]

Discomfort Blankets

By 1956 Britain stared once more into the abyss of financial ruin caused through weakening exports and a military budget overstretched by the Suez Canal escapade. The future for civil defence looked even more precarious. Rather than choosing between 'guns or butter', the country had followed the acquisition of both, the burgeoning welfare state increasingly weighed down by the post war baby boom that added to the financial woes. At the beginning of that year, the Cabinet received the unwelcome news deflationary measures had not worked which led Chancellor of the Exchequer Harold Macmillan to announce his intention to cut both civil and military expenditure by £100 million. The politics received a degree of adroit handling behind the introduction of Premium Bonds that sent up a smokescreen of opprobrium from certain church quarters about the sins of gambling. Cigarettes went up two pence and an outcry followed that a similar increase did not reflect in the cigarette vouchers afforded to old age pensioners.[46]

The predicament did not end there and played out with much pain inside the Cabinet. Harold Macmillan, again as Chancellor of Exchequer, announced his desire to make savings and suggested the budget for civil defence be cut down to £15 million and the volunteer forces stood down. On the opposing side against demobbing the civil defence volunteers, which included the Ambulance and Casualty Collection Section of the Civil Defence Corps and National Hospital Service Reserve, were the Prime Minister Sir Anthony Eden and the Defence Minister Sir Walter Monkton. Their prescription was to stay with civil defence and accept it should be maintained, but on the strict basis of affordability. Ideologically this meant home defence preparations could remain because their absence as a cultural expectation might undermine the deterrent, but expenditure designed to enable the country to survive a war and recover would disappear altogether. Tweaking the facade in such a way thus increased the nature of its hollowness by having to be designed with the explicit intent to convince local councils, hospitals and volunteers their services were still required which the narrative of deceit unashamedly promoted on the basis, 'purchases of equipment would be limited to keep the organisation going'.[47]

Of course, taken along this new policy route, all the weaknesses of the system began to be exposed in different ways. The political expediency applied to the original purchasing strategy of medical supplies emerged as an area where the rot began to set in and eat away dangerously at the overall stability of the medical facade. Equipment had simply ended up in 22 stores throughout the country. Therefore, along with the dubious nature of the contents, the geographical spread did not have a gram of strategic logic, but the result of a policy to use any Ministry of Works stores available when the purchases of the reserves occurred. Nor did the stockpile reflect a balanced holding of equipment since its history, as already described, reflected a political dimension such as the Northern Ireland situation and the curtailment of the programme meant some elements did not reach completion. Now faced by a war so different in kind, the stockpile valued at £16 million remained either useless functionally or because items were in the wrong place.[48]

For all its many flaws, the stockpile still represented a consummate political signal for the Ministry of Health which showed support for civil defence, particularly when it came to dealing with hospitals. Unfortunately, the Treasury did not see it in those terms and interpreted the political edict of no money on survival as an excuse to hit the stockpile itself and thereby achieve immediate savings. A budget ceiling of £150,000 p.a. was slapped on its annual maintenance, though according to the Ministry of Health it required at least £233,000 p.a. to bring the disaster into any meaningful strategic order through redistribution, and not much less to maintain it properly. However, the financial consequences of such a turnaround strategy were potentially highly damaging because it represented nearly a third of the total medical civil defence budget allocated amounting to £750,000 p.a.[49]

All the same, the Ministry of Health officials chose to hold their ground and the most sensitive areas of the stockpile selected as ammunition to aim at the Treasury where disposal either within the hospital system or on the open market would become politically embarrassing. The first involved items for which no day-to-day use existed.

2 million coloured blankets
128,000 pallets
42,000 hair mattresses
430,000 camp beds
90,000 stretchers
15,000 stretcher fitments
15,000 water containers

Added to this mountain, another of equal bulk included nearly 3.2 million yards of canvas with the potential of furnishing more tented hospital units, and large quantities of outmoded medical and surgical instruments stocked during the last war. The second element related to items issued to the hospital service, but were not at that time actually the subject of central supply arrangements by the Ministry of Health. The main items were:

½ million white blankets
1 ¼ million sheets
½ million draw sheets
350,000 pillows
1 ¾ million pillow slips
1 million towels
37,000 hospital beds[50]

Defending their corner, the Health Departments raised the first problem that would occur in respect of the bulky items having little day to day use in the National Health Service. The 2 million coloured blankets complied with the British Standard specification of the day, but not the specification demanded by the Services who were regarded as the only potential users due to their unpopularity with public. Consequently, the Ministry argued this white elephant would require disposal as surplus over a very long time with adverse consequences on the woollen industry. Bulky items represented by wooden camp beds, stretchers and stretcher fitments had no ready market and would need to be broken up and sold for their scrap value with a massive financial loss in prospect. As for the three million yards of canvas, although tents would not provide protection against fallout, arguments were raised that the material could be made up as tented annexes to existing hospitals or complete mobile tented hospitals thereby reducing the demands for requisitioned buildings. The second defensive move made against the Treasury related to the items not the subject of central supply. Requiring hospitals to purchase these also had immense political ramifications. Again, because of the amounts involved and the time needed for them to be absorbed into the hospital system, it provided further shots for the Ministry of Health to fire at the Treasury. The white blankets, sheets and pillowcases, in particular, represented three years supply and a complete halt on further orders would cause problems in the cotton and linen sectors of the very kind their original purchase had prompted. Finally, the Ministry argued that the conversion of the stockpile from a static to a continuous supply arrangement needed additional staff and thus negated any savings made on storage. By producing a list of political, economic and practical problems, the answer according to Ministry of Health added up to keeping the stockpile and managing it more carefully.[51]

All these arguments won the day, but the result in many respects turned out to be a hollow victory since the trade-off for keeping the stockpile caused problems to other areas of the Ministry's civil defence establishment. With an unbending Treasury, the costs of keeping the stockpile meant the budgetary axe had to fall elsewhere. The Ambulance and Casualty Collection Section especially took the brunt of the accounting consequences and began to face a fight for survival as it risked collapsing after already suffering years of having to live with second hand vehicles, or indeed no vehicles at all. A certain irony lay in the fact the problems were the result of stunning recruitment figures to the ambulance sector that had attracted a membership of 54,000 to its ranks. Much of the success, rather amusingly, had actually resulted because of recruits seeking free driving lessons a matter which caused its own headache. Though tuition involved a combination of using regular ambulance crew and local driving schools, the Ministry confessed the process had become tedious and costly, all of which aggravated the problems and in turn seriously affected morale.[52]

Reacting to the deteriorating situation, a special grant raised in 1955 allowed for the production of 50 ambulances so the needs of the most desperate authorities could be covered. In the event, only half the production run materialised because of funding problems thereby sending out the worst signal possible, even worse perhaps than doing nothing. The Ministry of Health attempted to mitigate the disaster by issuing a limited supply of 'soft' training equipment, primarily first aid haversacks, boots and anklets, plus a small pool of denims to members of the Ambulance and Casualty Collection Section. But the main deficiency of training ambulances still hung over the entire organisation, a matter which the Ministry admitted gave rise to a great deal of discontent to a point where the section rapidly came to regard itself as the 'Cinderella' of the Civil Defence Corps.[53]

Truly, the lot of the ambulance service had become untenable, particularly when compared to the Auxiliary Fire Service and their bespoke equipment developed to fight the nuclear conflagration. High on the jealousy list were the magnificent fire engines known as 'Green Goddesses' which aptly reflected their operational power and majestic presence.[54] Confronted by a crisis of confidence the Ministry of Health were forced to make an uncustomary admission to those supporting the hospital service:

> As you know, the shortage of training vehicles for ambulance and casualty collection training has been a matter of difficulty and has increasingly been a source of dissatisfaction locally and of embarrassment centrally. The difficulty which has been beyond our control is finance, but we are hopeful that a number of measures mentioned later in this letter will gradually improve the general position.[55]

The so-called 'measures' which did eventually emerge were not exactly a spectacular remedy and included the balance of the fifty new ambulances withdrawn earlier being reinstated in the form of new Bedford vans. Severely pruned of all embellishments, their designation as 'utility vehicles' came with a sales pitch they were 'quite handsome and manageable medium sized training vehicles'. In defence of their cheapness, the argument went they possessed an advantage over purpose built training ambulances and more closely resembled the type of vehicle likely to become available through requisitioning. Another move to bolster morale involved approval for authorities to spend their allowance for ambulances, raised from £350 to £500, on actually building their own vehicles by using an old chassis and constructing a new body. The London County Council were mentioned as being pioneers in this kind of recycling venture and an inspection of their workshop offered. Really, the package could not do much as it simply scratched the surface of a total disaster area. A further suggestion that a survey should also be conducted of the ambulance situation in itself precisely pointed to the scope of the problem, especially with authorities being asked to denote on the questionnaire whether their vehicles came into the 'derelict' category.[56]

Whilst the disintegration of the civil defence ambulance units appeared more and more to signify there would be little prospect of transporting nuclear casualties to hospital, the realisation also began to emerge there would not actually be much of a nuclear hospital service to take them to anyway. Stretching the distances out of reach of a hydrogen bomb blast to conserve staff and equipment resources now produced an even greater problem because of the numbers of new beds that had to be created outside the extended target areas. For a start, calculations suggested no fewer than 90,000 out of the 171,000 acute hospital beds would be lost in England and Wales.[57] With these needing replacement, plus expansion, some 369,000 acute beds alone were necessary to find, even before the formulation of plans for another 500,000 beds in auxiliary hospitals. If that was not challenging enough, the new hospital plan also persisted in its ethical pretentions by promising the chronic sick, mentally retarded and those with TB they would not be abandoned.[58] Regional Hospital Boards in England and Wales reckoned losses of beds in the numbers tabulated below would arise in each sector:

Chronic beds	13,500 out of 36,000
Mental beds	72,000 out of 145,000
Mental Deficiency beds	19,400 out of 53,000
TB and other beds	30,000 out of 65,000[59]

Logistically, the bed situation threatened to erupt into a fiasco of political incompetence on the grandest scale imaginable if the planning history of the atomic era was anything to go by. Ministry of Health calculations put a total of 150 million square feet now being dependent on requisitioning.[60] Plenty of sympathetic political noises echoed around Whitehall corridors about the casualty plan requiring support. Even the Official Committee on Civil Defence, representing the main ministries involved in planning, agreed in March 1956 'that the provision of accommodation for hospitals must receive first priority'.[61] But with a policy geared to simply keeping the thinnest veneer of civil defence in place, when it came to starting earmarking, particularly schools, nothing much materialised. Moreover, a number of options to add bed numbers were disappearing. Up to 100 tented hospitals, equipped and organised on the same lines as an Army Casualty Clearing Station were to be pitched by the Army once the fallout patterns were established.[62] Despite being a major plank in civil defence strategy, at the beginning of 1958 the Ministry of Defence unexpectedly announced the costs of such a facility, together with the attendant vehicles and storage, would need to be borne by the Ministry of Health. In the circumstances of the budgetary constraints, the news inevitably came as a terminal blow to the idea and left another gaping hole in the medical plan.[63]

Canvas especially left an uncomfortable legacy resulting from the purchase of a staggering 7.2 million square feet at a cost of £3 million. Nearly half had been made up at an additional cost of £1 million to provide the 100 tents. But it meant that a balance of some 3.5 million square feet of material still existed in bale form. The Ministry of Supply requested this balance also be used for the provision of more tents, mainly to prevent the last tent making firms in the country closing down due to decreasing orders by the army. When the Treasury applied their austerity logic, the arithmetic produced the fact the 100 canvas hospital units already in store occupied 52,000 square feet of storage space, whilst the remaining 88 units of unmade canvas occupied only 8,000 square feet.[64] Consequently any further tent making incurred the Treasury's displeasure and strictly forbidden, with the issue to be considered only on war being declared, a judgement which left a disbelieving Ministry of Supply to formally dissociate itself from the decision.[65] The canvas question, therefore, ended up with utilising the tents available as annexes to permanent buildings already in use, or earmarked for that purpose in an emergency.[66] Surviving records of hospital plans such as those prepared by the South-Eastern Board of Scotland, which covered the evacuation of Edinburgh, show the tented annexe concept still held good right up to 1968. Operationally it meant tents and equipment were due for release to the Board by the Scottish Home and Health Departments in the warning period, but the operational use of annexes through tentage would depend on the fallout patterns after the missiles had fallen.[67]

The extent to which Ministry of Health started to descend into a state of desperation about the hospital bed situation is reflected in the Department's machinations over its holding of old wartime hutted accommodation. Altogether, it held a portfolio of sixteen camps of which seven were Crown freeholds, one held on a lease and the other eight retained on land acquired under wartime requisition arrangements. Subjected to a tight rein on expenditure, the huts received only the minimal maintenance with the result the fabric of most of the premises had deteriorated badly. Those on requisitioned land had especially come in for criticism as 'presenting a sorry picture of neglect'. Undoubtedly the case for surrendering the entire holding was obvious, but the Ministry of Health felt that to diminish its symbolic artefacts would cause irreparable damage to the facade. Whilst it was agreed the buildings could offer no protection against radioactive fallout, the Ministry countered the point by suggesting a similar situation applied to many hutted buildings used by the National Health Service still left over from the war. Besides, in the Ministry's view, the retention of the camps was known for their potential use as casualty support centres amongst those involved in the planning and staffing of the wartime casualty service and any abrupt release would have 'a disheartening effect on the Civil Defence and Allied Services'.[68]

Eventually, the potentially disastrous course civil defence policy had taken began to trouble many in the Cabinet. Home Secretary Rab Butler found it necessary to plead with his colleagues for a change of heart, saying: 'The general inadequacy of our preparations will inevitably become apparent in the course of exercises and discussions with the various interests concerned such as local authorities, public utilities, trade and industry'. A meeting in April 1957 between ministers responsible for civil defence finally showed a distinct schism on the issue:

> In discussing other home defence preparations some ministers took the view that it was unrealistic to pretend that without very substantial expenditure anything effective could be done to temper the effects of nuclear attack on this country and that it seemed possible that the general public had themselves already reached this fatalistic conclusion. Other ministers thought that there was a clear responsibility on the government to take such action as were possible, within the limitations of our economic and financial resources; otherwise the

general public might not continue to support the government's policy of reliance on the deterrent.[69]

With no positive action in sight, civil defence lurched from crisis to crisis and eventually led Butler to remark in desperation: 'How are we to justify life and death economies such as those proposed in a home defence programme as low as that agreed for the current year?'[70] Probably regarded at first as internal posturing amongst colleagues, the question did not look so dismissible the following year when tensions over Berlin began to bubble up in 1958 as Soviet Premier Nikita Khrushchev delivered an ultimatum to the Western Powers to withdraw their garrisons in the city. The Defence Committee reacted by confirming a continuing need for the facade as a psychological comforter, even if it lacked any survival measures:

> The Defence Committee recognised that, although ideally survival measures should be taken as an essential part of home defence preparations, the additional expenditure involved could not be contemplated in present circumstances. It was, however, decided that it would be undesirable to abandon home defence preparations since this might undermine the credibility of the deterrent and would put us in an embarrassing position with our Allies. Home defence expenditure should, therefore, for the time being continue at about the current level, but that the main emphasis in the programme should be laid on those measures which provided a positive and visible indication of the Government's support for the voluntary civil defence services.[70]

Whilst the Defence Committee accepted the necessary evil of illogicality in their edict, it was by no means a unanimous decision in Whitehall circles. A summary of a meeting held the same year between various interested parties made that clear. The Treasury were perfectly happy about continuing with the whole facade although they felt their political master, the Chancellor, might seek even further cuts. Sir Norman Brook, the Cabinet Secretary was 'clearly bothered about the lack of logic' and in the circumstances he considered the entire charade should be terminated. The Chiefs of Staff recorded their views: 'The maintenance of the morale of the civilian population is an essential feature of the deterrent'. Conversely, Sir Richard Powell, Permanent Secretary of the Ministry of Defence, came out as an outright abolitionist, whilst the

Foreign Office said they were horrified at the thought of ending civil defence and felt it would harm relations with Britain's allies.[71] The idea of promoting civil defence at the Staff College without any survival measures was sufficiently troubling for General Sir Sidney Chevalier Kirkman, Director General of Civil Defence, to write to the Home Secretary Rab Butler. He expressed his misgivings by saying that he 'had a reasonable standard of honesty', adding, 'I should not however feel able to maintain the enthusiasm of those concerned if money, within the limits of what is available, were not devoted to certain projects essential to our survival in war'.[72] A note scribbled by Butler on the memo as an immediate response confirms just how the deception had run by October 1958. In this, he suggested: 'We must certainly render our facade as honourable and effective as possible. At present there is some ambiguity'.[73] For all that the 'ambiguity' persisted. Eroded by inflation, an attempt made in 1959 to increase the home defence budget by 23%, serves to draw attention to the degree with which the facade just continued to exist as a low cost expediency. The Financial Secretary to the Treasury advised ministers in charge of civil defence his department was satisfied about the situation and it could see no reason why any further funds were necessary to allocate:

> Our policy in recent years of keeping the voluntary civil defence services in being at a steady level of expenditure, with no attempt to provide for survival measures, seems to be serving its purpose of supporting the deterrent while avoiding any impression that precautions are being stepped up to meet a nuclear attack in the near future.[74]

In actual fact, the cost benefit statement as a road map of doctrine pointed the facade on a course towards destruction. To those in Whitehall who still maintained it had an important part to play in deterrence policy the situation was developing into an agonisingly intractable problem with much at stake. The medical side of the belief system, fundamental to projecting the caring and moral state, had actually entered dangerous dilemma ground. The organisation seemed in danger of collapse if no improvements were made, but equally at risk if the outstanding issue relating to the mobilisation and control of the general practitioners was brought to a head given the apoplectic reaction over the Skeleton Plan by the BMA. Moreover, in the post Coventry mutiny world, where civil defence had become a weapon to turn back on government, the uncomfortable possibility the NHS itself could be at risk also added a further issue to the growing list of toxic elements merging into one of the most sensitive socio political problems of the Cold War.

Chapter 5

ADMISSION IMPOSSIBLE

The budgetary stranglehold on civil defence expenditure saw the facade edging closer and closer to collapse with the possibility of dragging its medical component along with it. Keeping the image of mass compassion intact meant an increasing need for excluding corrosive pictures of medical neglect within the casualty chain, but with resources paired to the bone this no longer seemed possible to realise. Even if more funding were available, the question remained how the kind of marginal increases likely to be involved could ever achieve the level of credibility required. In their bid to win extra money, a view of how the Home Office saw a resolution to the problem reveals an extraordinary insight just where the evolutionary progress of the facade had reached since Churchill's decree it must provide political benefit and what might happen next if the political will existed to stop the rot:

> In the view of the Home Office, it is possible to give a positive and visible indication of the Government's support for the voluntary civil defence services without showing that their training has some relation to realistic preparations for a situation in which they might be called upon to function. We cannot hope to attract our customers – or convince other people that we are still in business – unless we have something in the shop window, and a little on the visible shelves, and are able to assure our customers that if necessary something can be provided from stock.[1]

Looking at this statement, which called for the extraction of high visibility political value but was disconnected from the new realities, it is easy to appreciate with such thoughts hanging in the political atmosphere the NHS could also succumb to this proposition. Making matters seemingly impossible, by 1960 Britain had become a nuclear fortress with bomber bases ready to take the bomb deep into the heart of the USSR. Along with dispersal airfields and THOR missile sites, the number of potential targets was making it increasingly difficult to justify the continuance of the civil defence charade. Home Secretary Rab Butler wrote to Harold Macmillan, by that time Prime Minister, about the difficulties of maintaining the facade and warned: 'It was fully recognised his policy could not be defended on logical grounds, and it is increasingly difficult to disguise its logicality from those outside government service on whom the implementation of keeping civil defence alive depends'.[2] Macmillan conceded that a committee should review the situation under the chairmanship of 'Freddie' Bishop, Deputy Secretary to the Cabinet. It seemed, in the circumstances, civil defence was finally on the list for closure.

Faith Healing

Contrary to all expectations, the committee's final judgement must have disappointed the Prime Minister's eagerness to cull the volunteer services. Instead Bishop strongly advocated the facade should be maintained in the national interest and secured in ways to ensure it appeared more logical and, therefore, believable. In reaching their decision, the review committee recognised precisely the nature of their actions. One background note on file could have come straight out of a Campaign for Nuclear Disarmament publication. This said: 'Civil defence policy in the UK is a sham, a facade of comparatively useless expenditure on non-essential purposes concealing an absence of any plans to minimise casualties in the event of nuclear attack or to prevent disease and starvation carrying off the bulk of any survivors'.[3] A split in the committee gave a choice that dug the proposed deception ever deeper into the realms of a conspiracy that has few counterparts in post war Britain. A majority view considered civil defence would steady public opinion at a vital time and must remain an integral part of deterrence policy. On the other side, a minority expressed their serious concern about the futility of continuing with the organisation since most people realised no protection against nuclear attack existed. Sir Norman Brook warned Macmillan of the decision on the grounds strong feelings had emerged that: 'The facade of a home defence policy (including the maintenance of a Civil Defence Corps and the cooperation of the local authorities in this field) would gradually crumble away unless expenditure were increased and certain gaps in our planning filled'.[4]

Presented to the Cabinet on the basis that the level of home defence preparations did not provide a reasonably coherent policy, it also came with the warning that these 'had for some time been insufficient to command the continuing support of the local authorities'. Put in this way, the situation especially had an unsettling resonance with the Coventry debacle and raised the politically dangerous possibility of a negative decision, confirming the left-wing agitators in the city had been right all along. Convincing local authorities and doctors was in the circumstances stressed as an essential move to show government was doing what it reasonably could within the inevitable limitations. Adopting such a philosophy, the argument went, demanded limited funds be carefully allocated on those measures which provided 'a positive and visible indication of the government's support of the voluntary civil defence services'.[5] Posing the problem in this way 'Freddie' Bishop and his 1960 Home Defence Review Committee successfully played to Whitehall's fears that something was better than nothing and approval duly given to bolster the 'something' part of the equation.

Where the situation left the medical planners was abundantly clear insofar as logicality depended on keeping out as much nuclear reality as possible. One problem immediately discarded underlines the depth of the illusion in its total sense. Until then, the hospital plans had assumed a city target attack by the Soviets. In the case of the hydrogen bomb, with its propensity to spew deadly radiation across the country and attacks likely to occur on military and city targets, the evacuation of many hospitals would be jeopardised. Bishop invited changes on the basis hospital resources should not just include movement to the periphery of target areas, but involve redistribution to a different area of the country altogether where the risks of radiation might be minimised. That precipitous change in strategic direction, of course, meant even less existing hospital beds being available with huge logistical problems in prospect. Unsurprisingly, the city target assumption stood as the preferred route for national planning purposes and at least provided a reassuring air of continuity.[6]

So the Bishop doctrine and a combination of war scares over the Berlin Wall in 1961 and the Cuban Missile Crisis in 1962 began a process whereby all the various pieces of the hospital plan, which had proved so elusive to accomplish during the late 1950s, began falling into place in compliance with the 'logicality' principle. One of the most important elements involved completing the earmarking of schools to secure the one million bed target. As far back as June 1959 Ministers had recognised the strategic consequences of a thermonuclear war meant education in its normal sense could not continue and a tentative list of some 2,000 schools deemed suitable for hospital use had been prepared.[7] Because the Bishop review of 1960 did not abandon the facade, but rather chose to strengthen it, this critical component needed attention without further delay.[8] Under these circumstances, Home Secretary Rab Butler ensured he threw the most cutting moral blackmail card when the final decision was at stake with the plea: 'The two paramount considerations are the maintenance of morale and the personal safety of the children. In time of emergency it is likely that parents would wish to keep their children near them as they do during the holidays; that the children would be at risk on their way to and from school; and that their schools may offer less protection than their homes.'[9]

With little room for further prevarication, Ministers agreed the earmarking policy in April 1962. It took another two years before becoming operational since it had to run the gauntlet of several involved parties and gain their support. These included not only local authority interests, but also the National Union of Teachers, the Headmasters' Conference representing public schools and many others.[10] The new Accommodation Clearance Register formally became operational on 30 June 1964.[11] Bids for buildings such as schools, supermarkets and department stores were due for submission to the appropriate Regional Director of the Ministry of Public Building and Works, the closing date set for 30 November 1964. In the event of more than one bid for a particular property occurring, this would trigger an adjudication process if the competing parties failed to reach agreement. Regional Hospital Boards did at last receive priority for acquiring educational premises, but on the understanding that a mutually-acceptable allocation was still required with local authorities in the case of those schools in their care.[12]

Caught by the new determination to progress matters, another operational element to receive urgent attention involved the area of transport planning which had drifted into obsolescence. During 1963, the Ministry of Health lodged a bid with the Ministry of Transport for the requisitioning of 3,000 single deck coaches to carry out inter hospital transfers in England and Wales. Specifications defined the number of stretchers per coach as eight, to be positioned four on each side with two above and two below. During the atomic era, stretcher fitments had been designed for this purpose with 3,000 held at Royston, Hertfordshire and 2,000 at York, altogether enough to convert 625 coaches to the desired specification.[13] Instead of indicating a piece of well executed forward planning further studies eventually showed the fitments had become outdated. Considerable problems had arisen because of coach operators changing their vehicles to designs no longer suiting the configuration of the stretcher racking. A review concluded that to modify everything and convert a coach in the few days now available in the pre attack phase could not be done. Instead, the stockpile moved into the 'no longer fit for purpose' category which meant the exercise having to fall back on improvisation with coach seats simply being ripped out and the installation of any kind of fitments abandoned altogether.[14]

High on the list of other outstanding issues came the lack of training vehicles for the ambulance sector that by then had gone through a further change into the Ambulance and First Aid Section. With all the anguish expended over the years, the results were spectacular and by 1963 no less than 800 'austerity' training ambulances had been supplied centrally.[15] The following year further deliveries started of 189 dual purpose vehicles capable of being used for training both ambulance and first aid party personnel.[16] Secondly, the Ambulance and First Aid volunteers were drawn into a review during 1961, which covered the entire Civil Defence Corps designed to change any public perceptions of the organisation being staid and ineffectual. It had originated against a background of concern that 'an undue number of ageing volunteers who served in civil defence in the last war: many of them, while retaining their enthusiasm, have found it difficult to adapt themselves to changes of outlook'.[17] Not only did this seem harsh and disparaging to the loyal members, in truth the attitudes described were as much to do with government policy and the reason why a Second World War mentality persisted at all. Nevertheless, the exercise led to bounty payments of £10 p.a. being introduced to the rank and file in return for stiffer training commitments. It probably in the end meant many of the 'ageing volunteers' actually receiving an allowance and their enthusiasm rewarded accordingly![18]

Behind the scenes, the vexed question of the medical stockpile also came into the spotlight. As at June 1960, its value amounted to a staggering £16 million pounds with an annual maintenance tag of £200,000, albeit Bishop noted even the most basic reserve supply for war would be of the order of £50 to £60 million.[19] At the very least, it required decentralisation to less vulnerable areas and preferably held at hospitals from where distribution could take place. During 1959, a transfer of some of the items to designated acute hospitals had begun on the basis little or no capital expenditure was necessary to create suitable storage space. Supplies ended up as bundles called 'composite units', each calculated to take up 2,500 cubic ft. of space. The inventory of a standard unit comprised bedsteads, coloured and white blankets, feather, hair or flock pillows, pillowslips, bed and draw sheets, roller and terry towels.[20] Bales of cloth were also included consisting of apron cloth, calico for dressing towels and surgical gowns, as well as white and coloured flannelette. Official arrangements mentioned receiving hospitals could expect notice when the items were due for despatch by rail, with crates identified by stencilled letters CD to denote their status as civil defence stocks. Hospitals could then turn the usable items over with their own supplies, on condition they provided replacements, the only exception being that white blankets needed substitution by the coloured variety due to these being regarded as unwanted by the public.[21]

Regional Hospital Boards were written to again in August 1964 and advised that because the available time for changing over to a war footing had been compressed to no more than two or three days, the dispersal of the stockpile was even more essential. Each RHB had notice of its outstanding stockpile allocation requiring decentralisation, with the request they conduct a further search for storage at their hospitals. Despite the good intentions, the project began to take on the appearance of an exercise in the impossible given the space requirement amounted to millions of cubic feet. Cramming all the supplies into spaces often quite unsuitable, such as old redundant coal cellars, raised a certain inevitability that a major drama would result and this duly erupted in June 1965. By then a point of exasperation arrived when the Ministry of Health felt compelled to write a stern letter to Regional Boards. The Department referred to what they called 'substantial losses' of dispersed items and in some areas described the conditions under which they were being stored as 'far from satisfactory'. Exhibiting signs of acute bureaucratic neurosis, the Ministry of Health suggested any losses amounted to a treasonable offence given the supplies were paid out of public funds for the public in war. Regions received strict orders to ensure better custodial arrangements and were required to designate people for the future wellbeing of the stockpile, their names to be sent for recording at the Ministry.[22]

An internal note referring to a meeting with the Regional Hospital Boards reveals just how deeply civil servants considered hospitals were not taking the nuclear war plan as seriously as they should:

> While we have no wish to offend the susceptibilities of professional people in the hospital service by interfering in their little kingdoms at the same time we have a duty to the taxpayer and even more to the potential victims of a nuclear attack to ensure that goods put into the stockpile either permanently or on a turnover basis are properly cared for, will be available if and when required, and are not being used as a sort of bonus or supplement to normal working reserves. If Hospital Management Committees resent interference of this kind, which we have tried to keep to a minimum consistent with responsibility to the taxpayer, they must, we feel, lay the blame at the doors of their fellows who in recent years lamentably failed to afford to the stockpile the same standard of care and protection they give to their normal peacetime reserves.[23]

Whilst creating an impression of prudent action, the dispersal exercise did nothing to improve the quality of the stockpile itself and certainly little else demonstrated any kind of joined up planning. No reserve of drugs existed. The only insurance cover, beyond saving or recovering any stocks in the pre and post attack period, came in a payment made by the Ministry of £7,000 a year to firms who maintained increased supplies of Dextran and a small stock of blood matching sera on a turnover basis for civil defence purposes. Many of the bandages and dressings in the stockpile were old. The Ministry also reported the stockpile remained seriously deficient in stretchers and altogether described the position as 'unsatisfactory', a typical civil service understatement of a much grimmer situation.[24] Furthermore, the only scheme to provide a substantive painkilling capability ended in disaster. Though a spend of £60,000 p.a. was planned for between 1961 and 1964 to process the raw opium stored in bonded warehouses, no manufacturing pharmacist could be found to undertake the work. Feelings about their logistical vulnerability, which all these shortcomings exposed, caused immense tensions to build up at the Ministry of Health. Unable to contain their fury, the medical mandarins prepared an internal battle plan to protect the political position of the Health Departments and instigated a review of the holding of drug supplies by manufacturers to assess where deficiencies might lie following an attack. A private note by a Parliamentary Secretary reflected their frustrations very directly:

> I take the view that lags and shortcomings in our Civil Defence preparations are acceptable if, but only if, they have been known to Ministers collectively and possible remedial steps-including extra expenditure-have been ruled out by Ministers collectively on political or economic grounds. We must feel sure that if we are caught short it is not our Minister's face, but the whole Government's which will be red.[25]

The ferocity of the Ministry's reactions had the desired effect and produced funding for a tactical gesture of considerable importance. Treasury approval materialised for the disposal of the raw opium and Regional Hospital Boards invited to increase their stockholding of analgesics by doubling normal working reserves as part of a new £400,000 initiative to bolster civil defence preparedness.[26] The first tranche of funds amounted to between £4,000 and £5,000, which Regional Hospital Boards received so they could acquire additional pain relieving drugs and hold these at acute hospitals outside evacuation areas for rotation with their normal stock.[27]

Amongst other innovations, a new vehicle-requisitioning regime to provide transport for evacuating patients and conveying equipment out from hospital evacuation areas resulted from the new determination to create working systems. Arrangements had subsisted, since the start of the hospital plan, whereby the Ministry of Transport would requisition vehicles and drivers on behalf of the casualty services. By the 1960s, a reality check showed the scale of need had reached an impossible level of complexity and caused the department to confess the exercise being too onerous for them to conduct alone. Admitting they simply did not have the resources for such an undertaking, the Ministry of Transport decided to proceed on the basis of supplying lists of transport requirements to each RHB, giving its share of vehicles and operators so they themselves could get in touch with the firms selected and finalise schemes in detail. Surviving hospital documents attest to the epic exercise this became. Hundreds of dormant hiring contracts were finalised with removal contractors throughout the country as a contribution to the new regime of constant readiness. As a result, the meticulous recording of the proposed allocation of vehicles to each hospital and the times of evacuating patients in stretcher and sitting case categories created a logistical web of incredible intricacy right across Britain. On the equipment side, the detail turned out to be as thorough and included the capacity of equipment scheduled for transfer, numbers of vehicles, numbers of journeys and again the hours to complete the transfer to the appropriate location.[28]

The important aspect of hospital food also developed further. Since 1952, feeding policy had centred on the use of any surviving food or food released from government stockpiles. Hospital catering staff had received training by the Women's Voluntary Service in various methods of improvised cooking designed to overcome the anticipated interruption of power supplies. Then, after years of prevarication, the printing of special ration cards was finally given the go-ahead to ensure a fair distribution of any available food supplies, the scheme also covering hospital patients. As part of the overall rationing strategy, certain foods received a special designation for hospital use only in recognition of the practical difficulties hospitals might encounter to provide sustenance for patients. Those establishments dealing with casualties attracted second priority in liquid milk distribution, after expectant mothers and infants, but before the 1–15 year old age group. Cereal such as sago and rice, tinned food and preserves would not be released from any wholesale stocks surviving for distribution to the general public, on account of such ingredients being considered ideal given the more limited requirement for cooking. Undoubtedly, the provisioning of the hospital system on the scale outlined raised the danger of the hospital becoming the focal point for survival, beyond just medical aid, a factor that did occur to the Ministry of Health. Discussing food policy with the Ministry of Agriculture, Fisheries and Food, new concerns were raised: 'We should want to avoid anything which would make the hospitals a focus for the hungry-eyed apart from their need for purely medical attention, and should indeed expect to set up a small unit outside the entrance to the hospital if this appeared necessary in order to prevent the showing up of in-patient admissions at the hospital itself'.[29] In a sense, these anxieties were a reflection of just how the hospital resembled a nuclear oasis in the minds of the planners. Outside its confines of contrived order and attentive care those outside might well consider themselves to be less fortunate than those inside. Logicality had simply reached a pinnacle of perfection to a degree that the result must rate as one of the most ambitious exercises ever to cocoon the British Isle, albeit a mythical cover of false expectation.

Saving Lives

Just because the hospital plan had taken on a more complete look did not mean the problem of logicality was by any means completely solved. The building blocks were largely asset-based and still left the problem of system or operational planning to be resolved. Quite simply, the wrong kind of instructions could compromise the positive imagery of those assets if the full reality of the nuclear environment appeared to constrain or nullify their usability. This became a matter of some painful consideration focussing on the need to reposition the casualty chain against the hugely increased power of the hydrogen bomb. Vital to circumventing that problem came the requirement for the ambulance and casualty collection sector to appear as a logical operation in dealing with greater numbers of casualties and equally the greater problems of access to them. Moreover, transferring hospitals further out and the probability ambulance crews would have less operational time due to exposure to radiation were all new elements militating against the idealised image of prompt individual care being achievable anymore.

In spite of the obvious need for change, the planners remained nervous of making any kind of material alteration to established procedures. Just how much so comes through the first study of the problem conducted at the Civil Defence Staff College at Sunningdale by the Ministry of Health in 1956. Based on a ten-megaton hydrogen bomb exploding above Birmingham, STUDY BULL RING included a review as to where casualties should actually be sorted given the new circumstances where the numbers demanded the introduction of some kind of holding pattern. Typically, the immediate reaction sent a message confirming a sorting process needed to take place at the casualty front line, but the preference remained for making better use of the organisational elements already in position:

> There was general agreement that the initial sorting process would be carried out by the 'the first aiders' of the Ambulance and Casualty Collecting Section, or other Civil Defence personnel. Some would be patched up and sent home. Obvious stretcher cases would be sent to hospital. Those not falling into these two obvious categories would be sent to Mobile First Aid Units.[30]

Produced as the first appraisal of the hydrogen bomb effect, the outcome shows the degree of reticence about making radical changes to the ethics of dealing with casualties, particularly the seriously injured. Perhaps looking comforting initially, the sorting position deteriorated dangerously in terms of keeping mass compassion as an ideology logically intact. Although a primary sieve by civil defence personnel on the basis of the 'obvious' casualty being hospitalised was all right up to a point, it did not represent a professional medical judgement. Fundamentally, a requirement for a further sorting mechanism remained, which sent the argument spinning into all kinds of irreconcilable directions. On the one side came a recommendation the final sorting process should take place after casualties had reached the acute hospital. On the other, a school of thought considered *Casualty Collection Points* ought to be located in forward areas where all casualties would end up, other than those needing initial first aid only. These collection points, the theory went, would be manned by the Mobile First Aid Units that could provide such sorting and those who did not need hospitalisation discharged, the remaining patients allocated to either acute or auxiliary hospitals. But the idea of a new system of this kind collapsed because of worries over the unnecessary loading and unloading of ambulances and the inability of the Mobile First Aid Units to know the admission status in acute or auxiliary hospital or between hospital areas because the pressure on beds might vary considerably. Fearful of starting any major departure from accepted protocols, the issue conveniently stayed with the philosophy sorting had to be hospital led as far as possible.[31] The first thermonuclear casualty plan thus reverted to the familiar and comforting principle that the seriously injured would end up in hospital and assessed there by a surgeon, in much the same way as would happen in peace.[32]

Nearly one year later, as the horrendous implications of the Strath report began seeping into the planning system, the sorting conundrum came under closer scrutiny. A key element in changing attitudes arose because of hospitals being located much further out. With longer ambulance hauls causing vehicles to disappear from the forward areas for long periods, it was felt the morale factor needed addressing. Other matters, such as capacity issues relating to the screening of casualties by first aiders together with the problem of the comparatively small Mobile First Aid Units working on their own, also became important aspects of the ongoing debate.[33] The sum total of these concerns suggested the medical facade urgently needed a new operational model in order to sustain a convincing statement of individualistic care. In other words, if casualties could not be conveyed quickly and in vast numbers to hospitals a means of bringing the hospital to the casualty needed development, at least as an intermediate stage.

A definite eureka moment when the solution to the problem appeared can be traced back to a study at the Civil Defence Staff College conducted between 10 to 12 April 1957 called 'MEDICAL CARAVAN'. Amongst those attending were the Ministry of Health and the Home Office, as well as their counterparts from Scotland and Northern Ireland, senior members of the hospital service, the armed forces and the voluntary aid societies. The centrepiece of the workshop, destined to have such a profound effect, came with a visit to the Field Training Centre of the Royal Army Medical Corps at Mytchett, near Aldershot where a live demonstration of a military Field Ambulance unit in action ran alongside two civilian Mobile First Aid Units. The study group were able to make a comparison, but saw the process used by the army, which had its origins in the First World War, as presenting the answer. Unlike the small MFAUs designed primarily to deliver limited first aid cover, the Field Ambulance concept could provide a higher level of primary medical attention to keep casualties alive or hold those whose injuries precluded their transfer to hospital. Consequently, an announcement indicating unanimous support for the arrangement as an ideal model for the conditions of nuclear warfare appeared with some exuberance this 'could provide the full answer if available in sufficient quantity'.[34]

The system promised a multifunctional process of casualty care capable of dealing with a range of medical conditions, but always based on the fundamental principle that initially a medical officer would carry out the sorting, albeit the decisions necessarily involved rapid assessments taken without diagnostic aids. In essence, the new set-up resembled a temporary field hospital with the most basic facilities. With that in mind, the only feasible solution suggested a need for bigger civilian units than the existing MFAUs, with a larger ratio of non-medical to medical personnel allocated to provide more nursing cover. Unsurprisingly, the conclusion of the study confirmed a general desire to bring together as close as possible the civilian and military patterns of sorting and holding.[35]

Structured on these principles, MEDICAL CARAVAN provided a pivotal moment in bringing to the nuclear arena a new medical formation called the Forward Medical Aid Unit. Albeit a revolutionary alteration, its introduction to Regional Hospital Boards appeared through an instruction both vague and short on detail and offered little more than a basic outline of operational principles. Using the allegory of a conveyor belt, the FMAU structure involved divisions by function starting at the reception and sorting headquarters where a system of colour-coded labels would denote the patient's medical status. Thereafter, the journey could take the casualty to the emergency and supportive areas pending transfer to hospital or the light treatment area for wounds capable of attention on the spot. Only the holding section remained as the final possibility where the dying would spend their last moments in horrendous conditions pending their eventual disposal. Staffing numbers of the FMAU confirmed its status as a major game changer with the assignment of four MOs, four trained nurses, thirty-six nursing auxiliaries and a support section of administrative personnel. Whilst dilution of medical expertise was tolerable to a certain extent by using dentists or medical students, ideally an experienced doctor or senior registrar from the hospital service remained the preferred solution.[36] Apart from that, one concession to medical protocol endured and the American approach to use veterinary surgeons in similar circumstances not adopted, their involvement in the post attack food chain considered more vital.[37]

While the FMAU provided a framework for coping with larger numbers of casualties, the continuing obsession with immediate medical attention raised a further alteration in the casualty system. The name of the Ambulance and Casualty Collection Section had changed to the Ambulance and First Aid Section. Organisationally this reflected an important addition to the ambulance drivers and auxiliary personnel dealing with stretcher parties and involved a dedicated First Aid Section operating as a parallel unit to render first aid before casualties reached the FMAU. Ironically, the importance of the move to show the immediacy of compassion also made it a focal point around which a medical debate began that would eventually corrode the very ideology the change intended to protect. This developed from a proposal to replace the simple first aid techniques, previously offered by the Casualty Collection Section, with more advanced medical procedures referred to as 'extended first aid' based on a twenty-four point lifesaving system used by the army. Subjects included the arrest of haemorrhages, use of the tourniquet, the bandaging and splinting of larger bones and the treatment of readily correctible mechanical respiratory defects, all aspects of first aid demanding a much higher level of training. Exemplary as the proposition might have appeared, more expansive medical knowledge at the sharp end raised the awkward question of whether the new first aid unit should then be turned into the means of establishing the first sieve to separate out the 'treatable' from the 'untreatable' so scarce medical resources could be utilised in the most beneficial way.[38]

Judged as a test of resolve to accept radical change, the outcome merely confirmed the inherent preference for conservatism. When the purpose of the new unit appeared as a civil defence instruction, it still held out its credentials as the bearer of universal compassion defined by three functions:

> To penetrate into the forward area allotted to them, with their first aid equipment and supply of stretchers. To render first aid to, and to care for, the more seriously injured until they are loaded on ambulances or otherwise reach medical aid. To ensure that stretcher cases are conveyed as speedily as possible to an ambulance loading point.[39]

Continuing to provide a mission statement of unbridled hope it could not have typified more just how the casualty chain remained encumbered with the fallacious idealism that the seriously injured would all receive attention.

Attempting to hide any trace of abandonment, the planners strove to project ever-greater numbers transported to hospitals, and as quickly as possible. Ambitious plans leveraged the perceived efficiency of the FMAU by the size and scale of the associated ambulance framework. The base operational unit consisted of an ambulance detachment and a first aid party equipped with six four berth ambulances and one vehicle to transport the first aiders whose equipment included a manifest of first aid haversacks, thirty-two stretchers, sixty four slings, sixty four blankets plus a reserve of first aid material. This unit then multiplied into platoons, companies, and finally the column, along with a column commander complete with staff car and motor cycle despatch riders. Made up to a total of seventy-two ambulances, each such column would serve one FMAU and provide a forward shuttle between the unit and the casualty collection points and a rear shuttle to and from the designated hospital, the whole working as a complete flow system.[40]

All such theorising about the efficacy of the casualty chain may have seemed a whimsical pastime confined to Whitehall. The fact is many sectors of the medical profession were willing to discuss publicly ways of dealing with the hydrogen bomb menace, thereby producing exactly the normalisation factor the Ministry of Health wanted. Those willing to embrace the medical problems of the nuclear battleground entered into quite emotional debates as to how mass casualties were possible to accommodate into some kind of ethical structure. Engagement with new spatial disciplines at the Royal Society of Medicine symposium held in 1957, called the 'Discussion on the Management of Mass Casualty Situations in a Time of War', demonstrated the potential of this kind of debate to divide and rule the medical profession, or at least parts of it.[41] Lieutenant General Sir Alexander Drummond, the Director General of the Army Medical Services, dismissed the crisis expansion of hospitals, describing it as a 'snare and delusion'. Considering the complex cross section of problems, he felt such a policy could only be considered medically viable if patients were suffering, as he put, it from 'skin disease, ingrown toenails or dyspepsia' and advised staff cover should determine intake and at some point suggested 'hospital gates should then be locked'. Readdressing the ethical balance, Colonel Timothy Ahern, also an army physician, explained the means of turning an unstructured position of medical chaos into one of order through casualty sorting. Focussing on the medical examination he advanced his view that in twenty-four hours one doctor's time expended on a unit shift basis might examine an average of 600 patients and operate on 100 of them by spending two minutes on each examination and nine minutes in undertaking basic lifesaving operations.[42]

The symposium fed the *British Medical Journal* with papers and correspondence reflecting the attitudes of the medical profession in a number of ways. A presidential address to the Bath, Bristol and West Somerset Branch of the British Medical Association by George Kersley, Consultant Physician at the National Hospital for Rheumatic Diseases, received extensive coverage under the title, 'Nuclear Warfare and the Treatment of Mass Casualties'. In admonishment, he began with the words: 'The apathy in this country, and perhaps especially among the medical profession, towards civil defence and education in protection from nuclear warfare is very evident'. A defence of the medical service in nuclear war followed, advocating the Royal School of Medicine conference held in June 1957 had offered positive ideas. According to Kersley, it had also correctly set out to recode the ethical structure at every level of treatment. A solution to surface burns of up to fifteen percent by a self-help initiative, as an example, proposed the following procedures:

> An interesting 'help yourself canteen' for the treatment of the less serious burns cases is

envisaged by Hunt (1957). Instead of a bun, the customer would collect the appropriate burns dressing', for a drink there would be saline and bicarbonate of soda; and at the cash desk would be some printed instructions.[43]

Morris Berenbaum, an eminent pathologist, vehemently opposed debate of that kind and expressed his anxieties this sustained the dangerous illusion nuclear war was survivable and acceptable. To drive the point home, he demolished Colonel Timothy Ahern's time and motion thesis because the doctor's job rate described had added up to thirty-six hours without pause and not the twenty-four hours claimed. Being drawn into the argument, Ahern defended his position by maintaining that instead of the two minutes quoted for the examination, this should have been 1.6 minutes and the injured would also have had 'their clothing removed and their injuries exposed'.[44] A third doctor congratulated the Home Office for shaking off their Second World War mentality and expressed feelings of a more pragmatic kind. He suggested doctors could well have to clear up the mess after a nuclear war and there was no point in pretending otherwise, however impossible or politically unpalatable the situation might appear. Even the usual starchy tone of *The British Medical Journal* narrative itself broke into an emotional appeal to all doctors stating: 'We, who believe in ourselves, must have faith that our essential values are worth saving and this saving can be effected'.[45]

Sometimes the theoretical turned more ominously into a question of actuality. The Department of Physics at the University of Bristol became the centre for delivering a challenge to senior hospital administrators of the South Western Region on a scale never before envisaged. Bristol councillor and Chairman of the Hospital Board, Sir Havergal Downes-Shaw, gave the opening address.[46] Then, set against a backdrop of the Suez Crisis and Khrushchev's threat to rain down nuclear missiles on Britain if it did not withdraw from the Canal Zone, an Assistant Senior Medical Officer of the Regional Board followed and gave a graphic picture as to how the internal layout of a wartime Bristol hospital might look very soon:

> The standard eight foot bed centres will have to be abandoned. Some space between beds will be maintained to allow nurses to pass between patients. It may be that by placing the beds head to tail further patients can be accommodated. Single or double lines of beds in the centre of the ward will help. If circumstances demand, it may be necessary to mix

> the sexes and group the cases but avoid too detailed distinction between medical and surgical cases. The question of double bunking of patients by putting patients under the beds is worth considering. Stretchers will be used as beds and they will litter every corner of the hospital - recreation and dining rooms, halls and stores.[47]

Whilst all these deliberations did indeed imply nuclear medicine to be negotiable rather than being untenable, or challengeable rather than impossible, discussions about the casualty problem began to narrow into uncomfortable territory. Combining the need to deal with as many casualties as possible whilst conserving resources under fallout conditions, slowly turned the argument towards the 'where' rather than 'whether' abandonment should actually come into the equation. On Sunday 13 July 1958, EXERCISE RELIANCE played an important part in the gradual move towards the unthinkable. Arranged in the South West, its purpose was to test the time taken to clear casualties from Ambulance Loading Points to their eventual reception and handling at hospitals. Based on a hydrogen bomb of unspecified power exploding over Avonmouth, near Bristol, the live exercise involved 650 'casualties' being transported to a civilian FMAU and a military field ambulance unit established at Keynsham on the outskirts of Bristol for sorting to be undertaken. Those chosen for further treatment were destined for transfer to Bath where members of the National Hospital Service Reserve staffed an acute hospital unit.[48]

When the exercise started, the urban scenery on a quiet Sunday morning hardly resembled the aftermath of a nuclear war. Yet the outcome confirmed the idea of modelling a sorting system using the military principles defined by MEDICAL CARAVAN looked sound. Secondly, and most crucially, general agreement was reached on the size of the FMAU which had appeared to work, although a suggestion added that the name should be changed to the Casualty Filter Unit. The time taken to treat the injured at the FMAU amounted to an average of ten minutes, the conclusion being, 'the speed with which casualties were disposed of was encouraging'. Further operational comfort came with the point underlined that the FMAU concept had not come undue pressure during the exercise and the official blessing given that it could operate under nuclear conditions without the danger of breaking down. Comically, what had actually completely broken down were the food arrangements under the control of the Women's Voluntary Service and their Food Flying Squad. Unfortunately, they were unable to distribute their usual feast of hot stew across such a wide field of operations with the attendant result many volunteers went hungry and the suggestion made that on future exercises volunteers bring their own packed lunches![49]

On the face of it, RELIANCE provided the medical facade with a spatial framework in which the mass casualty problem would provide a convenient hiding place for the attendant problem of abandonment. However, the exercise did reach another, more unnerving conclusion about the cavernous ethical gap in attitude requiring readjustment to make the system a workable proposition. This stressed the urgency for doctors to understand the function of the FMAU, a matter admitted requiring a considerable degree of reorientation from peacetime practice. Medical ethics of the past would be consigned to the impossible and involve many casualties who were dying or who could not stand the journey to hospital being left to face their fate within a holding unit provided by the FMAU. More radically, the study hinted that as sorting effectively meant abandonment by another name, the process should ideally start at the very beginning of the rescue chain that only the civil defence first aid personnel at the front line could achieve.[50] For the Ministry of Health this push at the sorting door to confirm a policy of outright abandonment started a journey of much anguish underlined by the fact the term 'Casualty Filter Unit' did not receive approval and the more assuring tone of the Forward Medical Aid Unit retained.

Just maintaining the reassuring title alone, however, could not forestall the problems banking up and fast eroding the appearance of logicality. Sustaining a workable system of mass compassion had become problematic given the constraining issue of radiological life that demanded limits placed on the exposure to radioactivity by all involved in civil defence operations.[51] Even more discomforting, the erstwhile symbol of medical hope found in the Blood Transfusion Service was no longer a logical symbol. Calculations undertaken for the Services showed the English and Scottish centres between them could only provide 1,400 bottles of blood in the first week of an emergency, enough to cope with just 4,500 wounded. After four weeks, the supply could be ramped up to just 3,500 bottles, enough to cover just 12,000 casualties as opposed to the millions of soldiers and civilians who would require attention.[52] Described as 'completely inadequate' arrangements for the Blood Transfusion Service to operate in the conditions of nuclear warfare were, therefore, diplomatically pronounced as being 'an uneconomic form of insurance' and no longer relevant to the casualty plan. With the life of whole blood being limited and the inability to build up sufficient supplies of dried plasma and plasma substitutes, only 'immediate transfusion' by collecting, grouping and matching blood at or near where blood transfusions were required appeared the only practicable alternative. As a result, new standing orders required all acute hospitals to prepare for this eventuality that meant stockpiles of equipment for the taking and giving of blood had to be sited at suitable locations for immediate dispersal. A constant state of readiness was to become part of the new Cold War routine and hospitals received further instructions to support that principle by establishing a nucleus of expertise consisting of at least one pathologist, registrar, technician and nurse who would be fully prepared to extend the service at a moment's notice.[53]

With all these changes that exposed the impossibilities of dealing with the thermonuclear environment in the old ways, it seemed an official abandonment policy simply had to be unveiled. A move towards introducing this new and unthinkable of ethical standards even received recognition in a lecture given at the Civil Defence Staff College on the *Initial Management of Mass Casualties* that proposed an ethical shift on the following basis:

> The object of civil defence planning was to ensure the survival of the race by what was termed the 'economic deployment' of limited resources and only selecting those likely to survive the holocaust. Lifesaving operations only were to be attempted and only later would definitive surgery take place. At the most brutal heart of this new ideology the sorting of casualties started with the rescue workers and the Ambulance and Casualty Collecting Service. Personnel needed to be trained not only in first aid, but also to make preliminary diagnosis.[54]

As logical as the new ethic was, it signified the very change the Ministry of Health quite simply did not want to escape into the public arena. The FMAU held immense value of delivering an indeterminate amount of mass compassion not only through its 'elastic' form, but also by offering a more robust healthcare system outside the environs of the hospital building. Wishing to bring those advantages into sharper focus, the Ministry established a working party to set out a common form of sorting structure and turn the somewhat vague FMAU framework originally published into a national model. On the face of it, the results did strengthen the perception of mass compassion through the physical layout of the FMAU, just as the Ministry of Health had wanted. (Appendix 3) The report even put numbers on the plan. It concluded that within a period of 24 hours a single unit was to anticipate the reception of between 2,000 and 2,500 casualties, but if admissions began to exceed those numbers over a prolonged period then a further unit or part would require deployment as support.[55]

The multiplier possibility of the FMAU must have been music to the Ministry of Health's ears in playing out the tune of increased hope. Inconveniently, however, in the midst of the optimism a discomforting note of dissonance sounded when the working party went far beyond their brief and commented on the need for the physical aspect of layout to work in tandem with firmer guidance on sorting. Radical changes to medical ethics were suggested which raised the ghost of RELIANCE and its recommendation that sorting be started at the coalface of the first aid exercise. Associated with that philosophy the working party raised the need for a policy to be clearly laid down regarding the quality of medical attention on the basis: 'All care and treatment (even in hospitals) in the early stages after an attack should be of the emergency life-saving variety; there should be no attempt at definitive treatment. The aim should be to prevent the patient getting any worse. Inevitably ill effects to the individual resulting from delay in instituting treatment must be accepted'. The second and most radical protocol change proposed that the right to medical resources should be related to a person's contributory capability to the post-attack position indicating: 'Treatment must aim to return the injured to duty as soon as possible so that they can make their contribution to the survival of the community'.[56] Critical to the whole thing, the working party categorically insisted that first aid personnel needed training to a higher standard of medical proficiency, a disturbing initiative that could deliver the first sieve of an abandonment policy.[57]

With the weight of logic stacking up against the Ministry of Health, the Department seemed finally to crumble and agreed some kind of priority system had to be introduced in the sorting of casualties. Changes duly appeared in a Ministry of Health circular published in 1960 as a basis on which hospitals and doctors could undertake training of Forward Medical Aid Units. Whilst the guidelines implied abandonment held a place in the medical effort, the protocol itself did not come in an overt and clear way, but announced as something hospitals had to work out for themselves. A further dilution of clear intent came with the view that producing lists of priorities and injuries could not deal with the problem alone and decisions would be subject to the varying opinions of doctors engaged in sorting, together with the changing circumstances that included the availability of hospital beds.[58] Characteristically, the circular did nothing at all to end the confusion and hospital authorities across the country proceeded to invest a great deal of time and energy into setting up large and ambitious casualty exercises to devise their own brand of casualty sorting.

Because of the Ministry's unusually ambivalent attitude towards this area of medical policy, the uncertainties it generated began to sow a great deal of confusion. Regional Hospital Boards started interpreting casualty sorting mechanisms in their own ways, with the result the rigour applied differed widely. Inconsistencies particularly surfaced between the more highly-regulated working procedures of the Ambulance and First Aid Section prescribed by the Home Office in their technical manuals and the much looser advisory memoranda issued by the Ministry of Health in connection with the Forward Medical Aid Units. Ambulance exercises showed first aid personnel often spending much too much time with casualties and using vast amounts of dressings on a burn involving more than one third of the body surface. After evacuating the casualty as a priority, the FMAU would then remove the dressings and consign the case to that of a moribund and untreatable category destined for the dreadful conditions of the holding area. At the other end of the scale, minor lacerations were being treated as ambulance cases which could more appropriately be passed on to a rest centre for simple first aid.[59]

Undoubtedly, a reason for exercise outcomes often descending into the realms of the bizarre, such as those described arose simply because of the need to bring down the standard of first aid to the lowest level of competency to maintain the interest of civil defence volunteers and encourage recruitment. The medical rituals might have provided good propaganda copy to reassure the public, but Regional Hospital Boards continued to express concerns at the increasing illogicality appearing in these ways and agreed on a joint approach to the Ministry to demand proper guidance. What should have been a watershed, the meeting held between ministry officials concluded with an impasse. The Department still refused to issue a manual claiming the advice on the functions, personnel, equipment, deployment, control and training already set out in circulars remained valid and did not require amendment. Once again, London stubbornly maintained that knowledge of the requirements of the FMAU could only come through studies and exercises and hospital authorities had necessarily to draw their own conclusions.[60]

Even when the Ministry of Health finally seemed ready to accept sorting at the front line and that 'extended first aid' required introduction, the reluctant approach adopted merely drove Regional Hospital Boards to further desperation. A somewhat half-hearted circular flirted with constructive abandonment by suggesting: 'Treatment must aim to enable the injured to make their contribution as soon as possible to the survival of the community'. Nonetheless, the Ministry still left the situation completely unclear as to what this meant in medical terms.[61] As a result, by 1964 an extraordinary position had arrived whereby the Ministry of Health were refusing to establish a coherent regime in a key area of medical ethics by confirming unambiguously that the seriously injured were no longer in the medical frame. The reasons for such reluctance were, of course, obvious. The FMAU represented an ideal format that envisioned care and attention to a broad range of casualties with further expansion possible as circumstances demanded. Furthermore, the loose instructions allowed the medical and ambulance domains to provide the elements of best practice which entirely suited their respective needs and expectations. What often developed reflected a challenge to show organisational perfection. The integration of police forces, hospitals, civil defence volunteers, and the army provided an outward sign of competent leadership. Swift conveyance of ambulances or the fast sorting of casualties could be ends in their own right. Much was at stake in the introduction of a new code of practice that dehumanised the decision making, especially if it then escaped into the public domain. Local initiatives completely diffused the abandonment problem rather than channelling it into a defined policy capable of destroying the imagery of the caring and moral state as well as handing over ideal ammunition to anti-nuclear groups on the one hand and alienating volunteers and the medical profession itself on the other.

Sieving Lives

The nature of the problem the Ministry of Health faced came down to just how far the sorting system was possible to keep in a state of ambiguity against the concerns of illogicality Regional Hospital Boards were increasingly expressing. A matter of some irony lay in the fact that the catalyst for change came from within the decision-making bureaucracy itself. Exasperated by the continued obfuscation over the sorting issue, the Scottish Department of Health decided to confront the Ministry of Health about the situation. Scotland could not have had a better secret weapon for this purpose in the illustrious Major General Frank Richardson who acted as their medical adviser. If a single event defined his character it was perhaps during the Battle of Keren in the Eritrean campaign of 1941. At great personal danger, he had played the bagpipes under fire to spur on his men at a crucial moment when the momentum was dangerously slipping away. His courageous act turned the tide of battle and earned him the Distinguished Service Order, though many considered the Victoria Cross would have been more appropriate.[62] This 'no nonsense' General now applied his prescription to the sorting situation. It is not difficult to appreciate from the exchanges that took place why the Ministry of Health had been slow to introduce a common code of practice. Getting to the crux of the problem Richardson suggested the familiar slogan, 'save the woman and children first', be turned into 'save able bodied men, children, pregnant women and those of child bearing age first'. He acknowledged this might cause a serious quandary in casualty sorting and gave a graphic example of rescue parties who might have to 'by-pass one old lady crying for help in favour of a simpler clearance task which would release several people to help in further clearance'.[63]

All the same, Richardson applied his blunt approach to a draft policy statement, but when he tested the new philosophy on eminent colleagues, not all were sure about the drastic nature of the guidelines it produced. Professor E J Wayne, Professor of Practice Medicine, Department of Practice Medicine, Gardiner Institute, Western Infirmary, Glasgow provided the most apposite comment on the psychological difficulties of abandonment in its most extreme forms which would face all medical support teams. Drawing on his wartime experience, he expressed severe reservations Richardson had left out references to the important role of the FMAU as a reliever of suffering and pain. Citing practical experience, Wayne spoke of his time as the officer on duty at the Sheffield Royal Infirmary during the city's first large air raid in November 1940. He indicated his ability to deal first with the relatively 'useful citizens', but unable to imagine he could have persuaded his assistants to agree not to ease the sufferings of the aged and those unlikely to recover. He, therefore, advised if this ethos received appropriate emphasis, then the memorandum would become much more acceptable.[64] The Professor's comment was taken on board and to 'tone down the aridity' of Richardson's slant, the following statement added:

> When medical resources are inadequate common sense will dictate that definitive treatment should be afforded only to those who will survive with treatment but would not survive without it, especially those with the best prospects of recovery of adequate function. For many other cases all that could be done in the circumstance may be the relief of pain and the best nursing which may be available.[65]

Eventually, the General's barrage of ethical revisionism did force the Ministry to reconsider their obstructive policy over codifying the casualty sorting system. Whitehall finally accepted the need for new rules and in October 1964 established a working party of medical experts to prepare a version for use in England and Wales. An internal memorandum self-righteously justified the many years of delay exclaiming: 'We knew that extended first aid would prove difficult and slow to get going. This has not altogether been a bad thing because revolutionary doctrines are best put across gradually'.[66] In spite of that, an appointment letter to those chosen also shows the Ministry's reluctance, even at that stage, remained as strong as ever:

> As you may know, we are under pressure from time to time, to issue some form of technical manual for the use of doctors in Forward Medical Aid Units: this we have strongly resisted, and for the moment shall continue to resist. It is, however, worth mentioning that there appears to be an increasing feeling that the younger generation of doctors, who have had no experience of any sort of war, might welcome some guidance, and would not consider it an attempt to interfere in their clinical judgement.[67]

For all the initial enthusiasm, the Ministry of Health's nervousness echoed in Scotland once Richardson's version appeared in draft form. The blue pencil appeared through some of the most acerbic of the General's commentaries. But what remained still had his essential philosophy of medical rejection throughout its pages. Not surprisingly, by the time the Scots finalised their treatise under the title of *Civil Defence, The Management of Mass Casualties* they were very much aware of how politically sensitive their document might be, the internal debate on the subject attracting a painfully circuitous argument:

> While the notes do not give clinical guidance (except for some details about radiation sickness), they do to some extent have a bearing on clinical decisions e.g. whether this patient should be treated as a priority over that. The Department are not in the habit of issuing generally material of this kind and we ought to consider whether it may be desirable at least to inform representatives of the profession in advance of our intentions. The BMA are not noticeably interested in civil defence and it may well be that if we merely proceeded to issue the document it would not excite their attention. But conceivably depending on the current mood of the profession, they might adduce the issue of such a document as an example of failure to consult the profession at the proper time.[68]

Any qualms about the politics of handling the new instructions disappeared when London requested Scotland defer issuing their manual until the English and Welsh version was ready to avoid embarrassment if the two countries came up with different standards. The request merely drove the Scots to show their independence with a senior official dismissively announcing: 'I don't think we need be committed to adopt all or anything that comes out of the working party'.[69] Striking a note of defiance, the booklet duly appeared in January 1965.[70]

Welsh Hospital Board files record that distribution of the English and Welsh equivalent took place in January 1967. A covering letter attached to the manual swept away years of prevarication indicating its preparation was due 'in answer to requests for more detailed advice than that contained in official memoranda'.[71] In Scotland, the document had gone into its second edition and although both versions said the same thing, they did so in different ways. Scotland's appeared in a shorter format but still included at least some of the picture-painting Richardson's vivid mental palette had produced. South of the border, the working party produced a longer document with scientific information added behind a nuclear explosion and a different title, *Civil Defence, Guidance Notes for Doctors Teaching Mass Casualty Care (Previously Extended First Aid)*. Notably, 'the Richardson factor' had been constrained in many areas. A noteworthy difference related to the public health consequences of irradiated casualties and their care, which the Scottish version kept as originally drafted by their irrepressible General, an extract indicating the kind of style Edinburgh embraced:

> Controllers and their medical advisers should be prepared at any time to organise improvised treatment centres, possibly under canvas, and must be aware of the hygienic problems involved. The frequent attacks of explosive and uncontrollable vomiting and diarrhoea which occur, especially in the acute severe early cases, would confront nursing staff most of whom will be unskilled, with a daunting task, which must be tackled somehow, for the patients in such centres when in the stage of bone marrow depression are very vulnerable to infection and it is at this stage that results from treatment may be expected. Disposable bags for vomit, plastic sheeting, disposable plastic liners for bedpans, urine bags (such as the portex type) colostomy bags, disposable paper blankets and sheets, and even the use of straw, heather, or

bracken for bedding might all have a place in the nursing of such cases; and if they should ever have to be nursed on stretchers under canvas, pits dug beside the stretchers and improvised scoops to cover vomited matter with earth might even have to be used. The situation would call for much improvisation, and it would be in such treatment centres that any available disinfectants might play a more useful role than if they were used as a screen of ineffective sanitation in areas of devastation, where the control of smell is of secondary importance to the control of flies, which the ritual scattering of strong smelling chemicals is unlikely to achieve.[72]

In London, Richardson provoked accusations he had gone too far. Not only did the cutting text depart from the medical order the Ministry of Health still preferred to project, the files showed the Ministry harboured a distaste for such macro disciplines, especially in the suggested use of disposables. Ministry procedure, the party line went, played down 'disposables'. Under no circumstances could they enter the realms of procedural advice in England and Wales. Any attempt to replicate such conditions in civil defence role play not only made the plight of radiation victims more evident than officially admitted, the cost of buying in equipment on the scale required stood to cripple the medical budget.[73] Whilst some differences in emphasis occurred, both documents for the first time introduced the cruel ideological imperative of national interest. If anything, the Ministry of Health underlined the point more aggressively by suggesting because some areas would be left undamaged, national regeneration would start from those centres and added: 'It is therefore worthwhile to plan for survival of the nation rather than to do nothing and thereby to achieve nothing'. Following the imperative of national survival, medical ethics changed beyond recognition with comparatively light injury being on the immediate list for treatment at the FMAU and/or carriage to hospital. The slogan 'keep them breathing' and 'stop the bleeding' defined the new mantra, but was to be administered against a new background which assumed a lack of qualified surgeons, a lack of drugs and other medical resources such as anaesthetics with the goal of saving the greatest numbers of lives. Serious injuries, once the passport to a hospital, were of necessity relegated to 'holding' and the likelihood of a lingering and painful death.[74]

An initial draft prepared by Richardson clearly spelled out the thinking behind the protocols in suggesting: 'Healthy young adults with the best chances of survival will naturally have a higher priority than the elderly and crippled who are poor risks, quite apart from considerations of national survival'.[75] However, the final advice turned out less explicit with the words changed to: 'In the interests of national survival, a high priority for hospital treatment must be given to cases in which useful lives can be saved and adequate function restored by relatively short surgical procedures, especially if they can be discharged from hospital very soon after treatment'.[76] Interestingly, the Ministry of Health's presentation of the medical judgement day provided more procedural depth and stressed sorting had to be instilled throughout the casualty chain starting at the ambulance loading points as there would not be enough ambulances to deal with all casualties. At the FMAU, the guideline demanded a 'ruthless' approach to sorting and added: 'It would often be necessary to give priority to the less severely injured casualties and have regard to the nation's need in the phase of regeneration'.[77] Ageism also subtly appeared with the advice on burns where the signal for abandonment came in the line that in serious cases 'age worsens the outlook' and that mortality in the over sixties could be ten times greater than in younger age groups.[78]

Psychiatric casualties that could be vast in number but with little chance of any kind of formal therapy being applied now came in for attention, having been a taboo subject in the realms of nuclear medicine for many years. The Ministry of Defence raised the problem after a NATO conference in 1957, under the dry heading of 'Psychological Problems in Nuclear War'. Looked at through the eyes of the Service situation, the issue had a critical implication as the front line of the British Army of the Rhine would be both the deliverers and receivers of tactical nuclear weapons. Nuclear 'fatigue' casualties were to be kept out of the regimental casualty chain to prevent contagion. Whereas such practices were possible to apply to a disciplined force, within a civilian population the report warned, the effects of nuclear war presented a daunting problem for civilian authorities especially through uncontrolled movement to the hospital areas with the consequent overloading of facilities and disruption to their work.[79]

The military analysis raised the sceptre of an impossible situation that could turn a medical problem into one of civilian control by force rather than sympathy. Nevertheless, in terms of medical practice both countries veered towards the sensitive approach, the Scottish narrative giving the following calming advice:

> In the management of these cases it is essential to adopt a confident attitude. One should never use any phrase which could be interpreted as meaning psychiatric illness. Such terms as neurosis,

nervous breakdown and mental shock should be avoided. If a description is required these terms should be replaced by 'fatigue and exhaustion' conveying the impression that it is nothing that a good rest or sleep will not put right. In dealing with relatives and friends, on whom much of the caring for these cases must fall, reference to temporary reactions to stress or to fear, with the emphasis on the temporary, might be appropriate. Such optimism would sometimes be stultified by events, but would do less harm than a pessimistic, or even unduly guarded, attitude.[80]

Richardson also stretched the issue into other areas. As an army man, he noted that the diagnosis of 'shell shock' during the First World War had been replaced in the Second World War by the term 'Combat or Battle Exhaustion'. He related this to the nuclear aftermath when people affected could become stunned, disorganised and obstructive unless firmly controlled and argued the loss of balanced judgement in such conditions needed recognition where disorientation and possible flight could be dangerous in conditions of fallout. Though admission to hospital might be confined to those cases that were psychotic and dangerous to the community, the creation of large centres should, he argued, be avoided. Instead, Richardson suggested that survival regimes be developed at different levels and so called 'rest rooms' established at FMAUs, auxiliary hospitals and at control centres where even trained individuals might be subjected to psychosomatic disorders caused by the awful scenes that they had witnessed and the heavy burden of their responsibilities.[81]

As a result of the recoding of medical ethics the term 'national health' finally took on a new and sinister meaning, but this position only emerged as the medical facade was in the last stages of delivering political comfort and its real impact never fully tested. However, some of new realities did percolate through and graphically appeared in one of the last regional studies, incongruously named STUDY SURVIVAL carried out on 19 October 1967 at the Northumberland County Council Civil Defence Centre. This depicted a very different post-nuclear attack scene to the ordered casualty regime conducted in EXERCISE RELIANCE some ten years earlier. The position turned into a struggle to make do with what had survived altogether producing a picture of hideous misery. Patients suffering radiation sickness would require antibiotics, whole blood, special food and intensive nursing, all resources likely to be unavailable. As for the promise of individualistic care, it was recognised casualties in holding areas requiring major surgery were equally unlikely to have much hope of admission. To prevent overcrowding and epidemics the study stressed the need for ruthless sorting, combined with an equally cold blooded discharge policy when faced by many who would not wish to leave the relatively sheltered conditions of the hospital. Water, the narrative stressed, would remain a critical concern with strict rationing, conservation and collection being vital. Hospitals were natural water guzzlers necessitating radical changes, including regulating the flushing of water closets along with baths and showers by patients totally banned. Other unsavoury practices might include the washing and rinsing of surgical instruments in basins and not under taps. New priorities would even demand water being given over to the functional sections of the hospital such as sterilisation and operating theatres and for that reason the use of bedpan washers prohibited. Equally important in the battle to cling on to vestiges of humanity by the fingertips, conserving precious heating fuel for generating steam to sterilise instruments might be considered necessary and very literally become a chilling prospect if imposed in the harsh winter months.[82]

The imagery of Hieronymus Bosch proportions appeared to have no end. Although the second stage role of the hospital system might be possible at some point to resume reconstructive surgery for selected survivors, the study warned conditions under which such work could be undertaken held equally bleak prospects. A lack of traditional anaesthetic materials would impose a serious constraint on the extent to which surgery was possible. It meant the indefinite use of surgical instruments with disposable scalpel blades and needles utilised for as long as possible. Dressings utilising, sheets, handkerchiefs or other available material were likely to be recycled by being washed over and over again, or made by using the clothing of the dead.[83]

The floodgates might have opened to the conceptualisation of the gruesome through the issue of the two training manuals, but both countries were clearly worried about the guidelines putting off people becoming involved in mass casualty care because of the brutality factor. To overcome that, both versions came with a comforter offering the idealistic possibility those assigned to the dreaded holding unit within the FMAU might eventually receive life-saving treatment. The form of nuclear hope in the Scottish version expressed the point through the following sentiment:

> It will be important for the morale of these patients, and also of their relatives and friends, and indeed also of the nursing staff, that it should be clearly implied that they too will receive hospital treatment

> as soon as possible ie when road transport is easier and pressure on hospitals is less severe. The rather prevalent tendency to refer to such cases as relegated to the holding department of the FMAU as 'moribund' etc is to be deplored. They are sometimes called the 'expectant' category, and must be dealt with as though expected to live, for it is no part of the function of members of the casualty service to extinguish hopes of survival.[84]

So despite the formalisation of mass abandonment the addendum brought back mass compassion in an anticipatory form as the final cosmetic application to the face of the caring state. The very need to do this exposes the tension that stubbornly persisted about dealing with the seriously injured and could be used to political advantage. Compassion remained the essential *zeitgeist* honed through two world wars. How deeply that commitment ran in terms of the Cold War is impossible to say, but it existed out there to the extent that it allowed the Ministry of Health to achieve its political remit and complete an operationally logical hospital plan defined by its own realities.

Chapter 6

BODY LANGUAGE

Taking a quick backward glance at the facade, its psychological thread was very much about ensuring that escape routes from the environment of impossibility were kept open. Nevertheless, with millions and millions of casualties in prospect during the hydrogen bomb age, a great deal of perceptual manoeuvring was necessary if the belief system could continue working for the secret state. Obviously, the greatest danger lay in the facade falling into institutional irrelevance by the sheer weight of numbers that medically defied all human comprehension. Censorship of various kinds therefore became essential to ensure the dilution of the real catastrophe. Delivery of that kind of emotional management necessarily required mechanisms where body language and information combined through a relationship that not only subdued the overwhelming nature of the nuclear conditions, but also brought back human dignity as part of the equation. This tantalising challenge, which faced Whitehall with growing intensity merits a closer look, albeit briefly, to gain an understanding as at to how that process developed. Providentially for history, the kinds of control factors applied both through omission and commission do become very apparent and add an idiosyncratic and very British flavour to the mythology constructed.

Pain Killers

Since the very early days of 'the nuclear health service' radiation injury had always been a medical curse. Offering intensive attention to radiation sickness, particularly by giving blood transfusions, held disastrous resource implications. Early symptoms of lethal exposure shared those of shock and non-lethal doses of radiation. Embarking on treatment could be immensely counterproductive. Without the means of individual radiation measurement a range of probabilities existed about the intensity of radiation a person may have suffered, the extent of attention necessary and in the worst case, whether it was likely to be successful. A working party on morale, as early as 1950 made attempts to find a solution to the problem and suggested that members of the public should be issued with dosimeters (small pen-type instruments) so they could tell whether they had received a light or lethal dose of radiation. In response, Wing Commander Sir John Hodsoll, Director

General of civil defence training, poured scorn on the idea adding in a state of considerable agitation: 'I think the whole idea is attributing a degree of intelligence and understanding of this problem to the general public which I do not think it possess at all, or is ever likely to possess'.[1] Instead, Hodsoll insisted the subject had to be managed by the civil defence services. This, of course, was fine by the Government who could control public awareness more easily and prevent the mechanics of mass compassion being spoilt by the radiation problem.

Whitehall did attempt to keep the issue low-key. With a public largely ignorant about the delicate sensitivities governing radiation and health, highly-generalised solutions to radiation control made out the procedures to be simple and effective. A decision to adopt 75 roentgens as the safe accumulated Wartime Emergency Dose represented only a small contribution in an enormously complex propaganda history. As the figures published by the Home Office in *Nuclear Weapons* show in Table 3, the wide bands indicating the relative effects of radiation levels for civil defence purposes (compared to the 0.4 roentgens permitted for atomic power workers) were ambiguous in the extreme.[2] Applying such basic assumptions could not predict physiological outcomes for individuals determined by age, gender, physical health or injury, nor adequately cover the whole, complex question of possible long-term effects.

Table 3: Possible Effects on People of a Single Exposure to Gamma Radiation.

Single dose / roentgens	Mortality in six weeks
0-25	0
25-75	0
75-100	Less than 0.1%
100-150	Less than 0.5%
150-200	Up to 5%
200-400	About a third
400-600	About a half
Over 800	Almost all

Source: Pamphlet No. 1, *Nuclear Weapons*, HMSO, 1956.

Despite the optimism applied to radiation injury levels, the undoubted medical disaster the hydrogen bomb now symbolised still had to be subdued. In this respect, the solution originally alluded to by Strath as good nursing by family and friends appeared to be the most satisfactory route to take. Keeping 'victims' under observation at home offered an efficient, not to mention, cheap way of bolstering the view of medical order by separating 'the problem' from the finite resource of the hospital bed. Initially, the idyllic vision of the nuclear carer fell victim to the 1956 squeeze on civil defence expenditure. Nonetheless, with the post Bishop financial settlement agreed to prevent the facade collapsing, home nursing surfaced as one of the most cost effective ways of delivering the message of nuclear survivability. With the sum of £5,000 allocated for the year 1960/61 to introduce the project, it seemed destined to become the most ambitious indoctrination exercises since the last war.[3] Yet, for all its innocent simplicity, the scheme still jangled political nerves to an unusual degree reflecting the inherent nervousness of Whitehall that accompanied any proposal that involved direct contact with the public. In this case, such anxiety especially stemmed from concerns that the exercise could become a harbinger of disaster capable of generating a counter climate of fear and in turn lead to demands for more civil defence spending. Alternatively, too much fear might cause the 'boomerang effect' and stop people listening to civil defence advice entirely. The prospect of millions ending up in utter degradation through lack of medical facilities also held perceptual dangers.

Creating comfort zones where the ideal patient could receive care in idealised surroundings seemed to provide the right answer. Originally, the title of the home nursing scheme was to be the 'Emergency Home Nursing Service' indicating it would be run by local health authorities along with their home help visitors and home nurses, plus reinforcements using general practitioners. The Ministry of Health, in the final event, believed the term 'service' needed playing down and the nuclear family preferred as the method of delivering compassion because the notion of regular visits by doctors possibly stretched credibility too far. The Scots, at first, expressed their anxieties about embarking on such a venture at all and considered it would prove unpopular with the public, but did agree that its introduction across the border would require them to follow. Backed by the empowerment principle termed 'self-help' the Ministry of Health, therefore, pronounced its social benefits to save the family as a unit and also its potential lifeline for the normal sick and the injured who in peace would have been hospitalised.[4]

Completely idealistic, the doubtful credentials of the project were apparent with the training syllabus that contained just two sections and the thinnest of time schedules to match. The first covered aspects of dealing with shock, haemorrhage, asphyxia and burns, including those received through radiation with four hours tuition time assigned to these subjects. Home nursing techniques formed the basis of the second section focussing on the bedridden patient and his or her comfort, as well as diet and hygiene; all subjects to be learnt in five hours overall. The entire course had to be undertaken in no more than five sessions with much of the advice consisting of the most basic practice thus presenting many opportunities to hide the real horrors of the medical after effects of a nuclear attack. Particularly diluted for public consumption were the terrible consequences of radiation sickness, the symptoms compared to those patients might suffer when treated by radium or deep X-ray. These included extreme lassitude, vomiting, and diarrhoea with rapid loss of weight, a sore mouth and symptoms of anaemia. Only references to the need for special nursing care to prevent bedsores, care of the mouth and to tempt appetite gave any hint of the exceptionally difficult conditions that would involve palliative care, but might still result in a lingering and unimaginably painful death.[5]

As planning progressed, attacks of serious self-doubt surfaced especially the inherently awkward prospect of dealing directly with the general public, and the possibility of handing further ammunition to the anti-nuclear lobby. The Ministry of Health only narrowly overcame their deep-rooted anxiety by persuading themselves no point existed in attempting a maximum effort from the outset and members of the public would only come forward in large numbers during a period when the international situation worsened. Instead, the view prevailed only one bite at the cherry was likely and so the best strategy would be to incubate interest in readiness for the right moment, at which time members of the public would flock freely to participate. To kick-start the process, local authority staff were chosen to become guinea pigs, but faced by opposition generated through the representative bodies of the councils the exercise eventually ended up by being using more 'sympathetic' sectors of the community such as the Senior Scouts and Girl Guides.[6]

Other organisations found it useful simply to boost their public profile. Looked at another way, 'home nursing' actually became a medium through which groups could use it to secure some domain advantage. The St Andrew's Ambulance Association were unhappy a fuller course under the direction of the voluntary societies had not been sealed. Even so they excused their dismay with the comforting view the scheme was 'aimed at creating greater interest with the hope that it will encourage the pupils to pursue the matter further'.[7] Similarly, the Association of County Councils in Scotland saw every advantage to slot home nursing into schools as part of an existing instruction in health education, although they did warn their Medical Officers of Health were highly critical of the content in trying to convey too much without actually producing little, if nothing, in the physiology behind the actions being applied. Fearful of being the odd-man-out, Scotland constructed its own syllabus to meet the time constraints, but in so doing quite extraordinarily left out the most crucial bit of the exercise relating to the palliative after-care of radiation sickness. Instead, the omission was glossed over with the excuse that because of the time factor 'persons who are anxious to acquire a more detailed knowledge can, of course, approach the Scottish Branch of the British Red Cross Society and the St Andrew's Ambulance Association'.[8]

Home nursing had already furthered the cause of the government funded Women's Voluntary Service. (Later the Women's Royal Voluntary Service) The topic of the nuclear sick was included in a programme of talks called *One-in-Five* whose wartime founder Lady Reading decreed should be delivered to a fifth of the women in Britain. What the public saw, therefore, involved mainly women being sympathetic to the idea of becoming nuclear carers. In the area of dulling the pain of nuclear war the WVS remedies often reached epic proportions. A 'women and home' page editor in the *Reynolds News* reported on a *One-in-Five* talk she had attended where the well-intentioned WVS lady concluded the proceedings commenting that nuclear war was nothing to worry about and reassuringly added: 'You see it's not going to be as bad as all that. There'll be simply lots of people to look after you'.[9] But a tendency by the WVS to make light of nuclear suffering did at times cause consternation even in their own backyard, the most notorious example being the production of a poster for local offices. Displaying a bright yellow door, a sign on it read 'Gone to WVS One-in-Five talks. Back with some idea to cope if nuclear war ever comes!' Many local organisers found such flippancy difficult to accept and, following an outcry nationally a sticky label was quickly produced and dispatched to cover over the offending words, which then changed the message entirely to 'Please come in WVS needs your help!'[10]

Occasionally the campaign did attract adverse attention that dangerously lifted the lid on the hidden political truths organisations such as the WVS were unwittingly fronting. Probably the most hurtful, given the highly gender orientated base of the message, came in the *Nursing Times* during 1958 in an exchange of correspondence between a senior official of the WVS and a female nurse who expressed apprehensions that she and many of her colleagues had about the *One-in-Five* scheme. Her words adroitly expressed the view the organisation was simply riding rough shod over the warnings given by two respected scientific activists about the medical consequences of nuclear war:

> May I explain to Marguerite M. Hammond why so many of us distrust and even feel disapproval of the Government-sponsored One-in-Five Scheme. We feel it is not purely a practical and Samaritan

> scheme but something of a propaganda stunt to get nuclear warfare, or at any rate the idea of it, accepted as part of our background. Moreover, since the scheme is sponsored and indeed was formed by a government which did everything they could to silence men like the late Joliot-Curie and the – happily still with us – Linus Pauling when they would warn us of the probable consequences of nuclear warfare, we look upon the One-in-Five Scheme as an attempt to play down intelligent, reasonable misgivings so that the politicians, unhindered by feminine opposition, can go ahead with their plans for dreary disaster.[11]

Behind the cosy imagery of prepared sick rooms more realistic truths were, however, being secretly considered that did indeed recognise the nature of the 'dreary disaster' as 'home nursing' became stretched into wider and wider operational applications. The concept provided a seemingly logical reference point for those grappling with the mass casualty problem and it expanded into all kinds of alternatives. Examples included the possibility of a sick bay for radiation casualties being organised under the management of a public health nurse and regular visits made by a doctor assigned from a medical pool of practitioners. Extending the ideology still further, local authorities began to consider the identification of a large number of sites for indefinite 'welfare/medical' purposes for holding the sick, casualties of all descriptions, isolation wards and even for accommodating mental patients. Ideologically home nursing, therefore, became far more wide-ranging than its somewhat timid introduction by the Ministry of Health might have suggested. As a principle it especially broke the peacetime imperative of the hospital providing the only treatment space and by the time of its introduction in 1962, had become an operational model capable of indefinite extension to hide the deficiencies in the traditional forms of care.[12]

Although home nursing strove to contain a great deal of wretchedness within its propagandised walls a need to sweep up still more remained, but raised another bout of political nervousness. This related to government giving general first aid advice to the wider public. Hitherto, teaching 'nuclear' first aid had been contained within safe institutional boundaries, especially the police which bolstered their 'Dixon' image and projected a benign support for the public in need as opposed to quelling the social violence likely to erupt in the wake of a nuclear war. However, allowing nuclear healthcare suddenly to enter the public arena unabridged and create psychological damage did not escape ministerial attention in 1962 when the kind of guidance possible to provide householders came under discussion. Nothing could have illustrated more the political fear still haunting Whitehall at the highest level. Yet again, the idea of publishing a compendium of advice directly to the public seemed a step too far. So when a pamphlet eventually appeared it was addressed to the civil defence services about the appropriate survival information they might have to give the public during the period of an alert. In the end the problem of whether it should also be made more widely available came down to a judgement made not against the document's public safety credentials, but on the grounds that 'It was standard practice for Civil Defence training pamphlets to be available on sale to the general public. Any departure from this practice might give rise to suspicion or alarm'.[13]

Attempts to quell 'alarm' by offering the booklet on sale, of course, meant the potential for 'alarm' then had to be controlled. As a training pamphlet, the Ministry of Health considered a section on first aid should be included, along with the other advice about building a refuge room as protection against fallout, and laying down stocks of food. But of all the pointers about the potential horrors of a nuclear conflagration the medical side probably held the most. The Ministry of Health had attempted to marginalise the medical affects by giving comforting messages of the type of injuries that might be sustained at the periphery of an explosion which suggested: 'Within a wide area round a nuclear explosion everyone out of doors or near unprotected windows may suffer some degree of burning to the exposed skin. Generally, the effects will be fairly superficial as in sunburn'.[14] Instead of producing the comfort intended, the assurance itself suddenly assumed the proportions of a 'somewhat alarming character'. Quite astonishingly, it led minsters responsible for civil defence preparations to indulge in one of the most incredible acts of censorship ever to befall a public document during this era of the Cold War. Gripped by a complete sense of insecurity it was not felt 'appropriate' to include the whole section that had been proposed on first aid, the offending text cited in Appendix 4.

Edited by such ultra-political caution, the pamphlet confined medical advice to the suggested contents of a first aid kit for keeping in the home, just in case the hydrogen bomb dropped. Included were the following items that appeared in the *Civil Defence Handbook No. 10 Advising the Householder on Protection against Nuclear Attack* which the Home Office prepared on the whole topic of refuge rooms and could be purchased at Her Majesty's Stationery Office for the princely sum of nine pence:

> Aspirin or codeine tablets
> Adhesive plaster

> Bandages, two-inch
> Clean cloths
> Dressings
> Safety pins and scissors
> Skin cream
>
> Cotton Wool
> Salt, household, one half pound
> Soda, bicarbonate (Baking Powder), four ounce packet
> Bowls, various sizes, three
> Hot water bottles and covers
> Teaspoons
> Vaseline
>
> Talcum powder
> Paper handkerchiefs
> Methylated or surgical spirit
>
> Clean cotton rags in plastic bags
> Disinfectant
> Packet of strong sewing needles
> Reel of white cotton.[15]

The degree of political obfuscation behind this so-called medical 'advice' may be gauged by the subsequent reactions by the NHS and their complete bewilderment about what it all meant in practice. For the purpose of instructing National Hospital Service Reserve nurses, hospitals had been asked to buy in copies of the pamphlet. Quite reasonably they complained that as a standalone statement of medical procurement it made no sense whatsoever and requested further details.[16] The response served up by the Ministry of Health, if nothing else, reveals the way the information had been carefully orchestrated directly by ministers as a political diversion:

> We realise that this is not entirely satisfactory both regarding the items noted and also the dividing of the items into various groups with no self-evident relation to each other. It has been suggested that we elaborate the appendix in any reprint but we do not propose to do this since in our view the only satisfactory way of explaining the uses of the various items in the first aid kit would be to publish in full the chapter on first aid and this we cannot do

as a matter of policy. We hope however that during a precautionary stage arrangements could be made to publish it in full.[17]

This statement confirming the relative uselessness of the medical advice certainly anchored the proposition as another element of the medical illusion. When a Parliamentary Committee on Estimates chose to look at the handbook it came to the more public conclusion the guide should be withdrawn immediately on the grounds of being useless and misleading. As luck would have it the censure of the document then became submerged under a general review of the Home Office, including immigration records, or rather the lack of them.[18] In its defence, the Government reiterated the original intent behind the pamphlet was only to provide loose guidelines for training purposes and promised all the details would be filled in during the course of time.[19] During 1964 some discussion did take place about enlarging the first aid advice during the threat of war whereby an extended version of the *Advising the Householder on Protection against Nuclear Attack* might be delivered through broadcasts and also published in the newspapers, but as usual nothing happened.[20]

Certainly, what the progress of the home nursing and first aid programmes does reveal is a very definable historical characteristic about the depth of fear that persisted within government when thoughts turned to disseminating nuclear information outside the civil defence organisations. Firstly, came a deep anxiety of approaching the public directly and secondly alarm about the entry level at which any kind of information should be provided, if that really became necessary. As the 'sunburn' factor in the medical advice illustrated, even the dilution of information in one direction could leave much to the imagination about the injuries likely to occur at the opposite end of the scale. In the event, the action by ministers is a most remarkable example of censorship, on a David and Goliath scale, but does show just how even the most minimal information was regarded as a threat to the deterrent.

Narrow Escapes

Home nursing in its various guises provided an incredibly pliable propaganda vehicle. For all that, although it produced an organisational sponge that could soak up a massive amount of the medical burden, the unforgiving developments in mass destruction progressively began to threaten the hospital system in its entirety. The hospital building and the hospital bed had become iconic symbols to provide security for the less fortunate members of society by transferring them from the target areas.

Whilst the hospital plan had always stuck with that moralistic perfection, the statement came under increasing pressure in view of the destruction creep covering the country. The first challenge to that classic iconography emerged in a most unexpected way. Evacuation of the priority classes had its origins in the Second World War with the transfer of children, expectant and nursing mothers and still very much resonated in the Cold War era as the face of a caring state. Reflecting that sentiment, the scheme had been enlarged during the atomic age with the wartime total of 1.5 million evacuees increasing to some 4.5 million. Thereafter the political link between greater destruction and greater evacuation showed no signs of weakening. In the 1956 Defence White Paper the Government announced it had approved a revised scheme in the light of new attack appreciations. No less than twelve million people in the priority classes were due for evacuation, and the moral message amplified still further by including the aged, the blind and crippled from 16 evacuation areas in England, Wales and Scotland.[21]

Discomfortingly for Whitehall, however, the ethical signal on the scale suggested was becoming logistically problematic. Deterrent bomber bases had occupied much of the eastern part of England, hitherto regarded as suitable reception country, which made the region a potential target and effectively put paid to the idea of decanting twelve million souls. Caught between the opposing forces of practicality and political convention, an alternative plan materialised involving a reduced movement of some six million of the priority classes, but limited to the larger conurbations. These included London, Birmingham, Manchester, Merseyside, Tyneside, Leeds, Bradford, Sheffield, Teesside and Hull. On further consideration, however, the list of arguments against this proposal began to mount. Quite apart from the problem of any scheme risking damage to the economy and the poor reception capacity in the South West, the difficulty of using the limited radial rail network routes placed a limit on the numbers possible to evacuate within seven days. In addition, the exclusion of cities such as Bristol and Plymouth, which had been bombed during the last war, looked politically unacceptable. For all these reasons, ministers persuaded themselves against advocating plans possessing no political value. Challenged by seemingly insuperable difficulties, a divergence of opinion began to grow inside the Cabinet as to whether an evacuation scheme could ever be politically advantageous and the matter left for further consideration. As a result, a 'stay put' policy came into force, and if an emergency were to occur the Government decided it would 'urge all members of the public, without exception, to 'stay put' and take such measures as were possible to deal with 'unorganised and unauthorised evacuation'.[22]

Delaying a decision on the issue then created another problem because the 'stay put' position actually conflicted with the need of the Government to implement its own survival measures. Included amongst these were the redeployment of key staffs to their nuclear bunkers across the country. Concern also grew that no evacuation would nullify the essential principles of the hospital plan to preserve skilled manpower and moveable equipment. For the first time, the ongoing debate shook out the conservation of medical resources as requiring a possible priority over the preservation of human life. Although the situation may have raised a string of ethical conundrums through sheer practicality, the real question came down to just how much practicality the public should see. First thoughts suggested that whilst all patients for whom hospital treatment was not essential were to be discharged, a quarter of those who were in no fit condition might have to remain in general hospitals. For special hospitals, the scope for evacuation would be less and in the case of institutions for the mentally deficient, the opportunity was likely to be non-existent. As a list of practicalities, however, the discourse went no further except to suggest that the pattern of prioritisation could somehow provide the means of using the medically vulnerable as a propagandist human shield. Controversially it meant the clearance of hospitals, whilst leaving enough patients behind to camouflage the evacuation of resources and in that way preserve the spirit of 'stay put'. The Health Departments were, however, mindful such a change would require hospital authorities to be informed well in advance to avoid confusion and equally nervously aware Ministerial approval was necessary for such 'disclosure'.[23]

Discussed at the beginning of the Berlin Crisis, the human shield idea never did cross over into the darker areas of policy making. Having said that, the concept of using the unfortunates of society in a scheme that created a form of megaton martyrdom had made its appearance, which disconcertingly raised the possibility that any prioritisation plan could be construed as a covert arrangement to avoid panic. Thereafter, the Ministry of Health certainly took every opportunity to prevent that assumption ever happening and fought hard to maintain the integrity of mass compassion as an absolute ideological commitment that might fall to unavoidable circumstances, but not through policy. The defence of that medical corner began as Berlin and the Bishop Committee nudged the 'stay put' policy from its slumber and brought the issue of patient prioritisation to the surface. The evacuation of the priority classes might have become quite impractical on the one hand, on the other, feelings hardened in Whitehall that without such a scheme the British public would regard it as a signal that nothing was being done to reduce casualties. But the change of heart still came with fears about introducing evacuation which might start a chain reaction and end up with a demand for public shelter building.[24]

Whilst the public disclosure of an evacuation policy generated more nervousness about the consequences, the final jolt came two years later when Cuba eventually added the catalyst for action. The Home Secretary, the Secretary of State for Scotland and the Minister of Local Housing made a joint plea to the Cabinet: 'As a Government we cannot take the easy course of remaining silent indefinitely,' a move which at last brought the scheme to life.[25]

Eventually the strategy adopted involved 9.5 million people, to use the new terminology, being 'dispersed' from 19 centres of population in England and Wales. Hiding spaces against the ravages of nuclear war in Great Britain were becoming ever more limited and except for Sussex and parts of Kent, areas in England to the east of a line drawn from Middlesbrough to Southampton no longer provided sanctuary for reception purposes. In Scotland, the transfer involved people being moved out from the central areas to the northern and southern areas of the country. However, even though the practicality of this scheme looked highly questionable because of the shrinking warning time and the likely panic movement of unofficial evacuation, the production of billeting notices, bus and railway timetables all provided a comparatively cheap reassurance to councils some preparations were in hand. That said, the plan introduced a major change regarding the priority issue. In the new scheme the future generation were again the main benefactors with those under eighteen and expectant mothers included, but the blind, crippled, aged and infirm were struck out of the equation, unless they were dependant on the care of someone taking part in the dispersal as a chaperone.[26]

With the problem changing to instigating a new dispersal policy, focus on the issue of evacuating special hospital patients began to attract attention. Many hospital Regional Hospital Boards, unable to find answers to the evacuation of their special hospitals and chronic sick, pounced on the new priority list for dispersal to deal with their difficulty and pressed the Ministry of Health to apply similar exclusions to the hospital evacuation scheme. Regional Hospital Board Secretaries faced the Department's usual contortions in July 1962, which put the onus on whether and how abandonment ought to take place squarely at their feet. Hospital Boards received advice that the evacuation of all hospitals, including mental and psychiatric establishments, must stand in absolute terms:

> After considering the matter we have come to the conclusion that the principle underlying the hospital evacuation plan should not be changed. We think therefore that the aim should be to continue to

> evacuate all types of hospitals in the Hospital Evacuation Areas except those required for home cover and that the Board's plans and their requirements for premises and transport should be based on that intention.[27]

Then again, the statement went on to say it would be 'unrealistic' for hospitals not to give priority to the needs of acute hospitals that would be at the front line of casualty treatment. It was, therefore, 'realistic' to assume if evacuation could not be completed in time the chronic sick, psychiatric long-stay and mentally subnormal patients would, in the circumstances, place them below acute hospitals.[28]

This contortion between the 'realistic' and 'unrealistic' represented a minor, if roundabout, shift in policy, particularly for the 'special' case category that had festered as an issue since 1956.[29] Inconclusive debates had raged about what should be done in the face of the resolve of government not to have any trace of desertion of the sick and weak on its hands. Scotland attempted to come to terms with the problem on the basis it would be better to send home as many tuberculosis patients as possible and simply risk the incidence of the disease increasing rather than try to raise beds that might be critical to national survival. Pragmatic as ever, the Scots once more hounded the Ministry of Health in London for more guidance on the issue of hospital evacuation, including the scale of equipment to be considered for transfer as well as staff/patient ratios. For all the pestering, even by May 1963, London remained obstinately quiet and refused to give any formal guidance.[30]

Finally, on the 23 October 1964, as a direct result of the intense pressure exerted, the Ministry of Health acquiesced to making some kind of move to define how all hospitals should approach the clearance problem. Described only as a 'guideline', the proposals indicated that as many patients as possible were still to be discharged not only in target areas but throughout the country, with appropriate discharge percentages suggested if decisions linked to social expendability had to be made quickly:

Acute Hospitals – 75%
Geriatric and Chronic Sick – Nil
Maternity – 85% (of patients after delivery)
Infectious diseases – Nil
Mental Hospitals – 20% (perhaps higher in peripheral areas)
Mental Deficiency Hospitals – Nil
Children – 75% (as many as possible of the remaining 25%

should be evacuated from hospitals in target areas, because it should be a primary aim to ensure the survival of the children).[31]

For all that, the Ministry of Health still resisted making any kind of absolute policy announcement, even refusing to come clean about the abandonment issue within Whitehall itself. A statement concerning the status of the hospital plans to the Home Defence Review Committee on 27 November 1964 by the Ministry conspicuously failed to report the existence of the advice it had given just a month earlier to Regional Hospital Boards. Instead, the Department confined their comments to the problems that might occur in the transfer of patients through traffic congestion, and indicated some Boards felt at least fourteen days would be required to undertake an evacuation plan, let alone five. The Review Committee were, therefore, informed: 'Whether or not to move chronic sick and psychiatric patients from hospitals in likely target areas was a difficult question which, had not yet been resolved'. The Ministry thus left the matter on the basis they were reviewing the arrangements for providing medical services in the post attack period and promised a further paper on the subject in due course.[32]

As usual, the situation drifted without any progress, but during 1966 it appeared the Ministry of Health had at last run out of excuses to keep the pretence of saving everyone continuing any longer. Home defence plans were now to be capable of completion within two to three days to take account of the shrinking attack times as missiles fired from submarines replaced traditional forms of delivering mass destruction. Regional Boards were, therefore asked to undertake a review of what they considered they could do in the way of evacuation under such conditions. The results showed the obvious that hospitals could only hope to achieve five steps:

To restrict admissions.
To discharge home as many patients as possible.
To move from other hospitals in hospital evacuation areas as much staff and equipment as could be spared, again leaving behind the patients with skeleton cover.
To move from acute hospitals in hospital evacuation areas as much of the staff and equipment.
To provide extra beds outside the target areas by overcrowding existing hospitals (with beds, not patients) and setting up beds in requisitioned premises.[33]

The writing had now shown up on every hospital wall that apart from discharging patients, saving staff and some equipment not much else was possible. Yet even then, the Ministry of Health still refused to acknowledge defeat by agreeing to any kind of blanket abandonment policy, but did disclose their innermost thoughts about the reasons behind their intransigence:

> It is not proposed to suggest that the possibility of evacuating residual patients should be completely abandoned, as such a decision taken in peace-time might prove unacceptable. But all the emphasis would be placed on the need to phase evacuation, and Boards would be told to restrict their present planning to (a) the measures set out (above) which would help to provide the additional staff and equipment needed for the wartime hospital service and (b) the evacuation of any children and expectant and nursing mothers remaining in hospital (because they would have qualified for evacuation under the official dispersal scheme if they had been sent home).
>
> If in the event there proved to be time to proceed to a more general evacuation of patients, this would be improvised in the light of circumstances at the time without having been planned in advance.[34]

Quite plainly, the 'moral signal' still held considerable value in the minds of the Ministry and there was no intention to move it officially from the realms of the possible into the impossible. The unease about not antagonising public susceptibility illustrates the predisposition towards the 'hidden truth', subscribed to as a means of ensuring the integrity of mass compassion. But the 'hidden truth' was becoming ever more difficult to manage with the prospect all patients would become megaton martyrs, not just those left in target areas. For hospitals, the Government scheme offering a possible escape route to avoid high levels of radiation devised under the title of *Radioactive Fall-out, Provisional Scheme of Public Control* provided some reassurance of escape, at least in theory. First published in 1956 at the time of Suez, the manual setting out the procedures had been initially restricted for use by civil defence officials only. It represented the lifesaving bible that laid down survival regimes for people in undamaged areas who might find themselves caught in fallout plumes of different intensity. These were designated W, X, Y and Z zones, the last being the most dangerous which would be cleared as the radioactivity contracted to a safe level. Within less contaminated zones people were to be advised how long they could exit any refuges they might have prepared over the period of radioactive decay. In that way the scheme provided an important, albeit dubious representation of both escape and limiting the disruption to everyday life.[35]

Typically, the arrangements were not made publicly available until 1958, conveniently coinciding with the ending of a major series of British nuclear tests, followed by the ratification of the test ban treaty.[36] By then it could be said to have quite literally passed its sell-by date. Contemporary records released to The National Archives show how the fundamental flaws of the scheme received a purposeful layer of glossing over to keep it in the public arena as a tactical utopia. Background documents admit to serious failings making it inherently unsafe. Many assumptions were simply no longer true, including the presentation of a post raid environment with neatly-formed radioactive plumes of the right intensity and size coupled with sufficient buffer areas into which flight from contamination would be possible. Further optimism included nuclear hits taken within a narrow time frame to avoid the complication of evacuees running into fallout caused by subsequent strikes.[37]

Looking at the raid evaluations made inside the secret sanctuaries of defence planning, the escape protocols should have been withdrawn by 1958. A 'Top-Secret' appreciation of that year, the *Form and Duration of a Major War,* coldly forecast that a Soviet attack could be aimed at up to 40-50 nuclear bomber bases and missile sites as prime counterforce targets, followed by secondary countervalue strikes on key industrial and population centres.[38] Home Office records provide additional detail drawn out of minutes recording a meeting at the Air Ministry on 12 February 1958 which further advised that the attack predicated on military objectives be interpreted as a strike by medium jet bomber forces to ensure one nuclear weapon hit each site. On civilian and industrial centres, with an allowance taken into account for the Circular Error of Probability, (aiming error) the assessment suggested three ten-megaton hydrogen bombs would be detonated as ground bursts to ensure complete obliteration of the chosen targets. Counting the grizzly mathematics of radioactive fallout likely to result, scientific advisers concluded such a target strategy would mean the eastern half of England being shrouded in a deadly blanket of radiation. Unless able to construct home refuges in time to the recommended Protective Factor, the outcome would be fatal to some twenty-two million people.[39]

Notwithstanding this growing environment of utter impossibility acknowledged by the secret state, the hospital structure continued to rely on the optimism prescribed by the public control scheme. A report of a study at Taymouth Castle, the Scottish Civil Defence School, held in October 1957 usefully illustrates the kind of procedures that were being promoted should a hospital find itself in a lethal radioactive Z Belt. The sequence of suggested arrangements included the issue of warm clothing and blankets to patients with everyone then transferred to the ground floor and crammed into the centre of the building as far as possible. In theory, this would provide the maximum radiation shield where they could remain until evacuated. Guidance on protection included sealing off the wards against radioactive dust with wet sheets and hospital staff relocated to places where they could work that meant restrictions on internal traffic with emergency arrangements made for services and sanitation. Precious water needed decanting into containers with food, drugs and dressings also protected. Rather highlighting the difficulties of the situation, roofs would require hosing down where the structure afforded little defence against the penetrating deadliness of radiation. All this activity ultimately anticipated the arrival of transport once radiation levels had reduced to safe levels in a decay period that might last 48 hours or more. If there was a reality side to the package, it came with the final advice that emergency mortuary arrangements should also be prepared. Predictably, the pessimistic side was duly balanced by the last and ever optimistic submission that patients once extracted from of the lethal Z zone would eventually find a Forward Medical Aid Unit at some point along their exit route where they could stay until final arrangements were possible to make.[40]

Any comfort these theoretical exercises may have given hospital authorities eventually eroded when they started to discover some discomforting truths. A review undertaken by the Western Regional Hospital Board in Scotland during 1960 with the intention of evaluating the performance of their buildings against radiation showed just how difficult in practice finding refuge really was. The Royal Infirmary in Dumfries constructed of stone provided a reasonable Protective Factor, but their temporary wooden wards and certain surgical wards offered no defence whatsoever. Cresswell Maternity Hospital, built in 1959, with a frontage largely made up of windows could not be considered in any way suitable. Finally, the Lochmaben Hospital consisted of wooden huts introduced during the First World War which had protection described as 'derisory'. The conclusion was that none of these hospitals, even with the enclosure of windows by 9-inch brickwork, offered any kind of realistic resistance against radiation. Effectively the exercise proved the mix of buildings, which made up the typical hospital in the National Health Service, could not provide any kind of nuclear retreat as portrayed in the past.[41]

At a meeting with Regional Hospital Boards in May 1962 the Ministry of Health conceded that the whole issue of managing radioactivity had been 'underestimated', a rare admission made with uncustomary clarity:

> The Department recognised that the problem of clearing hospitals in Z-Zones had not been fully explored and that problems set at exercises and studies under-estimated the difficulties. It had also to be recognised, however, that multiple fallout plumes of irregular pattern and intensity which were now assumed to be a more realistic expectation than a few widely separately cigar-shaped plumes of regularly zoned intensity, immensely complicated not only the mechanics of clearance but also the question of whether or not to clear.[42]

A year later Regional Hospital Boards were advised that:

> The subject is under consideration with the Home Office but we do not see an easy solution. There may be a case for a radical change to ensure that hospitals and staff are re-deployed to the civil reception areas in the West and the extreme South East of the country to a greater extent that we envisage at present but at present we are inclined to think that we must adhere to our present plans even though they may involve risks to hospital staffs and patients and we hope that some hospitals will be useable by the dispersal of hospital facilities in accordance with our present plans.[43]

Pressing their point, Regional Hospital Boards strongly maintained some guidance must be given on the principles and mechanics of clearance of hospitals in Z zones, and that a study into the problems be undertaken. Finding itself totally beleaguered, the Ministry of Health closed down the discussion on the basis that they could offer no further assistance. The party line demanded responsibility for the clearance of an area rested entirely with the civil defence authorities outside the area. In a final washing of hands over the whole issue, the Ministry advised the boards that their responsibility only related to preparing patients for evacuation. The hospital medical officer would, as part of that process, inform the Civil Defence Controller as to what transport was needed for the operation.[44] Falling back on official protocols undoubtedly sought to destroy any possibility of a formal study that could reveal the real situation of utter hopelessness. Instead, the ideology of escape was bolstered when the Home Office informed Regional Hospital Boards of their allocation of operational radiation measuring instruments and asked them to appoint officers who would be responsible for the collection and subsequent distribution of such equipment. As ever, the exercise became nothing more than a further step in gesture politics. The medical service had been at the end of the list for years when it came to distributions of training equipment, let alone operational instruments for reading radiation levels. Limited expenditure meant the first allocation went only to acute hospitals and FMAUs conveniently underwriting the focus on frontline support, but equally hiding the fact fallout would not respect the distinction between acute and auxiliary hospitals.[45]

Typical of the false morale-building techniques that underwrote the facade, the possession of such instruments, even if they had been available in larger quantities would do little to lessen the dangers within the nuclear reality secretly acknowledged about the sheer size and intensity of the radioactive pall that would hang over the entire country. EXERCISE MINERVA 65, conducted at the Civil Defence Staff College in 1965 tested the thesis that in such circumstances the clearance of the public from the deadly Z Zones made any kind of escape impossible. The study assumed Northampton County Borough survived as a physical entity following a nuclear strike, but sited on the edge of such a Z Zone. Local authorities were excluded from participating and the event limited to some ninety senior officials representing the Home Office, Nationalised Industries, Fire Service, Government Ministries, the Police, WVS, as well as representatives from the United States Civil Defense and the Canadian Emergency Measures Organisation.[46]

The whole tone of the occasion was set with a startling admission made by the Home Office that for 'some time' it had not felt entirely happy about the public control scheme as a realistic lifesaving opportunity. The post-raid environment they expected to build up involved fallout patterns of lethal intensity caused by a landscape of merged and overlapping plumes and across areas hundreds of miles long and hundreds of miles wide. Against that background, the study concluded with cold precision that any clearance of those caught in most deadly zone would actually become a danger to the unaffected zone itself. It was apparent, for example, that stocks of food in accessible areas would be so limited that attempting such operations 'would be to transfer a disaster from one geographical area to another at the cost of many radiological lives and the wasting of thousands of gallons of precious fuel'. What the study essentially distilled was nothing less than total hopelessness. It also elicited the secretive mind of officialdom that demanded the public must never be presented with such a picture of futility in any kind of direct way. Albeit a statement of intent, it actually confirmed a policy that had already been put into place many years before.[48]

Dead Ends

External symbolism signalled both the aim to uphold ethical values and government having control over the post-raid environment. Just as the living had to be found spaces that held the preferred ideology intact, mortality also became a part of this equation. Responsibility for the Civilian War Dead, as they were officially known, rested with the Medical Officers of Health and in a sense represented the extreme end of the abandonment of humaneness. Accordingly, the belief system grappled with the continuation of keeping it an individualistic process that would not be overwhelmed by the sheer weight of numbers. When the *Civil Defence (Burial) Regulations 1949* were quietly created under a Statutory Instrument they gave little away about the gruesome journey the subject would take. As with all legal documents of this kind, it remained short on detail and admitted the action suggested was limited to what it called 'essentials' and further guidance would be given when the Home Secretary thought it appropriate.[49] Though the 'appropriate' moment ostensibly arrived on 20 September, 1950 with the publication of a circular this notoriously became the only substantive advice on the subject ever to be made publicly available.

The very first statement as to the scope and scale of any arrangements which the authorities were to adopt provided as its benchmark the Second World War experience which ensured the political safety catch could be kept switched on:

> Experience of the war of 1939 to 1945 will be a reliable guide as to the arrangements to be planned since, in any future war, the Councils will be responsible as they were then for the collection, registration and where necessary, the preparation for the identification burial (or cremation of the bodies or persons killed in their area as the result of war operations). It is realised that if a mass destruction attack were made on a largely densely populated area the number of persons might be so great that the preparation of the bodies for identification and burial in the ordinary way would take too long and would, therefore, have to be abandoned. The Council should, however, plan on the basis that the 1939 to 1945 procedure would be followed in its entirety until authorisation is given to departures from it.[50]

By promoting the Second World War protocols used in Britain, the individualisation of the person in death appeared secure by creating the impression of a controlled containment of the problem in all kinds of different ways. Peacetime mortuaries had to be utilised first before adding more. All grades of council staff were to be formed into a burial authority and the circular envisaged the burial system itself would become integrated into the civil defence service. Councils, it was suggested, should encourage employees of local funeral undertakers to join up and provide the appropriate expertise. Talk of this kind was, of course, cheap and no action actually allowed to build up stocks of equipment to run the expanded mortuary service. Even the economic plight of the country preparing for World War Three managed to permeate the instructions as to the provision of body racks. They recommended these be planned with the 'utmost economy' due to the limited amount of timber available and wherever possible, the use of home grown wood preferred. Premises with sufficient floor space to permit bodies being placed in rows were considered ideal to prevent a waste of such a valuable resource, but a warning given against earmarking premises that might be more suitable for the needs of the living through extra hospital space.[51]

As enthusiastic as the circular had been to deal with the subject, a review of progress in England and Wales conducted across local councils produced results that were to say the least 'patchy'. These showed 87% of authorities had conformed by designating a responsible officer to deal with the civilian war dead, although Oxford and Middlesbrough were singled out for non-compliance. Thereafter, the picture looked less encouraging with only 41% actually identifying premises for additional mortuaries. Where the remit had been followed, a popular choice proved to be municipal swimming baths from which the water could be drained and the space refilled with the dead. Worst of all came the recruitment issue, which the survey admitted was 'not going well'. Many councils were said to have established contact with local undertakers, but few of their own men wished to join the Civil Defence Corps. In Scotland, however the project had received a more favourable response and all the authorities requested to make appointments and earmark premises had completed their arrangements.[52]

With little prospect of the Ministry's vision coming together as planned, the civil service route of convening a working party took its inevitable course 'to consider problems relating to the disposal of civilian dead in any future war'. As with many transitional arrangements, the study clung on to the principle that the old ways of doing things still had their place and should continue. Atomic bombing, according to the new thesis, needed to be approached by supplementary procedures, a philosophical thread reflected in its submission: 'We do not believe that weapons of mass destruction make such conventional methods entirely out of date, and they must in any case be the foundation on which to plan any further measures'.[53] So the tenet of the working party's recommendation came on the basis of creating a scheme to deal with a possible attack of the kind experienced in the last war, with the comment that it could also deal with an even larger number of casualties if the service was well organised.

To unblock the malaise, which had beset the planning of the burial side of things, the report suggested a special section should be created for this purpose as part of the Civil Defence Corps rather than relying on the vague responsibilities set out in circular 98/50. Given proper training, went the theory, a centre of expertise could be established and become an integral part of civil defence exercises with proper chains of command established between civil defence controllers and civilian war dead officers.[54] Of course, well founded as the objectives might have appeared, publicly showing the portrayal of death in an organisation intended to propagandise the prospect of survival did not bode well. Worse still, it would visibly show scarce facilities such as vehicles being used to transport the dead instead of transporting the injured to hospitals.[55]

Further suggestions appeared on the doom agenda. One singularly gruesome one came in the recommendation that local authorities in key areas should dig mass graves in advance so the demands on heavy machinery in the form of trench diggers could be evened out across the country. Timing was acknowledged as difficult and a string of supplementary detailing suggested. This included trenches requiring shoring if left open for a long time and, if prepared beforehand, the first cuts should be made some distance apart so that the space in between could be utilised later on to achieve maximum capacity. Calculations suggested burial for between 5,000 to 7,000 corpses per acre might be possible in this way depending on water lines and the nature of the subsoil. In the case of a stacking system, the coffin at the top was not to be less than three feet below the surface. Furthermore, in places such as London, the problems of finding space on this scale meant provisional schemes might involve arrangements with neighbouring authorities to export the corpse problem elsewhere if necessary.[56]

All these ideas inescapably pointed to the continuing obsession with keeping to the protocols of normal burial, but extended on a mass scale. The ideological disquiet about departing from that line even stretched to keeping the illusion going by the use of special coffins given the experience of the Second World War during which there had sometimes been problems of securing enough supplies. Three types of substitutes for normal coffins received consideration, two at least having all the attributes of an end-of-pier magical show. The first was a design with a hinged bottom, said to be used in Holland, which could be lowered into the grave and the body released by opening the hinges with a cord thus allowing the entire coffin to be used ad infinitum. Second on the list of possibilities came a coffin with a detachable bottom or tray designed to be left with the body, the rest of the coffin then brought up for reuse. Finally, a container made using a strong fabric of a suitable kind, but non-reusable, ended the list of macabre paraphernalia. The problem with such props was that the illusions might become evident and damage the dignity of the ceremony. Nonetheless, the working party felt all these were valid alternatives local authorities might consider and use in dealing with the dead.[57]

Recognition of some of the problems sometimes did surface in the report. For example, mention was made of the Civilian War Dead Department acting as leaders and supervisors needing to organise the process in appropriate ways. Due to the sheer scale of death, bodies might have to lie for a long time in situ. Appropriate equipment including respirators, rubber clothing shovels, wheelbarrows and chloride of lime, insecticides and deodorants joined the list of any future local stockpile. Because of the possibility of many pre-selected burial sites being destroyed, further suggestions included the preparation of special local authority 'war books' identifying burial sites and equipment locations so the information could be shared with neighbours and arrangements adapted to meet each situation as it developed. The Hamburg raid method came into the procedures for the first time recommending that bodies were to be cleared from streets first, then from the edges of debris. However, even in all this, the point still endured that until it was actually physically impossible to afford the dead due decorum the 'basic' burial protocols should continue which meant the transfer of bodies to temporary mortuaries, the use of coffins and identification by relatives.[58]

For all the logic the report might have professed in organisational terms, no further action ever resulted and the issue of the civilian war dead was itself buried in the atomic era with nothing added to circular 98/50. Only in a long list of anticipatory arrangements for a possible war over Berlin did the true horrors emerge. At the time, ministries prepared instructions for local councils to mobilise their civil defence authorities. The Ministry of Housing and Local Government, on its part issued advice on the burial of dead, admitting 'we had not issued any advice on these functions for years'. The Home Office held these in addressed envelopes ready for dispatch by hand to county and county borough councils. Directions for district councils were to be delivered under special arrangements by the General Post Office stamped 'Emergency Instructions–Urgent'.[59] Inside those envelopes the advice amply indicated the reasons why there had been no rush to produce the real procedures of death management in the nuclear aftermath:

> Wherever possible, local authorities should continue normal burial and cremation arrangements for disposal of the dead. After attack, however, there would be places where the numbers of dead were such that special steps would have to be taken to dispose of the bodies. In these places all that can be suggested is that mechanical equipment should be used for digging pits into which bodies would be tipped from lorries. If no equipment were available to the Council, they should contact the Area Leader of the Works and Buildings Emergency Organisation, who could be approached through the civil defence organisation at Area Level. It is of the utmost importance that advice should be obtained from a suitably qualified engineer before pits are dug, to ensure that sites are chosen which will not cause contamination to a water supply. Authorities are requested to select suitable sites before attack, so far as possible. If mass burial of this sort became necessary, it would clearly be impossible to conduct burial services of any kind. If time could be spared to list the names and addresses of the persons buried, assuming that means of identification were available, this should be done.[60]

Since the grisly instructions were never released, the reality of death based on unceremonious necessity did not formally intrude into the civil defence domain. Indeed, the degree to which patience had run out over the issue is evident in a letter written on 1 February, 1961 by Captain Harkness, the Civil Defence Officer of London, to his bosses at the Home Office. This stressed the degree of dissatisfaction building up at local level, the complaint being: 'From time to time, a few of our London Town Clerks express the strongest views about the continuing lack of guidance on this rather macabre subject. One or two of them served on a working party in the atomic era and are rather hurt that nothing emerged then and there has been no re-appraisal to the meet the megaton menace'.[61] A bizarre twist occurred when the Captain's letter was mislaid at the Home Office. On its eventual discovery, the loss served to underline the lack of urgency in the Department and came with the reaction to match: 'We cannot go on stalling for ever and, with the fresh impetus that had been given to civil defence generally following the acceptance of the Home Defence Review Committee's recommendations, I fear we must expect to be prodded on this subject quite frequently'. To pacify the situation the usual route of setting up another working party seemed the only way forward.[62]

There is little doubt Whitehall wanted this sleeping dog to lie permanently and nothing further transpired. The only policy directive ever to reach any kind of realistic statement on the subject was confined to the secret Defence Regulations to be triggered in the event of a nuclear war. This allowed local authorities to forbid private funerals or cremations and prevent relatives attending what were termed 'disposal' places. Disposal by burning outside crematoria and of unidentified bodies, as well as being able to raise new burial grounds without formal government approval attested to the horrors that would ensue a nuclear war.[63] Yet, amongst them the attempted mitigation of the undignified ending remained, with prior preparations preferred as had been outlined by the 1953 working party. This included trench digging, secluded burial grounds, with any religious service being confined to the committal service. Even a technical nicety about the design of coffins managed to seep through in the following advice:

> A container made from strong textile fabric of a suitable kind, consumable and not for re-use, would have to be substituted for coffins. The material would need to be impermeable and a 3rd and 4th handle and cord provided to overcome the lack of rigidity for carrying and lowering. Local authorities in key areas should, if possible, have supplies of these containers. It is also essential that there should be a central system of supply.[64]

Concerns over coffin handles when dealing with the greatest catastrophe ever to confront mankind shows an inexplicable attempt to define some kind of last 'ethical handle' to hold on to as the remaining vestige of decency. For all their harrowing detail, the regulations were not part of the public picture. On that side, the facade continued the process of normalisation and provided new symbols of care through home nursing and first aid whilst at the same time defending established protocols. The public, though theoretically empowered to become proficient in nuclear nursing or first aid, were never involved *en masse* and specially targeted groups, particularly women, were chosen for the purpose. Training notes suffered censorship and sanitisation to hide the extent of nuclear injury, especially radiation sickness and altogether the system strove to portray and sustain an environment of medical care. Furthermore, the journey to the promised land of survival meant social expendability never emerged publicly and all escape routes from hospitals were kept open for normal and 'special' patients despite the barriers building up. In a quite extraordinary production of pretentious hope, the entire medical plan ensured that megaton martyrdom and its scale lay hidden underneath the complex framework that supported the ideology of mass compassion.

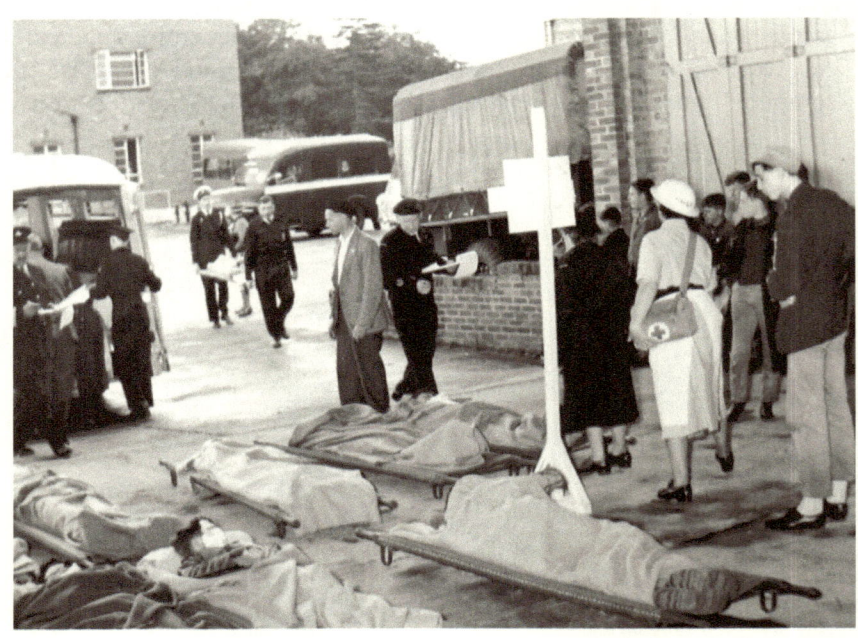

28. & 29. EXERCISE RELIANCE. Casualties await their turn before the initial critical medical examination by a Medical Officer.

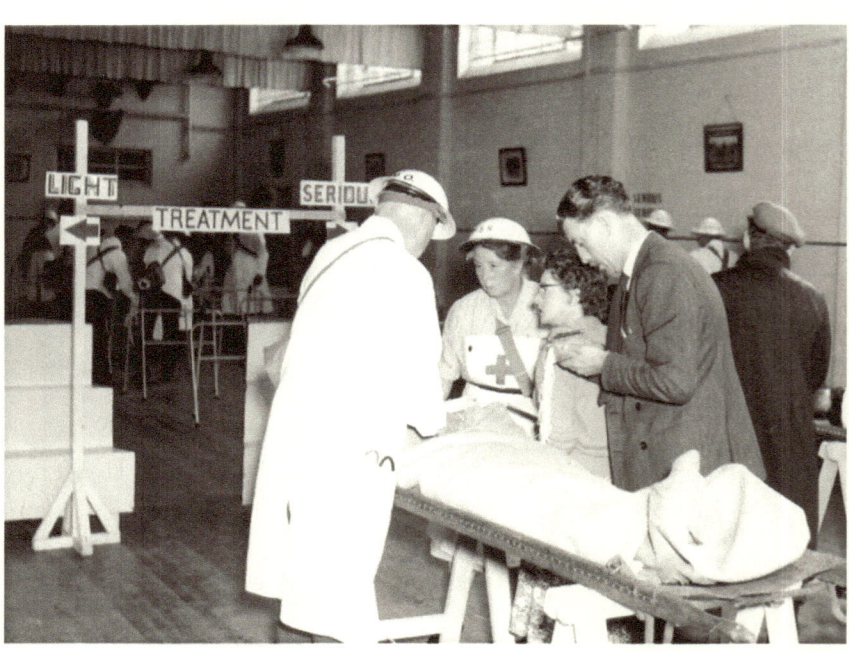

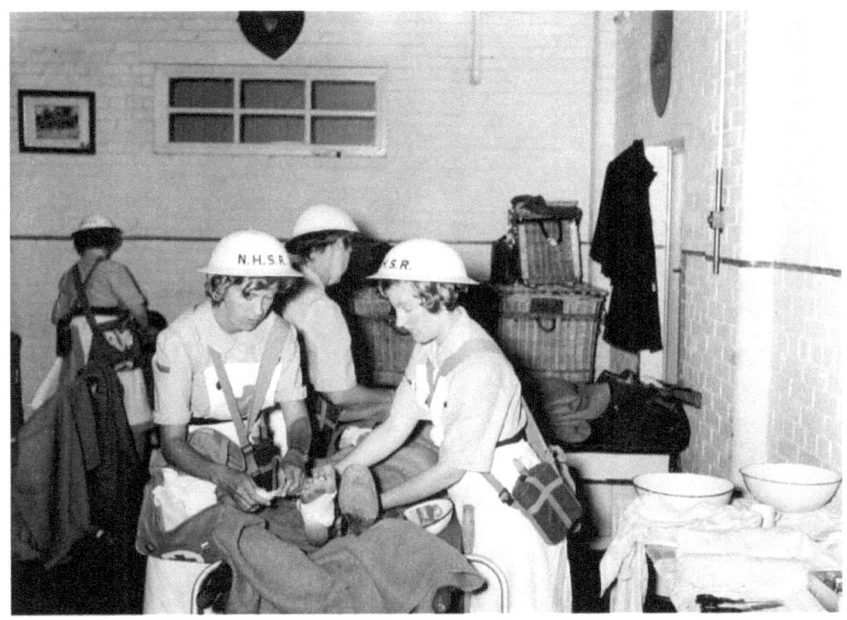

30. & 31. EXERCISE RELIANCE. Red Cross nurses of the NHSR and the serious case area of the FMAU.

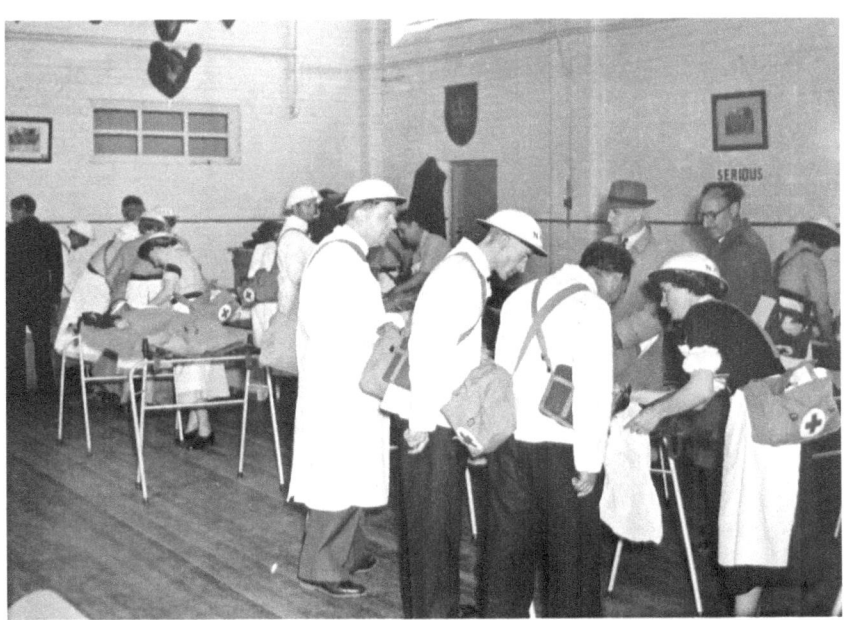

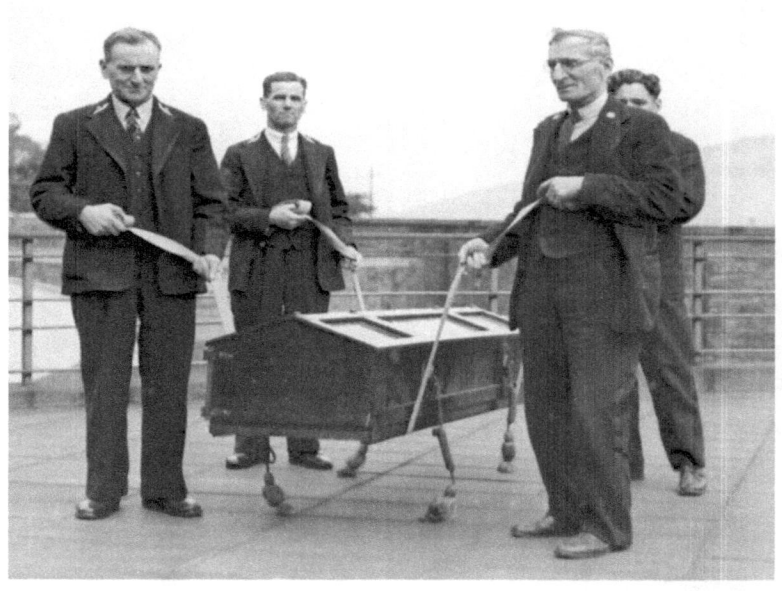

32. & 33. Demonstration of a reusable collapsible coffin by Scottish Office messengers outside St Andrew's House, Edinburgh, c. 1951.

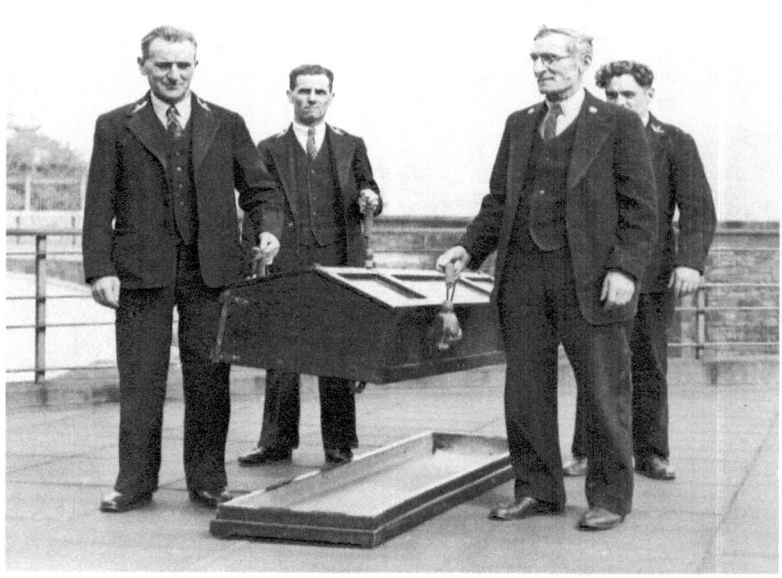

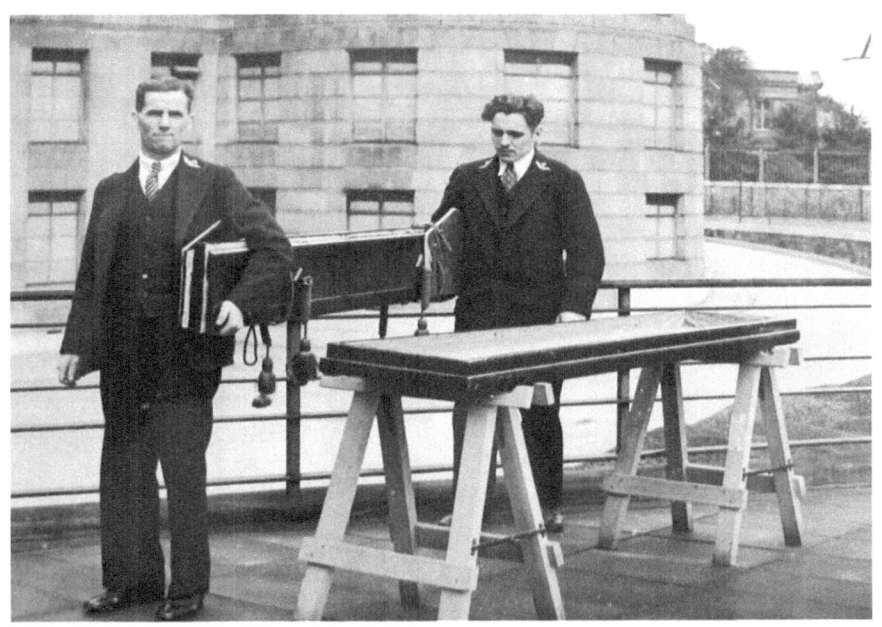

34. Recycling Decorum. The main coffin structure is completely folded for further use.

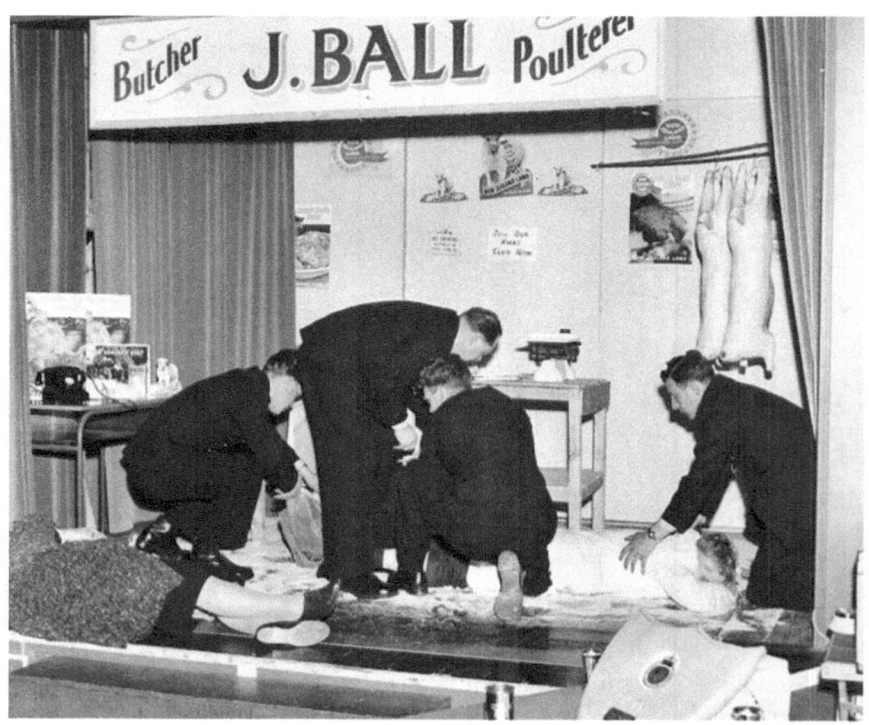

35. Police constables exhibit their first aid skills during a civil defence first aid competition set against the backcloth of a local butcher's shop. Involvement in civil defence first aid projected a humanitarian side to the police and hid the prospect of the constabulary having to carry arms in the event of social disorder following a nuclear attack.

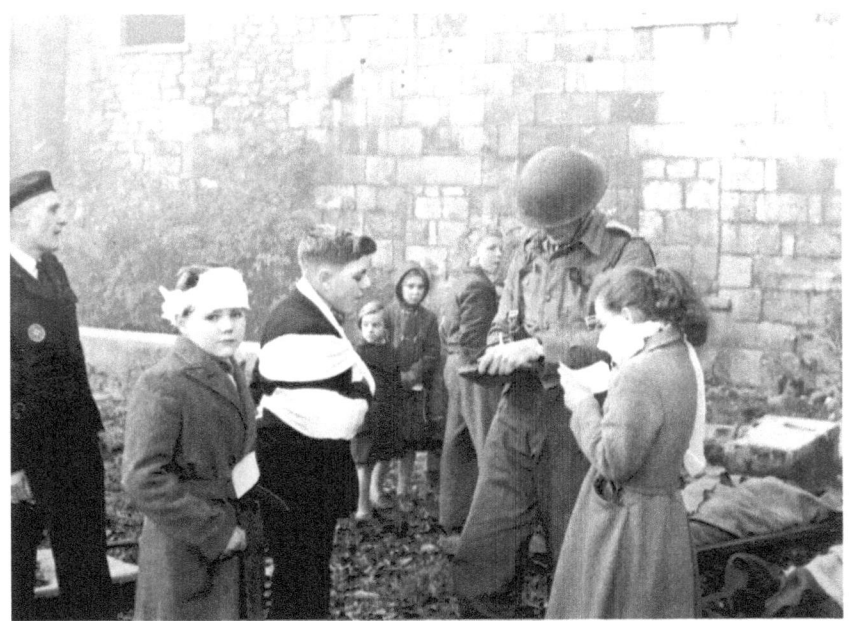

36. & 37. Children living with the bomb. Taking part in a civil defence exercise and shown the latest CD walkie-talkie equipment.

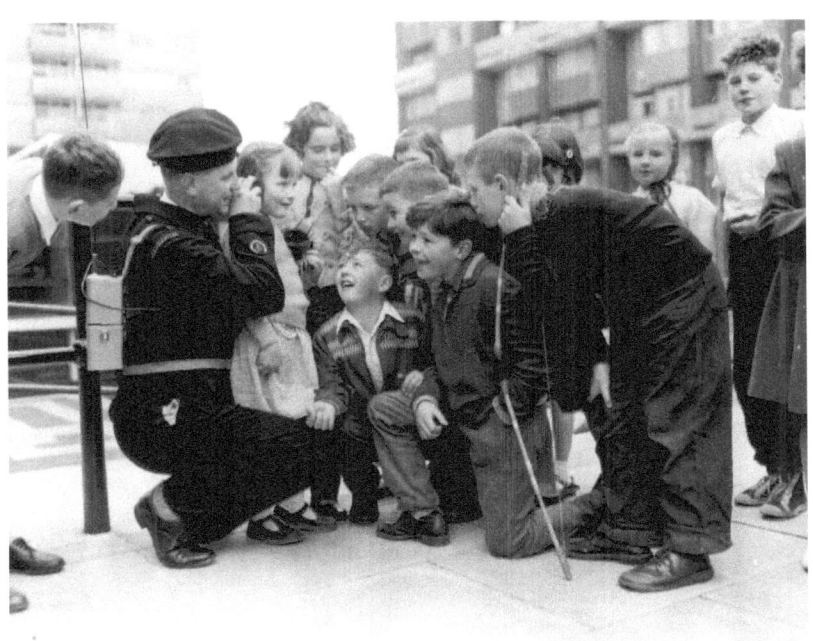

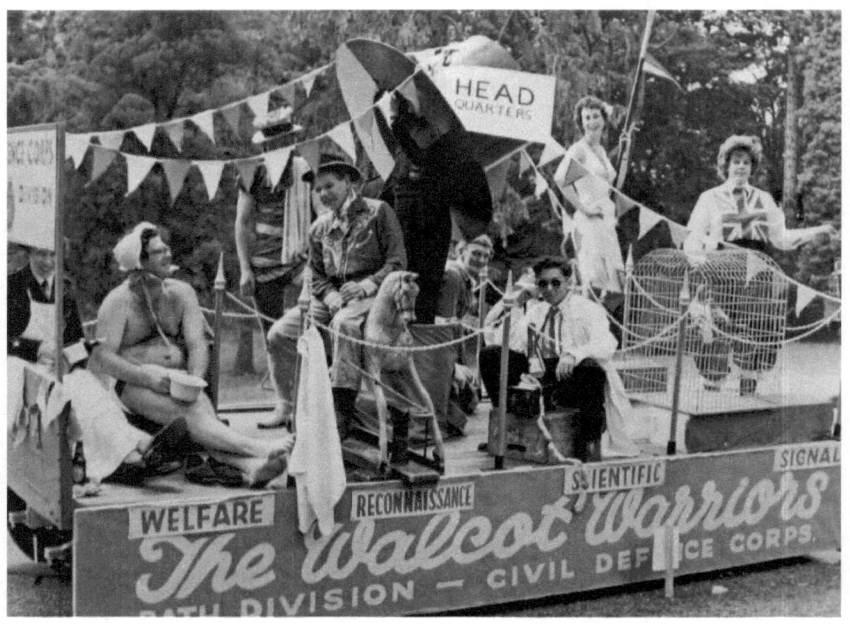

38. & 39. Carnival float depicting the Headquarters Section of the Civil Defence Corps whilst in their civic bunker HQ staff plot radiation fields.

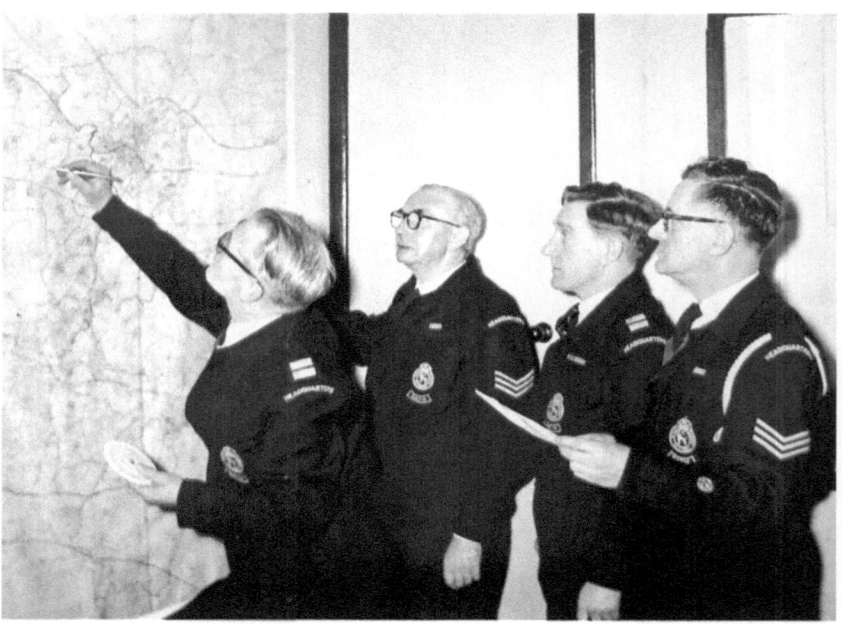

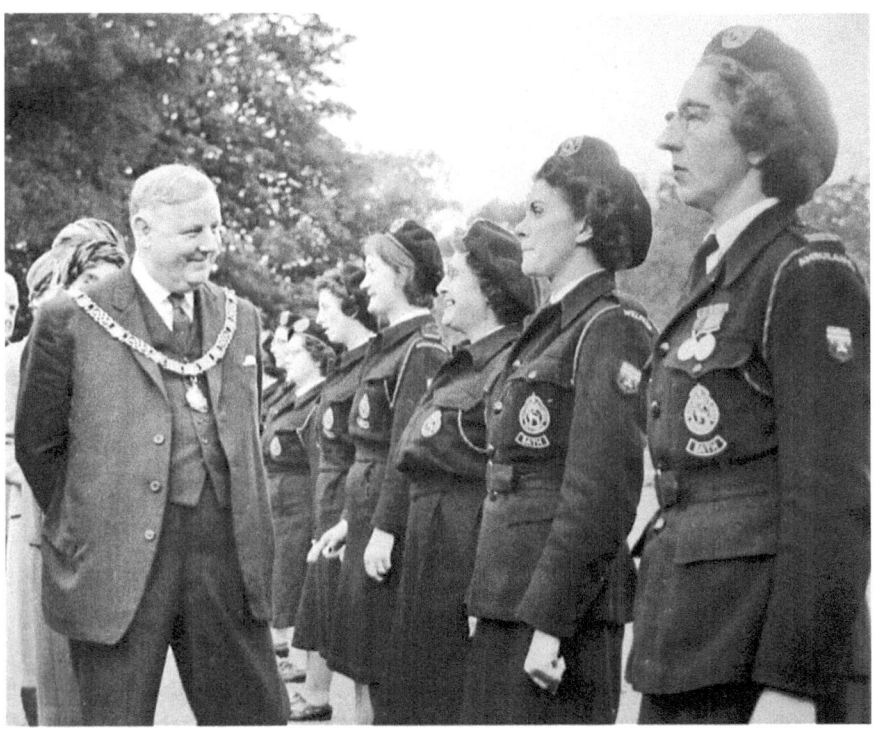

40. Civil defence allowed local politicians to use the organisation as a means of showing their communities how they were to be cared for in the event of nuclear war. Civic pride played its part with the mayor of Bath inspecting the Ambulance and Welfare sections of the Civil Defence Corps during a local pageant.

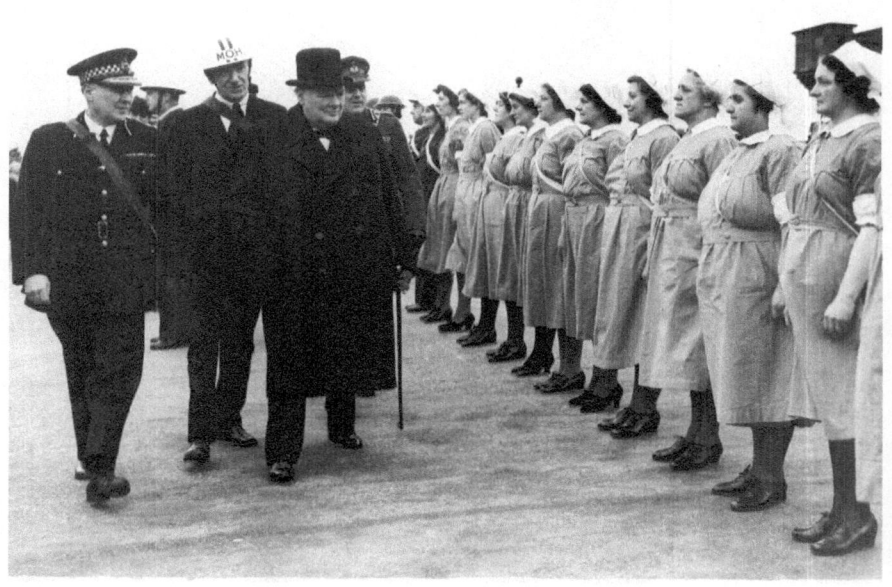

41. Sir Winston Churchill inspects auxiliary nurses when visiting Edinburgh during 1942 with the Medical Officer of Health behind him. Concerns over the general lack of fitness of women in the wartime organisation led to the introduction of stringent medical tests when a new voluntary service appeared in the post war era.

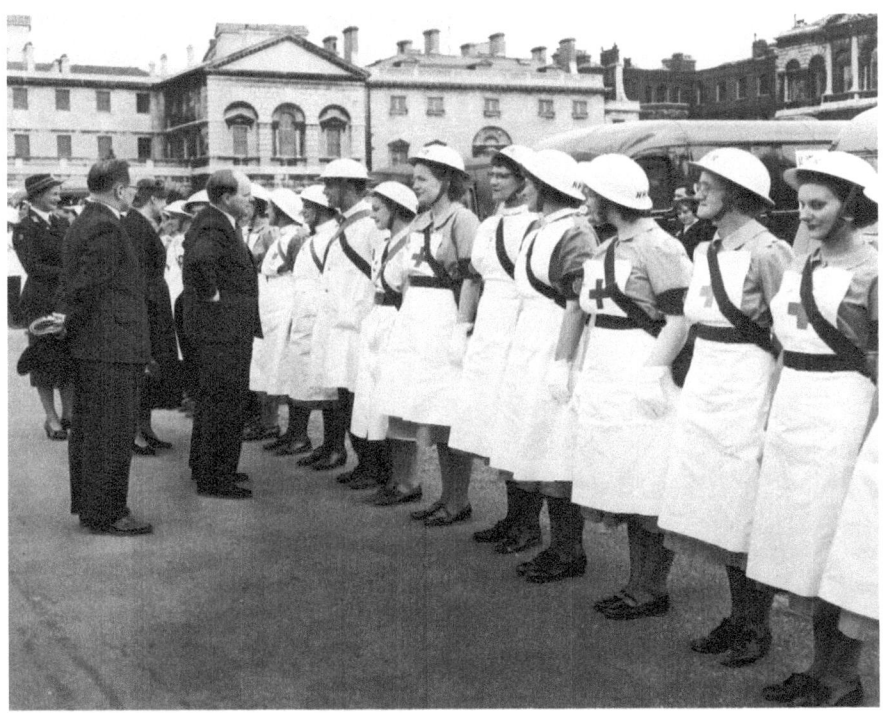

42. Finalists in the NHSR Minister's Cup competition are inspected by the Minister of Health Iain Macleod on Horse Guards Parade, Whitehall, during the early 1950s.

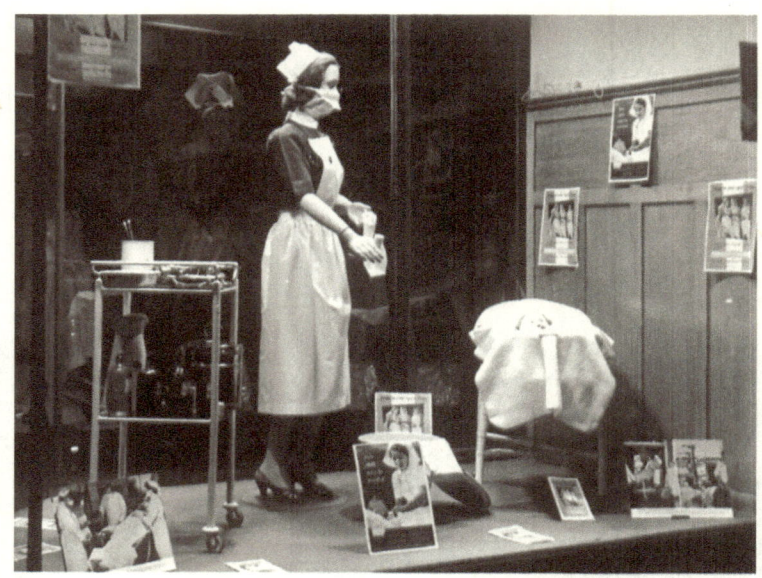

43. & 44. Shop window displays emphasising the attractions of the NHSR as a peacetime civilian organisation.

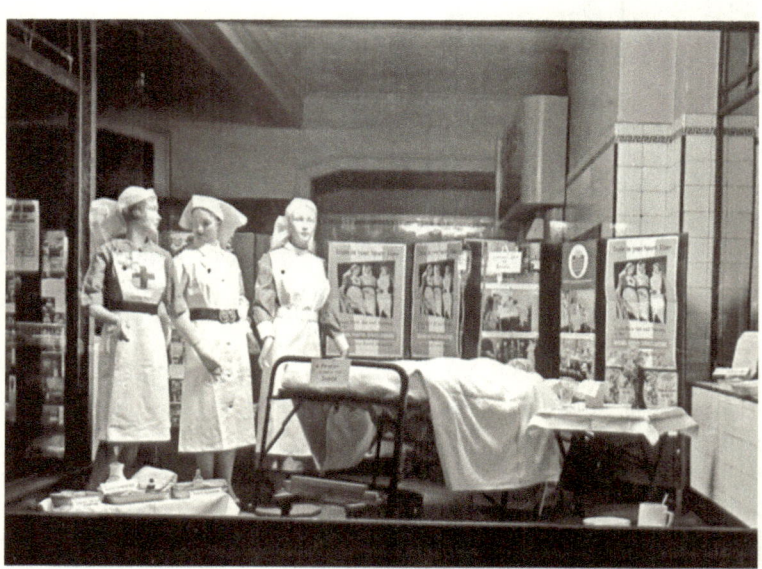

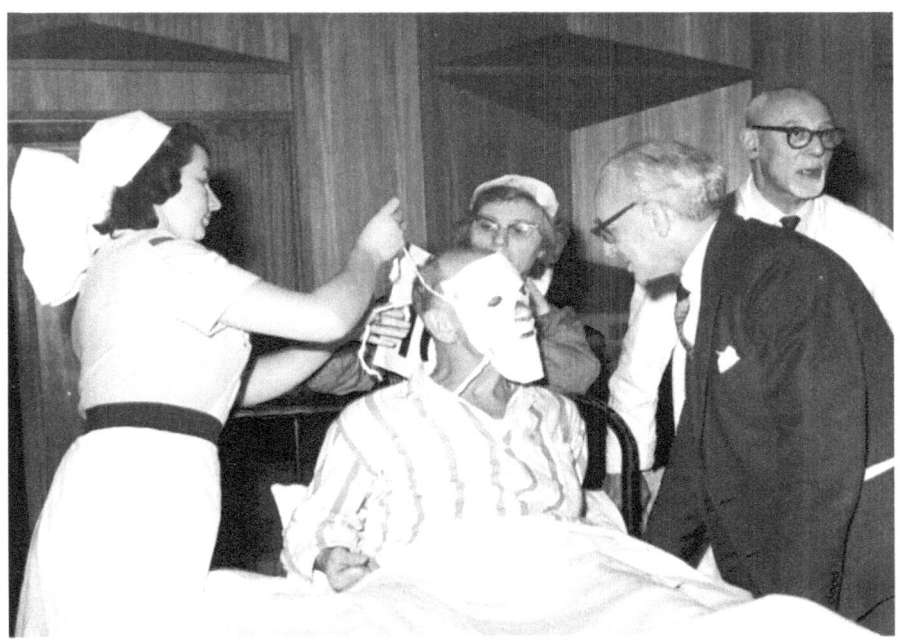

45. Sir Barnett Stross, Parliamentary Secretary to the Ministry of Health, talks to a pretend-facial burns casualty being prepared for the NHSR national finals of the Minister of Health's Cup held at the Fairfield Halls Croydon in 1964. The picture of a senior government representative staring at the mask is very symbolic of the time as the sheer hopelessness of establishing a nuclear casualty service became hidden more and more by a contrived policy of mass compassion.

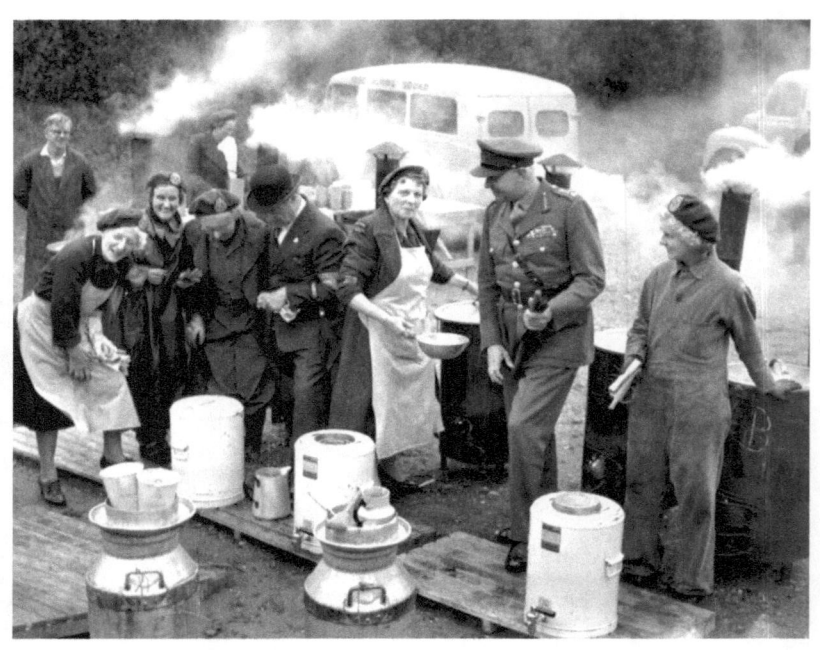

46. & 47. Nuclear Dinners. WVS support for nuclear exercises.

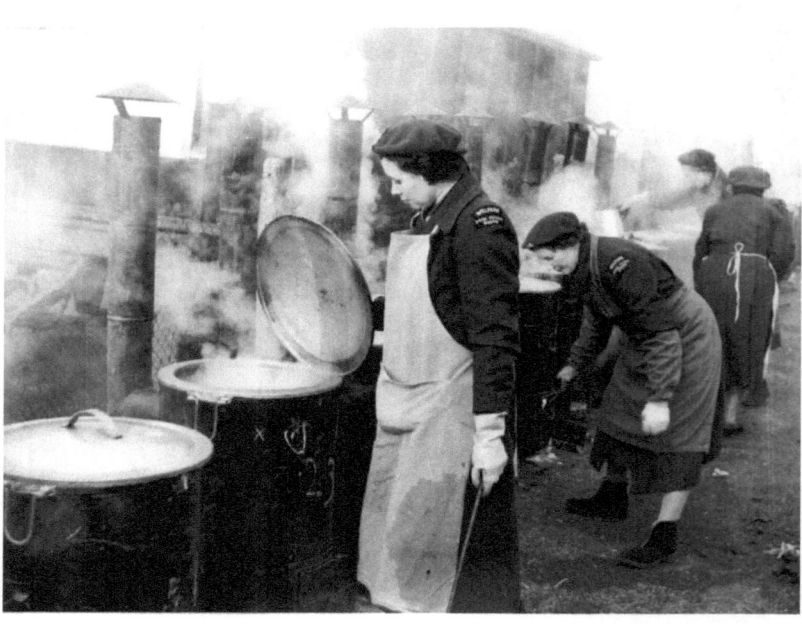

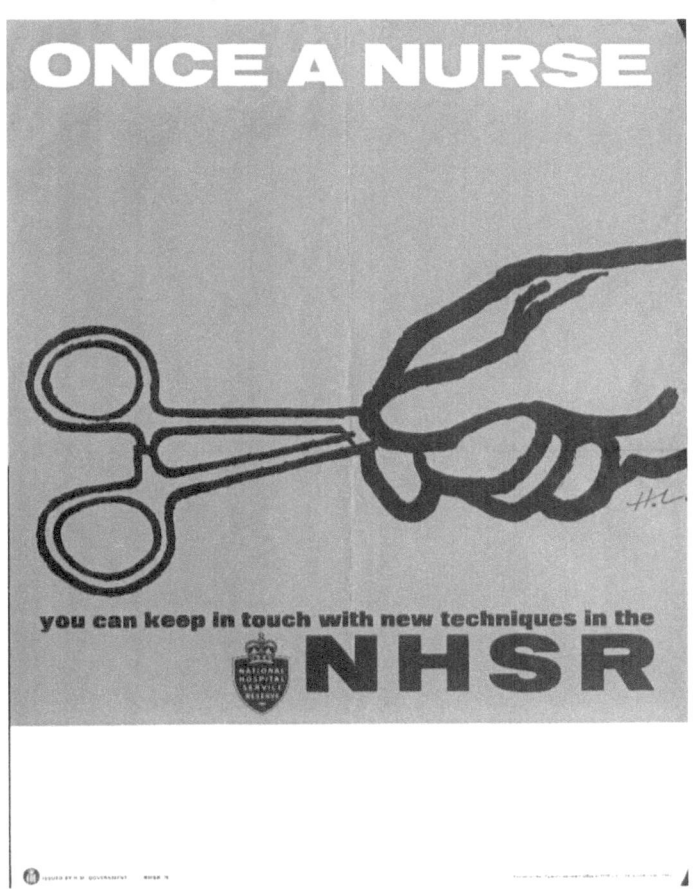

48. 1960s NHSR recruitment poster for trained nurses who had left the profession.

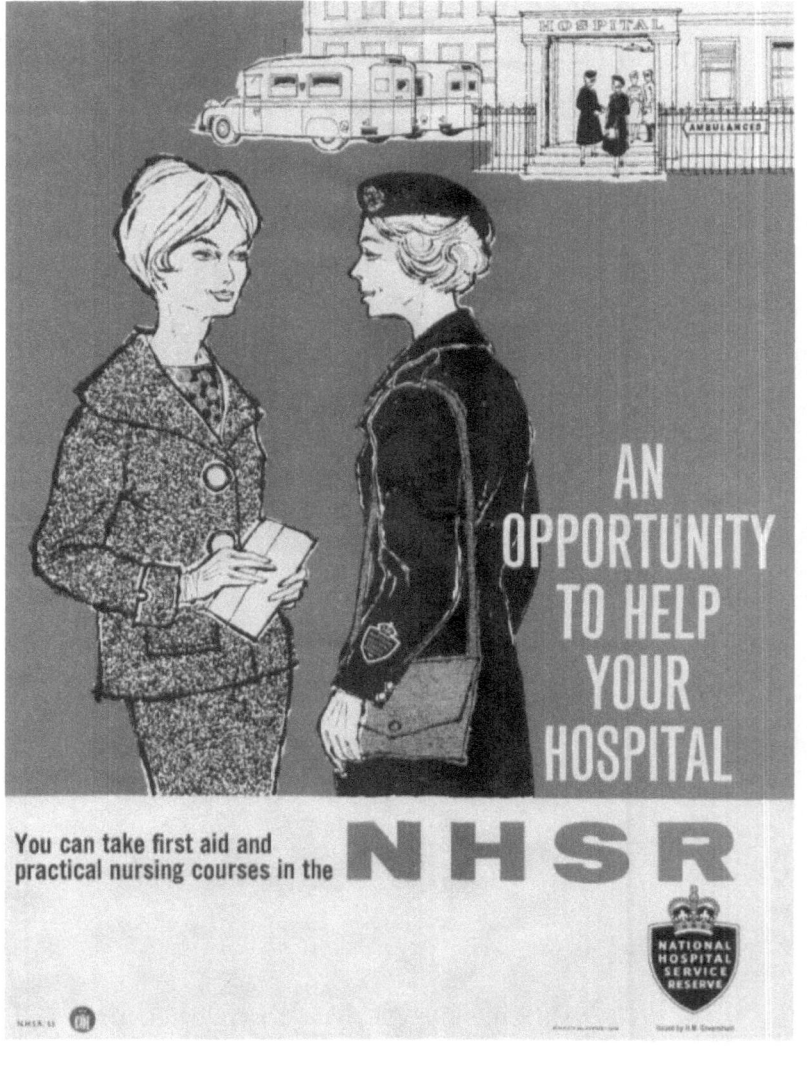

49. 1960s recruitment poster for volunteer nurses to help the local hospital, but no reference made to the civil defence role or nuclear war.

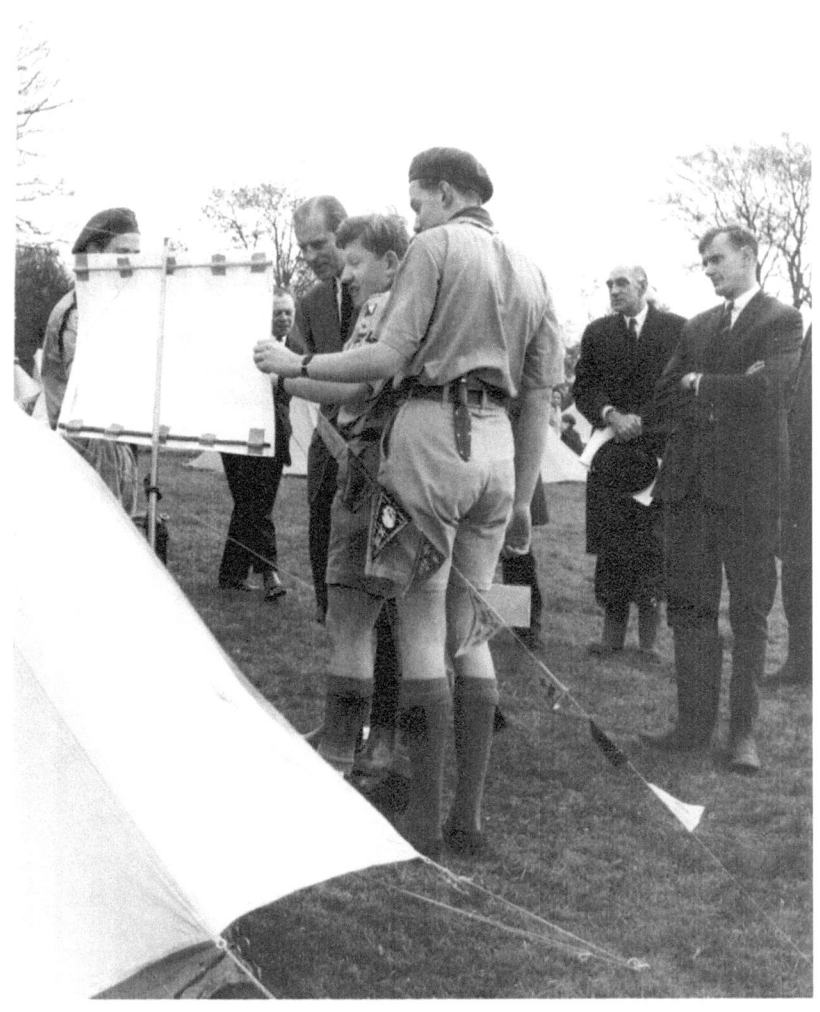

50. The author as a Senior Scout talks to Prince Phillip during a Duke of Edinburgh's award jamboree during 1963.

DOCTORS WANT

A BETTER NATIONAL HEALTH SERVICE FOR YOUR FAMILY

THIS MEANS

- well equipped surgeries
- more staff
- more time to study
- more time for each patient
- more doctors to meet the present shortage
- a new fairer system of payment for your doctor

to achieve these aims more money is needed for general practice and to provide new medical schools — to remedy the neglect of the family doctor service by successive governments for the past 17 years

your family doctor is working for this through the B.M.A.

51. Issued by the British Medical Association this poster reveals the strong feelings about the NHS that exploded during 1965. The depth of dissatisfaction caused the plans for a formal contract to mobilise general practitioners under the control of local councils to be abandoned.

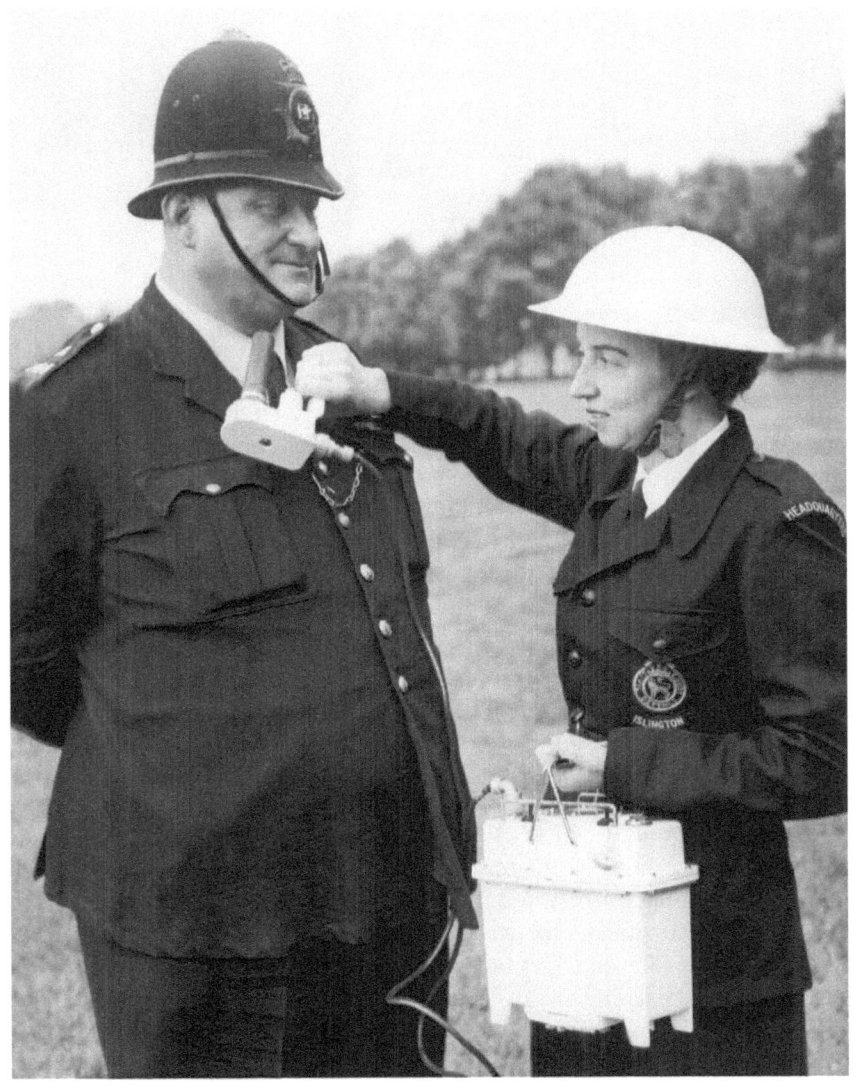

52. A demonstration of radiation monitoring during the late 1950s. The benign image typically hides the fact that such iconic symbols represented by the police and the Headquarters Section of the Civil Defence Corps would ultimately decompose into the means of controlling doctors through the Defence Regulations.

Chapter 7

NURSING NUMBERS

Fully exploiting the propaganda value of the National Health Service as a nuclear medical service provider was never going to be an easy matter. During 1948 the medical working party at only its second meeting took the decision to exclude nursing staff in hospitals from becoming directly involved in civil defence.[1] Somehow the contrived promise of mass compassion the NHS could deliver had to be transmitted through other means. Fortuitously, an answer existed in the surrogate use of nursing volunteers and linking hospitals with a new organisation called the National Hospital Service Reserve. Sustaining a kind of parasitic advantage in such a way meant keeping recruitment to the NHSR up to reasonable levels and ideally increasing the numbers in line with the growth in destruction. When the popularity of the civil defence volunteer services declined with the advent of the hydrogen bomb, 'the nuclear health service', encountered a singularly problematic situation given the critical propaganda relationship described. Yet, against all odds, the NHSR managed to sustain and even enlarge its membership. (Table 4) The achievement was so extraordinary that it raises one of the most intriguing questions of the early Cold War period as to whether the pattern actually reflected a genuine concern for the nuclear casualty by the public, especially women, or resulted through official manipulation.

The Ministry of Health were fortunate that creating an organisational framework for the voluntary nurses did not come with the kind of political machinations that shrouded other sectors of the medical territory. The Government had appointed a working party in June 1949 consisting of representatives from the Ministry of Health, Regional Hospital Boards, Teaching Hospitals as well as the Red Cross and St John Ambulance. Within just five months, this group produced a blueprint for an organisation that it named the National Hospital Service Reserve and worked out that for the hospital plan devised by Carling's working party an additional 100,000 nurses would be required. Though presenting a rounded and memorable figure, it did still raise the problem about how it could ever be delivered through voluntarism in a country settling into a new peace and rebuilding lives shattered by war.[2] Yet, for nearly twenty years it was conveniently used to beat the Regional Hospital Boards with as the definitive recruitment panacea.

Table 4: National Hospital Service Reserve Recruitment 1950 – 66.

Year	Trained Nurses	Auxiliary Nurses	Total
1950*	1006	9427	10,433
1951	1767	17,293	19,060
1952	2184	27,081	29,265
1953	2702	32,241	34,943
1954	3115	37,738	40,853
1955	3412	39,288	42,700
1956	3437	40,007	43,444
1957	3470	39,895	43,365
1958	4061	45,603	49,664
1959	4518	50,017	54,535
1960	4821	54,203	59,024
1961	4889	56,868	61,757
1962	5016	62,230	65,246
1963	5126	60,733	65,859
1964	4900	59,900	64,800
1965	4900	58,600	63,500
1966	4700	58,700	63,400

* From National Archives file TNA, MH 55/983

Source: Annual Reports of the Ministry of Health.

Subtracting War

Unusually, the National Hospital Service Reserve actually existed as a hybrid organisation. Although created under the *Civil Defence Act 1948,* it did not come under the control of the Home Office as did the Civil Defence Corps, Auxiliary Fire Service and Special Constabulary, and its natural affiliation lay with the Ministry of Health. With regard to the volunteer structure, this also ran counter to the arrangements in the other civil defence units since part of it could be regarded as 'professional' in nature. The position arose because the NHSR in England and Wales consisted of just two sections, one that included trained nurses who had retired or left the profession and the other which contained the auxiliaries recruited directly from the general public or the St John Ambulance (St Andrew's in Scotland) and the British Red Cross. Together these formed a volunteer force ready for integration with the NHS in a war situation and possessed no ranks or hierarchies to reflect its amorphous status.

Arrangements of this kind might have suggested the organisation being a simple and somewhat mundane grouping where not much could possibly go wrong. Circumstances had, nevertheless, conspired to endow its management with complexities that were never anticipated at its formation. The gestation of the NHSR, and indeed its eventual birth, took place through a time of exceptional difficulty within the nursing profession. Combined with Cold War pressures to deliver an auxiliary service quickly, the environment produced a scheme that had a profound effect on its shape and form. For a start, the timing to recruit more nurses, even auxiliaries, could not have been more inauspicious. Post war Britain faced a nursing crisis both on the supply and distribution side to the extent that in February 1947, *The Lancet* observed: 'Many of our hospitals are now in dire straits. In London, the LCC is reduced to less than half its pre-war complement of beds and all over the country local authorities are in a similar plight'.[3] The introduction of part-time nursing, coupled with revolutionary changes in training and service conditions only just averted a disaster, but the process needed time to catch up. The total strength of the nursing profession, which also included mental nurses, as at December 1950 amounted to 150,000 whole-time and part-time staff, but hospital returns suggested the shortage still came to a whole time equivalent of 39,000 nurses.[4]

Every possible pocket of nursing resource was wrung out of the system so it could then be applied in some way to avoid hospitals, chiefly mental institutions, from literally being closed down. Probably the most notable in this exercise related to the wartime nursing organisation established to support regular nurses. Known as the Civil Nursing Reserve it did not disband because of the peacetime shortage. At its peak in 1941, the CNR membership amounted to 107,000 nurses including 78,000 auxiliaries, 60% of whom were members of the two voluntary societies though its numbers at the end of the war declined sharply and amounted to a drop in the ocean as far as any long term solution was concerned. Yet, some hospitals were entirely reliant on the support of this unit and its usefulness stretched in other directions. One advantage, in particular, still subsisted linked to the organisation's wartime function whereby CNR nurses were duty bound to serve in any part of the country which made it an ideal emergency force to be sent anywhere at a moment's notice as a stop gap measure.[5]

Because of the difficult background, especially the conditions described in London, Sir Allen Daley, the head of the London County Council, promoted the idea of establishing a permanent nursing reserve. The Ministry of Health were agreeable and convened a committee delegated to form a new organisation called the National Nursing Reserve for possible use in national disasters or epidemics. Due to the urgency, the St John Ambulance and British Red Cross received requests from the Ministry to support the NNR through their own ranks, in addition to taking on its administration and the recruitment of other auxiliaries. Whilst the two societies were willing to cooperate, their grandee guardians had quite differing views about how such support should materialise. Lady Louis Mountbatten voiced her unease that unless the terms of this new service were very attractive, it would not secure many recruits and warned of possible unfortunate consequences on the recruitment to the Brigade itself. She also expressed a preference for St John Ambulance to be called up only when an emergency arose from the ordinary membership. Nor was she keen on the idea that they and the Red Cross should run the Reserve. Lady Mountbatten did, however, give her undertaking that if the Committee recommended such a route, the Brigade would willingly cooperate in every respect. By contrast, Lady Oliver supported the whole idea more robustly in its entirety, even to the extent of promising the BRCS were prepared to come into the scheme and deliver about 10,000 nursing auxiliaries immediately.[6] Anyhow, before this organisation got off the ground, the hospitals feared a flu epidemic would occur during the winter and began to advertise directly to the public for support. In the light of the initiative, the Ministry took the decision to shelve the National Nursing Reserve plan to avoid confusing the public with what would have become competing claims for nursing resources.[7]

The rather abrupt end of the National Nursing Reserve idea coincided with the start of planning for the Cold War.[8] Proposals to provide a parallel hospital service to NHS hospitals had been prepared with two levels of membership that would extend its capability to meet the new threats posed by mass destruction. The first included a volunteer army of trained and auxiliary nurses that after a time would also assimilate radiographers, medical laboratory technicians, biochemists, physicists, physiotherapists and even remedial gymnasts. At the second level, cooks, ward orderlies and every manner of other back up was also to be thrown into this eclectic mix of functions on the basis a separate corps incorporating the title 'domestics' would not prove an attractive recruitment draw. With a much grander scheme in prospect, the title of the National Nursing Reserve no longer seemed appropriate so it became the National Hospital Service Reserve to reflect the wider scope of support planned.[9] Of course, the incredibly complex model turned out to be nothing more than a pipe dream of the planners. The NHSR never did expand its horizons beyond the nursing side and left it with a title hardly appropriate when set against its founding objective.

As the National Health Service went through the throes of being established, a general feeling existed at the Ministry of Health that it would be unable to cope with the induction of a large number of auxiliaries. The British Red Cross and St John Ambulance once more were called in to kick-start this new initiative through their own membership. Additionally, the template they had agreed for the National Nursing Reserve already existed on the shelf, complete with all the terms and conditions prepared and ready for immediate use. The hectic circumstances surrounding the scheme even hit a politically sensitive note. Much to the dismay of the Ministry of Health, a whiff of discontent managed to surface before the recruitment campaign started for the NHSR. Described as a 'bad leak', the recruitment plan had been secretly handed over to the communist *Daily Worker* newspaper, the disclosure giving an opportunity to embarrass the Government by suggesting it had been unable to sort out the peacetime nursing situation and yet was preparing a nursing organisation for war.[10]

No inquiry followed the revelation for the fear of creating an unnecessary diversion and generating publicity damaging to the timely establishment of the organisation. The incident was though a bad omen. The real damage that would threaten the organisation was far more insidious and arose through two factors that embedded an organisational disaster waiting to happen. The first related to the way the NHSR had inherited an organisational framework of considerable complexity. Responsibility for recruitment and training ended up scattered across many of the institutions involved. Hospitals held the responsibility to recruit trained nurses, midwives, assistant nurses and nursing assistants by attracting the retired or early leavers and keep their records. When it came to dealing with the volunteer auxiliaries, the St John Ambulance and the British Red Cross were to provide these through their own ranks or recruit members of the public who (subject to certain exemptions) had to be trained in two qualifying subjects, one in first aid and the other in home nursing. Adding further potential for muddle, the administration of this group also fell to the societies, albeit the recruits themselves did not actually have to become members of their sponsoring organisation. After gaining certificates in the two subjects, hospitals were to receive the trainees for immersion into 'the hospital experience', the final requirement towards full accreditation. Thereafter, it was expected hospitals themselves would arrange refresher courses for both trained and auxiliary members.

The second factor that militated against a satisfactory outcome was the social environment itself that the recruitment process faced. The Reserve had resulted through the fusion of two quite separate plans in the way described. One had sought to provide the country with a relatively small, well-qualified reserve for civil emergencies whilst the other concerned itself with the delivery of numbers with the sole purpose of active engagement in war. In their wisdom, the Ministry of Health decided to pursue both quality and numbers, primarily because the terms for the former were readily available from the attempted formation of the National Nursing Reserve. Women between 17½ and 60 and men between the ages of 30 and 60 could join. In the case of trained nurses holding formal qualifications, the deal remained straightforward with no initial training liability, but hospital service of 48 hours minimum a year required by attending a refresher course.[11] For those volunteering as nursing auxiliaries the time obligation differed considerably because of the training element. It involved a part-time commitment of 100 hours over a period of 9 months, for which loss of earnings of up to twenty shillings a day was claimable. Once nursing auxiliaries had completed their training programme they were then required to give at least 48 hours service whole-time or part-time in a hospital each year remunerated at the appropriate scales applied to the regular nursing profession.[12]

However, viewed from the perspective of the immediate post-war world, the terms simply furthered both the uncertainty and state intrusion most people were attempting to forget. The awkward conflict between peace and war particularly arose with all recruits subjected to a medical examination, the only civil defence service with this requirement. Although representations complained that the standard of the examinations should not be the same as for permanent staff entrants, the Ministry of Health stood firm on the issue. This decision not to compromise came about because of adverse experiences in the Second World War when considerable numbers of the Civil Nursing Reserve could not undertake their hospital duties due unfitness. Encompassed by that stiff regime, both categories of nurse were also required to undergo X-ray and Mantoux tests to assess possible latent tuberculosis and to check their resistance.[13]

Initially, the underlying need for the NHSR as a war organisation received an impetus with the onset of the Korean War. Presenting a risk the war would spill over into another global conflict brought the appeal for nurses into a sudden reality. Campaign slogans asked, 'How long have we got?' and 'Suppose there is a next time?' Linked to catch phrases lifted from speeches by the Prime Minister, Home Secretary and the Parliamentary Under-Secretary of State for the Home Office these appeals left little doubt the word missing related to 'war'. Prime Minister Atlee's warning 'The fire that has been started in Korea may burn down your house' represented some of the starkest rhetoric since the Second World War.[14] By the time the campaign themes filtered down into the local scene the war message could be harsh. For example, the Wrexham, Powys and Mawddach Hospital Management Committee agreed a letter should be handed out to hospital visitors and outpatients during their recruitment campaign expressing the following sentiments:

> Dear Visitor
> <u>National Hospital Service Reserve</u>
> Can you picture what would happen in this Hospital if we were again at War?
> Civilian casualties from aerial attacks would make such big demands on the staff that only the worst cases might be attended to. Others could end fatally through lack of early treatment. It is, therefore, essential that you should volunteer as a part-time helper for training in First Aid and Home Nursing. Don't wait till hostilities have started, you may reproach yourself if you do.
> See the Matron or one of the Sisters now.[15]

Certainly, the Korean War fought between 27 June 1950 and 27 July 1953 provided patriotic capital towards mustering some support towards the 100,000 figure. Despite its influence and intense campaigning on a scale impossible to sustain under normal peacetime conditions, the results amounted to not much more than a third of the target. Many hospitals caught the spirit of enthusiasm prescribed by the Ministry, but a distinct problem developed between the effort expended and results achieved.

Illustrating how painfully unproductive even the most strong and high profile campaign could be is borne out by the plan South Warwickshire Hospital Group, as part of the Birmingham Regional Hospital Board, put in place. To break what was called the 'marked apathy' of the public, Lady Louis Mountbatten was invited to speak at the Town Hall Leamington Spa on 31 October, 1950 as a prelude to a comprehensive civil defence campaign.[16] Set up to be in every sense a community project, it could not have been more aggressively promoted and represents a typical social trail of how such efforts developed. Six cinemas: the Regal, Leamington Spa; Picture House, Stratford-on-Avon; Warwick Cinema; Regent Cinema, Warwick and the Alexandra Theatre, also in Warwick all agreed to show slides advertising the meeting. The Bishop of Coventry cooperated and asked his ministers to publicise the event during their services. Advertisements were placed in five local newspapers, posters distributed to the pubs of all the major brewers including Mitchells and Butlers, Ansells, Flowers, Atkinsons and Thornleys. Senior girls' schools and the Mothers' Union were targeted with notices advertising lectures on first aid at the Pump Room, Leamington Spa which were to run for nearly two weeks.[17] Only one departure from the schedule occurred which involved changing the film to be shown at the opening of the campaign. A documentary about Hiroshima did not seem appropriate to the occasion and duly replaced by the 'Hamburg Fire Storm'! It mattered not and although no greater effort could have been expended, the exercise only managed to attract 23 recruits, an outcome that merely reinforced the inherent problem of apathy.[18]

Concerns inevitably began to grow about the future prospects of promoting the NHSR under peacetime conditions as a civil defence organisation being prepared for war. Worryingly, even reducing the training time to 80 hours in 9 months for nursing auxiliaries seemed to have no effect.[19] A senior official of the Government's Central Office of Information had no doubts about the approach demanded. In a truly prophetic plea to his superiors he suggested remedial action must be taken and gave his reasons:

> To state my case for the last time - nursing and First Aid has quite a strong appeal to women, and as has been said many times the training they receive with both the St John's and the Red Cross, is of considerable value in peacetime. On the other hand an appeal to become part of the C.D. Organisation is not particularly attractive at the present time. People worry about whether they are being committed to take a particular course of action in the event of war, and because they do not know where they will be, or what their home conditions will be should a war break out at some indeterminate date in the future, they are repelled by the idea of taking part.[20]

Forced by a realisation women were positively troubled, if not frightened, about the war issue, the spin doctors pondered how the recruitment message ought to slanted more towards peacetime priorities. Growing evidence suggested good results were possible for NHSR recruitment purposes by focussing on first aid and home nursing to meet everyday emergencies. The psychological profile of women and their potential attraction to joining the Reserve was being increasingly seen as a connected system of thought starting off with the assumption they had a hatred of war and everything to do with it, so the idea for preparing for it could not be entertained. But if women could be persuaded that learning first aid and home nursing were useful peacetime skills for dealing with everyday emergencies involving family or friends and when trained women could also help at the local hospital, then they would eventually be more amenable to changing their stance on the war issue.[21]

In sympathy with that philosophy, two slogans emerged which became iconic sentiments associated with the NHSR. The first involved the 'would you know what to do' campaign that played on accidents in the home, on the roads and at work. Eventually, this approach focussed on calamities involving children such as falling off a tree or scalded by a saucepan tipping over from a stove. The second referred to the 'help your local hospital' theme with its distinctive moralistic connotation of tending the local sick. Exhortations of this kind promised personal empowerment in the family and community that possessed woman appeal, though acknowledged they did little to attract male nurses. As to the 'war' problem, Regional Hospital Boards were given complete discretion to emphasise the need for helping local hospitals without direct reference to wartime functions on the basis the Ministry felt 'that a decision on this point be left to local committees in the light of local needs and conditions'.[22] With the possibility of the war message being subdued, a new kind of pseudo social violence appeared to gain ground based on a theme of domestic vulnerability that played, with increasing intensity, on the insecurity of women in the home often through quite horrific images.

A growing air of crisis about the recruitment position also pushed the conditions for service towards a revamp for a third time. As part of the new psychology, the rules for joining the Reserve became more accessible to 'busy' women. Hospital training reduced to just 60 hours, nearly half of the original obligation for raw recruits.[23] Terms associated with wartime service were purged, at the top of the list being a mobility questionnaire requiring recruits to indicate their potential capability for wartime service, although the medical examination stubbornly persisted. Then, the message to underwrite the 'civilianisation' process came with a policy of intrusion which at times bordered on social harassment.[24] Local exercises as near to hospitals as possible were to be undertaken and everyday life suddenly became confronted by a rash of new social imagery. Special cut-out display units showing first aid and home nursing scenes in action were designed intended for use at departmental store counters. The popularity of the cinema did not escape attention. Special cinema slides presenting local information and trailer films for showing during intervals became an important component of the persuasion process.[25]

Women were the main target of the campaigns: the use of a women to women appeal adopted in the early 1950s through the glamourous Miss Pat Hornsby-Smith, the Parliamentary Secretary to the Minister of Health. She took on the role of arch-seductress by weaving the message in all kinds of ways, even recording a gramophone record for broadcasting at public gatherings, including football matches. An internal note on the approach admitted: 'The point on which we are now laying the greatest stress is the usefulness of the training to the ordinary citizen in peacetime as we feel that this likely to be a greater draw than preparation for the war which everyone hopes will never come'.[26]

Every speech Hornsby-Smith delivered linked something with the first aid theme whether it involved the NHSR helping in the flood relief operations or the flu epidemic of the 1950s. During the Korean War, she particularly attempted to isolate women as potential shirkers. National Servicemen were doing their bit so it was right, she reasoned, women should take their share of the burden through national service in the NHSR. Not an opportunity went by to draw such inferences. Speaking at a recruitment drive at Reigate, Surrey on 2 February 1953, the day after the North Sea Flood disaster killed 307 people in the counties of Lincolnshire, Norfolk, Suffolk and Essex, she wove war, natural disaster and home emergencies into a single propaganda bundle with the speech notes being titled 'Let Women Combat Apathy':

> Once again I am appealing to the women of Britain to give a lead against apathy. So often people say 'of course I'd do my bit in an emergency' and by emergency they mean war. But how wrong they are to think of emergencies only in terms of war. On this tragic day when many families are mourning the loss of loved ones: when the fury of nature has killed or injured hundreds and rendered thousands of unfortunate people homeless, we have a savage reminder that danger and destruction can overtake us without warning and how valuable it is to know what to do and how to do it until such time as skilled medical aid arrives. Our best defence against all emergencies is to be ready. Our slogan is: 'We can't be certain but we can and must be ready.' Now is the time to join.[27]

Hornsby-Smith added the usual theme that there were about one and a half million accidents in the home and another half a million on the roads, so learning first aid in the Reserve might provide the means of saving or preventing serious injury. Her audacity probably reached its most brash point when she suggested the NHSR logo actually represented a peace symbol when she made presentations of membership badges at Lambeth Hospital, London:

> These badges are an outward symbol that you are doing something active and practical in the cause of peace. By sacrificing a little of your leisure you are setting a fine example to your fellow citizens. And in helping the cause of peace – I am convinced that the surest way of preventing war is to be prepared – you are also learning nursing skills that may save life or relieve pain amid the hazards of everyday life, whether in the home, street, factory or office.[28]

Extending the psychological war game further, the Ministry of Health especially wanted the high street to become a campaign arena and devised a new marketing strategy to tempt the British public accordingly. This came with the theme 'Peace has its emergencies no less than war' and began with a Mobile First Aid Unit driven through the streets of London before arriving outside Fortress House, an imposing building occupied the Ministry in Savile Row. The MFAU team were inspected by the Minister of Health and then undertook a twenty-minute demonstration called EXCERCISE SAVILE in front of BBC television and radio, as well as newsreel cameras. The site became the edge of an atom bomb explosion with the ensuing action illustrating three serious casualties receiving treatment before being loaded onto an ambulance and two lightly-injured casualties given first aid and cups of tea and told to report to their local doctor, if necessary. A woman with hysteria ended the performance by being diagnosed as unfit to go home and also bundled into the ambulance for hospital attention.[29] Apart from the scale of optimism that even hysterics would be treated, such an intrusion into the street scene actually represented a good allegory of the way the campaign was to assail people in their everyday lives.

This single spark of promotional exuberance was to ignite the whole country and cause a blaze of social intrusion of a kind never seen before. A typical 'incident', which characterised the new urban scenery, raised Wrexham Church Street to the status of a nuclear battlefield. The war started with the explosion of a firework to attract the attention of startled passers-by. They then witnessed three casualties suddenly falling to the ground and within ninety seconds saw the arrival of a first aid unit duly summoned by a Civil Defence Corps warden who had been on the spot. Presented as live theatre on the streets, the public became an unwitting audience to nurses and doctors springing out of vans and giving treatment to a variety of wounds that included facial burns, concussion and a deep gash in the leg. Twelve minutes after the detonation of the firework, the wounded and the nurses were gone, but not before the onlookers were then harangued by an NHSR salesman who appealed for the need for everyone being prepared for an emergency explaining that, 'by emergency we mean war, pit disasters, rail or road accidents'.[30]

Seeking out every opportunity to deliver the civilian side of the NHSR story, the shop window display became a popular format and the nationalised industries with a high street presence offered help and made their gas or electricity showrooms available. Shop owners, equally anxious to express their patriotic duty, also volunteered retail space, a notable example evident in displays the Hackney, London Group of Hospital planned on two days in May 1952. Importantly, the theme showed the value of the NHSR to hospitals in times of peace and the point stressed, 'there was as little reference as possible to emergency, crisis and war'. Exploiting this tactical line to the full, one window display took the form of an operating theatre with mock operations performed whilst a ward scene demonstrated the bedside training of nurses and auxiliaries. Another tableau included a display of a premature babies unit together with a nursing mother and live baby. In a summary of the campaign the results, which amounted to gaining 103 recruits, were described as 'surprisingly good' and drew attention to the formula applied of no war with stress laid on the direct association to local hospitals. Moreover, the conclusion also suggested the exercise had disproved the general view subsisting that the East End of London represented barren recruiting territory.[31]

During 1952, the year of the Queen's accession, over 10,000 recruits had joined, the highest number for any year since the establishment of the Reserve with the membership increasing from 19,060 to 29,265. By 1954, the Ministry felt there was an opportunity to emphasise the companionship that the Reserve also offered. The Ministry's advertising agents translated this into a campaign by introducing a 'coupon' appeal with a booklet sent out written by 'a popular figure well known to and respected by women'.[32] Marian Cutler, a prominent journalist and broadcaster of the day, became the anchor for this purpose and the pamphlet given the title 'In good company' chosen to convey the usefulness and social benefits of the Reserve.[33] Advertised widely in women's magazines, the initiative produced what were considered very good results. 'Good results' by this time clearly had taken on a new meaning since by the end of the year the membership rose to 40,853, not even half the target. The only consolation in the figures lay in the fact they represented stable, if not spectacular growth and altogether much preferable to a position of decline.

Unfortunately, the somewhat pragmatic sounding principle of stable growth turned out to be short-lived. Attempting to improve the situation a shift away from the classless and ageless message occurred and moved the target audience towards the younger single women, men, to let them know they were needed, and finally the older woman whose family had grown up. However, in the background lurked a distinct nervousness about the need for nothing to go wrong, given the pressure to achieve better results. Already embarrassing mistakes had occurred. Trained nurses, for example, had resented a leaflet used to target retired colleagues with a banner heading 'Train in your spare time'. Unfortunately, more trouble was waiting in the wings and in the marketing push that had so much riding on it, a booklet on first aid sent free to those responding shook the NHSR administration close to destruction. Thousands of replies came in which added to the shock. The response mainly reflected the desire of people simply to obtain the first aid information without any intention of joining the Reserve. Many of the respondents, particularly men over 65, had sought to get hints on medical matters and over the age to join. The consequences were almost the last straw on account of the volume of follow up enquiries that were quite unrelated to gaining recruits and described as an 'unwarrantable burden' on the goodwill of volunteers. Publicly the NSHR were criticised as 'wastepaper' generators as the following complaint by a woman living in Bedford attested:

> I filled up the little advertisement as it said it would give hints for people who had accidents in the home. As I am 73 and a diabetic, I have had several bad black outs and live alone, I thought it would be useful to me as burns and scalds are treated in the same way as they were before. I had a very bad accident last year and was severely burnt and scalded, and my wounds were not allowed to be covered up, so I thought your information might be useful, but I found it was nothing but a recruitment drive. I naturally did not answer it, and I thought you would grasp from that I was not interested and I have had 3 lots of literature from you, it seems a great waste of stamps.[34]

Furthermore, the failure to make any great impact on the recruiting figures caused massive tensions between the various organisational factions that started a blame game rolling which never stopped. The figure of suspicion was menacingly pointed in the direction of hospital matrons. In less-than-amenable terms the Ministry of Health suggested: 'The poor results so far achieved in many areas have been attributed to a number of causes, and frequently to lack of knowledge of or interest in the Reserve on the part of matrons and other officers who may be called upon to take an active part in the enrolment or training of members'. Matrons, however, were in an invidious position, often accused of causing students to lose interest by confining training duties to minor nursing techniques and the serving of meals. Naturally, they did come out fighting to defend their professional integrity by pointing out where students only attended in the evenings as patients were settling down for the night they could not participate in procedures begun earlier in the day. Nursing seriously-ill patients needed continuity and also in their defence, matrons mentioned nursing auxiliaries would often more than not turn up after work which coincided with visiting times that all made it difficult to create an environment conducive to tuition.[35] Conversely, the official list of training duties for auxiliaries did not exactly represent spare time interest material. It included all aspects of bed making, giving bedpans, observation of stools and urine, preparing simple meals and cooking in ward kitchens.[36]

The voluntary societies also attracted a great deal of criticism. Their manifest of wickedness mentioned losing recruits by keeping them waiting for courses, or simply not bothering to recruit at all. Without a shadow of a doubt, however, the most insidious and damaging situation related to the 'bolshie' air of discontent which prevailed in some quarters over the thorny question of uniform. A deep-seated attitude problem particularly arose from one of the principles enshrined in the founding charter of the NHSR that it was not to have its own special outfit. Trained nurses received the normal uniform attire of the hospital they served on loan, an arrangement that did not attract controversy. Really the major problem came from the auxiliary side where members of the public had to borrow the uniform of either the St John Ambulance or Red Cross, depending on which they were attached to for training purposes.[37] The main, and indeed only, distinction of civil defence service was an armband with a special NHSR logo attached. At first, it had been felt the use of uniforms in this way might have discouraged recruitment in some regions of the country, particularly in working-class areas in the north-west as well as in Durham and West Riding. Soon it appeared the society members themselves actually represented the main antagonists against the arrangement. Long-standing trained first aiders were seeing their uniforms issued to untrained individuals who were not required to respect their ranks and in the final instance had no obligation to take up formal membership.[38]

During 1954 the Ministry announced the issue of personal uniforms at a cost of £300,000, but the change did nothing to improve the underlying resentments festering within the societies.[39] The new arrangement did not alter the fact nursing auxiliaries still wore the uniform of the voluntary society through which they were receiving their training. Within the Ministry, a great debate had ensued about the advocacy of continuing to issue society uniforms, or whether an entirely new uniform should be created to show greater allegiance to the Reserve. No answer was ever found. The issue simply left an emotive uncertainty hanging over the organisation summed up in the following few words pulled out of the thousands written on the subject:

> The arguments against the Reserve being dressed in voluntary organisation uniforms are that the absence of a special uniform is a great obstacle to our building up a corporate spirit in the Reserve. This lack of a corporate spirit means, inter alia, that Reserve members who are also voluntary organisation members often tend to treat their voluntary organisation commitments as having priority.[40]

Essentially, the Ministry of Health was hostage to an impossible situation. Having no common uniform continuously ate away at the cohesion of the Reserve, but introducing a standard design then seriously risked destroying the organisation through a possible backlash by the 14,000 regular voluntary society members.

Another issue also took its toll on the cohesion of the organisation. A competition called the Minster's Challenge Cup appeared in 1953 intended to stress the national credentials of the NHSR and test the skills of those interested in war gaming. After regional competitions, winners would fight for the national accolade, the first event of this kind staged on Horse Guards Parade in London, with the appropriate silverware presented by the Minister of Health. It continued there for the next two years, but in 1956 moved to an indoor venue for the first time at the Friends House in the Euston Road, London. The transfer could not have been more symbolic between the military connotations of Horse Guards Parade and the Friends House run by the Quakers, a religious organisation opposed to war! For these events the format involved hospital teams consisting of a doctor, a trained nurse and eight NHSR auxiliaries driving into the arena with their equipment van and then setting up a temporary first aid post in a mock building where they would proceed to treat a number of casualties brought to them by civil defence wardens and stretcher-bearers. The first such event under cover involved a hydrogen attack centred on Woolwich with spreading fires, extensive damage and heavy casualties assumed. The teams had to deal with ten casualties within ten minutes and at twenty minutes ordered to evacuate their post because of fire. An unscripted diversion at five minutes erupted when a man rushed in calling for help to rescue some people who were actually trapped nearby, the moment turning into a comic farce when a team mistook him for a case of hysteria.[41]

Appearance rather than substance accounted for much in this kind of display to show medical efficacy on the nuclear battleground, or at least, the nuclear battleground defined by the Ministry of Health. Making up the nuclear victim established an important ritual requiring an organisation called the Casualties Union to apply their expertise on volunteer casualties. Founded on the back of the rescue training arrangements in the Second World War, its members would simulate injuries and instruct the casualty how to react.[42] There seemed something invidious that the expenses of such theatrical application were permissible, whilst doctors did not qualify for any payment towards the considerable time and effort necessary to prepare their hospital teams. Of course, in many respects, the exercise did resemble a theatrical production and local newspapers loved it and led to headlines such as 'Tomato Sauce Adds Flavour to CD Display – Injuries Made to Order'.[43]

Because of the situation described, the success of hospitals to participate in competitions depended very much on their ability to secure the services of sympathetic doctors to give up their time without charge. Some areas were lucky enough to gain that important support, whilst others failed, a factor that could have a demoralising effect on NHSR members to see a lack of commitment from the top.[44] On the other side, the task for medical professionals more often than not became thankless where the contrived circumstances of the competition could lead to embarrassing situations, well-illustrated by the following report to the Ministry made after an incident:

> Our Medical Officer, who is a Registrar in the Westminster Group, has asked me to make a mild protest about the asphyxia case – there was a similar one last year where the circumstances were also the same. He did not order artificial respiration in either year – because the patient was obviously breathing – and the team lost all their marks last year and most of them this year. He contends that makeup in such cases is not a sufficient indication that breathing is inhibited or difficult, and as this cannot be faked, there should be some marking such as is always done when a pulse rate has to be drawn attention to. The M.O. says that in real life there would be no possibility of error to a doctor, and the makeup signs are ambiguous. In any case, he points out that even if there were a fault, it was due to him personally, and not to his team. Presumably it was not his capabilities as a doctor which were being judged.[45]

Even the image of team building suffered as the competitive spirit turned into open warfare between the voluntary societies themselves. Manchester noted the tendency existed for hospitals to choose the most proficient St John or Red Cross members for Mobile First Aid Unit duties because they were the highly qualified. So endemic had the problem become that even Whitehall recognised this as an idiosyncrasy where the breach between the two organisations actually risked alienating the interest of non-voluntary organisation personnel who had become to feel 'out of it'.[46]

Continually balancing such sensitivities, coupled with the disparate system of recruitment and membership, was not conducive to the creation of a strong and confident organisation. Underneath the propagandised picture of the NHSR as a cohesive social club, yet medically capable, was nothing more than a myth. Pockets of exceptional devotion, skill and motivation, of course, existed. To some women it meant escaping loneliness; one hospital in reporting the death of an NHSR member noted: 'Miss R.J.Solomon was a loyal and conscientious member for two and a half years and assisted the organiser in every way. She attended all meetings in the area and was in charge of refreshments: she used her holidays for recruitment'.[47] However, such devotion to duty was not consistently spread throughout the organisation. Many Regional Hospital Boards confessed to including nurses in their membership returns who had lost interest, or had even left. The system was in many respects off-kilter with the new age. Volunteers were leaving because of increased domestic responsibilities, particularly if pressure had been applied to take part in exercises or competitions. In rural areas, the usual difficulties of transport and getting courses together came high on the list of excuses. Voluntary societies stood accused of undue preoccupation with their own interests, whilst hospitals maintained they did not have the equipment or doctors to build up a properly trained medical organisation consistent with the aim of the Reserve as a national organisation. Everything amounted to the indisputable fact the NHSR had degenerated into a dysfunctional institution heading quickly towards self-destruction.

Chaos Rules

What became an extraordinary piece of historical theatre is the way senior Ministry of Health officials reacted to the problem of the hydrogen bomb, which slowly turned into a tragic farce when attempts to pull the organisation out of its spiral of decline actually created greater chaos. Like all other civil defence organisations, the NHSR endured its own a phase of introspection so the implications of the new weapon could be fully considered. A distinctly problematic situation confronting the disparate state of the NHSR concerned the changing face of war that really demanded ever more swathes of nursing staff gathered up to comply with the principle of logic. But even the target figure of 100,000 additional nurses and nursing auxiliaries seemed unattainable. For more than two years the membership of the Reserve stood between 43,000 and 44,000 and showed little sign of increasing very much beyond this. More and more reliance had been placed on recruitment campaigns to cover losses, but even this revolving-door policy appeared to reach a dangerous tipping point where it only just worked. Neither did the training statistics offer much encouragement. Only a quarter of the membership had actually gone through the whole process of training and the hospital experience. Instead, thousands were still waiting to start their initial programme. Most damning of all was the fact that up to 60% of the auxiliary membership had no hospital background experience whatsoever under their belt. The results, therefore, not only fell far short of the recruitment target by some 60,000, but they also lacked the skilled nucleus the arrangements had always intended to provide.[48]

Against this lacklustre picture, Regional Hospital Board officials received a summons to attend a special meeting in London on 24 May 1957. They faced a Ministry of Health in a rare state of self-criticism and more to the point self-doubt about the whole NHSR arrangement, which represented half the Ministry's total civil defence budget.[49] A senior civil servant expressed his view about the organisation being a culture based on 'bed pan rounds' and even went further to suggest: 'He had never believed that under the present set-up any hospital organisation in the hurly-burly of civilian and hospital evacuation would be able to get hold of more than a small proportion of the NHSR and there would be much administrative advantage of the Ministry ending this charade'.[50] Notwithstanding the rare wobble, the one thing not going to happen was any kind of public acknowledgment about the true state of play. New rules of the game had to be made up, and as quickly as possible.

The Ministry of Health first considered a change that would mean relying entirely on the voluntary societies for the provision of auxiliaries from their own ranks and scrapping the recruitment of the public altogether. The UK was one of the few countries where a separate nursing organisation had been trained for civil defence purposes, but the grass also looked particularly greener on the other side. The total adult membership of the St. John Ambulance Brigade and the British Red Cross Society stood at somewhere in the region of 110,000 people. Of this total only 13,000 had joined the National Hospital Service Reserve and 6,000 were members of the Civil Defence Corps giving support to the Ambulance and First Aid Sections. Some of the remainder, the theorising went, may have been precluded because of their society commitments, but there still remained a considerable balance of some 50,000 to 60,000 members who were fully trained in first aid and home nursing, plus having practical experience. Furthermore, the societies had a strong following in junior members that amounted to some 107,000, an impressive figure and a source of great potential.[51]

Acknowledging the old regime could never deliver the target of 100,000, the only way out of the problem seemed to point in the direction of waiving the requirement of compulsory hospital training and the membership of a separate organisation. As a means of removing these perceived obstacles an idea that the two voluntary aid societies might create a 'wartime only' membership emerged as the best way to structure the illusion of further growth. With a solution of this nature in mind, the Ministry persuaded themselves: 'We would be reasonably certain of having 100,000 bodies on the day. It is considered that this would constitute a much more realistic answer to the problem of the staffing of our hospitals in wartime. On paper we would be reducing our standards of training but in practice, having regard to the present training returns, it is doubtful whether we would lose much, if anything at all'. Grasping at every possible straw why this should work, the Ministry also felt that in a nuclear emergency it would be difficult anyway to make a transition to war and muster all the auxiliaries into the hospitals sufficiently quickly. In respect of trained nurses, the importance of scrapping training was also felt essential if it meant such a move could provide lists of those retired nurses willing to come forward in an emergency.[52]

To convert those ideas into practice, the Ministry of Health proposed the membership of the National Hospital Service Reserve 'should be thrown open'. Openness was to be unconditional and extended to all suitable members of the two societies who would no longer have to undergo compulsory training, but hospital and Mobile First Aid Unit training could be offered by hospitals if the societies wished it. Conceptually the idea moved towards the creation of a 'nursing cooperative' from which Regional Hospital Boards would be able to take up their requirements. Something vaguely referred to as 'special arrangements' were proposed for those auxiliaries not members of the societies that probably meant an ultimatum to join them. In the final semantic contortion, it was felt such a package had a place without abandoning the principles behind the nursing concept by producing 'a' National Hospital Service Reserve rather than reliance on 'the' National Hospital Service Reserve.[53]

Scotland reacted unfavourably and considered they were not open to the same criticism since the societies in their country purged at regular intervals those recruits who had not proceeded with their training. There were also other concerns. Citing their experiences with the Civil Nursing Reserve during the last war, the Scottish Department expressed its reluctance to hand over any more responsibility to the Red Cross on social grounds. They maintained: 'Up here at any rate there is a snob element in the voluntary aid detachments and we have some reason to think that not everyone who applies to join them gets accepted or rejected solely on merit.'[54] The idea also came under the scrutiny of an informal committee which brought together Dame Elizabeth Cockayne, Chief Nursing Officer, General William Dimond from Whitehall (an ex-Indian Army physician) and representatives from the Ministry of Health. Crucially, all those involved signed the minutes of the meeting that contained a collective unease encapsulated in a joint statement saying: 'Our main fear was that if we rushed into this without more information as the likely response we would run the risk of exchanging the substance for the shadow'. Worries especially arose about the proposed scheme alienating the independent volunteers of the NHSR who were not actually members of a society and the societies themselves then being uncooperative. A distinct nervousness also remained about the operational value of the societies themselves. Rather disparagingly it was felt their service potential might have to be quite heavily discounted on account of the numbers in the 'varicose veins' and 'flat footed' category who would find it difficult to keep up to the rigours of nuclear war.[55]

Any remaining doubts about keeping a cadre of NHSR volunteers linked to hospitals independently from the voluntary societies dissolved completely when the Regional Hospital Boards themselves added their concerns about the prospect of jeopardising future control over the recruitment message and its delivery:

> There is also clear evidence in the success of recruitment by hospitals on the theme 'help in your local hospital and gain valuable personal training at the same time.' This insures against failure through the dis-attractions of the Societies, and the C.D. theme. Civil Defence aspects are apparent enough to the member after the initial approach has been overcome, and are then accepted as subordinate to the members' main desired to help in the hospital.[56]

Observations of this kind vividly illustrate the emotional trickery women had suffered whereby war had been hidden to secure their allegiance through local hospitals and what the control factor meant. Confronted by the situation described, the Ministry of Health proceeded instead to coax the most out of the existing convoluted system towards gaining the magic figure of 100,000 nurses. The main thrust of their strategy involved a bulk membership deal with the two societies, but with the unattached class provided by the public retained as a precaution against failure.[57] To this end, the voluntary aid societies were absolved of their past sins, the two most mortally significant relating to their belligerence over uniforms and a reluctance to join the NHSR in large numbers.[58]

The new rules allowed society members to enrol in the Reserve as complete units or detachments and on the basis of lists furnished to local NHSR committees. Admission of trained nurses no longer demanded any requirement to undertake refresher courses, or for that matter any other commitments. As for training, the idealistic strictures of the past were removed and everything came down to the flimsy word 'encouragement' in the hope that lectures and exercises would be undertaken voluntarily to maintain interest. Basically, the change amounted to a secretly acknowledged ruse to build up potential contacts and numbers by attracting those no longer active in nursing, but who would come forward in war as they did in peacetime emergencies. Changes for the auxiliary not wishing to become a member of a society were especially illuminating for the way they attempted to pull the non-society auxiliaries more into the hospital system. They still had to submit to initial training in home nursing and first aid, but the new arrangements laid great stress that courses should be held at hospital premises, rather than at those of the societies. Secondly, and even more vital to the hospital connection, recruits in this category were to take a short introductory course totalling 6 hours, possible to complete simultaneously with the initial training programme. Obviously, the intention was to end the long time that often elapsed before a recruit might see the inside of a hospital. On the flip side, further hospital training afterwards remained purely discretionary and left again to the realm of 'encouragement'.[59]

Embraced by a new spirit of leniency wartime service for all, members received a further measure of watering-down and redefined as an obligation to be undertaken to 'the best of their ability', a sugary phrase that had little in common with the protocols previously imposed. Even the medical examination finally disappeared although authorities had the right to exclude those whom they considered to be medically unfit and an overriding right to demand it if circumstances seemed appropriate. Apart from that, the package bordering on the permissive was glued together by a preference for a club tie atmosphere to prevail which hospitals were asked to support in the following way:

> Links with the hospital should be fostered by every means----National Hospital Service Reserve Associations, social activities, etc. Members must be made to feel that they are truly a 'reserve' of the hospital and it is particularly important that the St

John and Red Cross Divisions and Detachments whose members join under the new arrangements should be made to feel part of the family.[60]

Notwithstanding the membership rules being diluted to the point of absurdity, the promise of great numbers flooding never did materialise and over two years only some 10,000 additional society members were recruited. The outcome completely justified the earlier suggestion that the recruitment of the general public to serve in an independent capacity should not be abandoned. Worse still, what should have been a simplification of the system creating harmony, actually led to greater divisions. It is fair to say that by 1960 the illusion of increased membership started to unravel. Time exposed serious flaws with the new system eventually described as 'unduly complicated and confusing'. The new rules merely served to create a complete rift between hospitals and the societies. On the one hand they drove the lack of liaison between the voluntary aid societies and hospitals ever further, and on the other those concerned in hospitals found fewer and fewer hospital staff willing to help with the training of the NHSR.[61]

Exasperatingly, even the figure of a 10,000 increase in numbers since the new arrangements began was considered largely fictional, much blame put at the feet of the British Red Cross Society, the Ministry of Health itself remarking that the BRCS 'did not fully appreciate the problems of hospital authorities'.[62] Using the term 'sponsored' for the self-certified members of the societies particularly irritated the Regional Hospital Boards more and more because they felt the societies had too much power and virtually everything to do with the Reserve required approval by them. Moreover, the sponsored designation had in many cases severed any kind of direct communication between such members and hospitals to the extent their recruitment statistics were stated to be 'far from reliable as an indication of either the strength or state of qualification of the Reserve'.[63] Without a shred of doubt, the organisation exhibited all the signs of drowning in a sea of ineptitude as it struggled harder to save itself. Accusations made in some areas that local society officers were intentionally sabotaging the scheme by starving Regional Hospital Boards of any information about membership numbers indicated the inherent nature of the problems that the rules could never overcome.[64]

The Home and Health Department in Scotland, which for many years claimed it had maintained control of the situation, proved to be equally vulnerable. When Mary Macdonald, Assistant Secretary, took a forensic look at the position in her department during 1963, the extent to which the organisation had been allowed to deteriorate is illustrated in her acerbic reaction to the situation she had uncovered:

> I have heard the term 'malaise' used of the NHSR, but to me it seems that the root of the trouble is not disaffection, but organisational weakness. In the first place, we - and I include the Department in this - have simply not faced up to the demands which an organisation of this kind makes in terms of day-to-day work, and we have not provided for the required number of paid appointments. Secondly, the organisation itself creaks. I have been appalled, in looking over the files, to see the amount of time and labour that has been put into devising reorganisations of the NHSR without commensurate success in improving recruitment or training. If any lesson is to be learned, it is surely that we must simplify and lay down as clearly as possible the respective fields of responsibility of everyone concerned.[65]

From the Scottish meltdown, the sheer sense of frustration about the attitude of the Ministry of Health becomes all too evident. To the Scots' minds, London also had a lot to answer for in the manipulation of the nuclear message and suggested the Ministry had been devious to a point where the situation urgently demanded more transparency:

> We do not doubt that the emphasis in the existing posters on the immediate and practical uses of NHSR training, e.g. in dealing with home accidents, is an effective line with many people. There is nothing in this, however, which an interested member of the public cannot equally well get as a member of one of the voluntary aid societies, and we are wondering if there is not something to be said for making freer use of the appeal of the more advanced training given to FMAU teams to which the voluntary aid societies can offer no counterpart. In other words could we not perhaps in one trial poster, relax our strict refusal to admit the NHSR has anything to do with war? I note that the leaflets at present in use, certainly in Scotland, are perfectly frank about the wartime angle and the kind of obligations that NHSR members might have to accept in war.[66]

Scotland's reaction to the governance of the Ministry of Health confirms the degree to which the stealth factor had become endemic in the whole approach to managing the National Hospital Service Reserve and its nuclear war connection. Even in 1966 and 1967 the recruiting campaign theme 'Would you know what to do' used for many years only slightly altered to 'Would you know how to help'. Learning first aid and 'practical' nursing still underpinned everything, including the means of helping the local hospital. Furthermore, the NHSR treatment became the route for dealing with an increasing list of situations including panic and road injuries, but never the real terror of nuclear war. If these themes bordered on moral blackmail, the spin-doctors crossed the line in 1965 with a poster to attract trained nurses with the slogan 'once a nurse' showing a hand holding a pair of surgical scissors, but still no mention of war.[67]

For all that, the drudgery issue refused to go away. An article published in the *Nursing Times* during 1961 titled 'Nurses Galore!' summed up the situation that existed in a great many places. Written by a ward sister, she admitted her reaction to Red Cross and St John's nurses had originally been unenthusiastic, but acknowledged with the right encouragement and involvement in nursing they had become useful in the life of the hospital and certainly made her life a lot easier:

> I had no thought at all of improving my own ward conditions. The motive was simply to ensure that what I had taught would stay put, and in fact I had so many doubts that I apologized to my staff nurses for burdening them with these novices. But a week or two later all misgivings were forgotten. Life in the ward was sheer bliss! The staff complement had gone up by 30! Although these women (some of them were in their fifties) only came for two hours each week it meant that we could all relax a little - the pressure of work was eased.[68]

However, the punch-line added that on seeing life becoming less stressful in one section, the assistant matron transferred the auxiliaries to hard pressed wards where they were then set what the writer referred to as 'the old tasks of washing up, seeing to flowers, and cutting bread and butter', after which they stopped attending.[69]

Quite simply, when it came down to a choice between projecting domestic drudgery and nuclear carnage, the predisposition of the Ministry of Health always veered towards the former and unsurprisingly so. During

1959 *Operation Shuttlecock* was introduced as a high-adrenalin, high-impact training film showing the support given by the NHSR to a Forward Medical Aid Unit. It presented a large scale exercise held at Sandown Park in Surrey that involved the setting up and operation of a FMAU linked to a forward and rear shuttle of ambulances conveying the nuclear injured chosen for hospitalisation. Naturally, the contrived speed and efficiency of the drills set out to illustrate how the casualty problem could be hoovered up with little difficulty. For all its optimism, the display did still visualise the medical position with an uncomfortable message a world away from the kind of recruitment imagery that oozed compassion. Casualty abandonment entered the frame more literally with the commentary describing the mechanics of the unit:

> The casualties are received in this area, stretchers placed on trestles for examination and diagnosis by a doctor. Those who need to be sent to hospital but require no immediate treatment will go straight through to 'Disposal'. Those who need some kind of treatment before evacuation will be moved into Treatment Bays. Those who do not need hospital treatment will be discharged to a rest centre, with or without treatment as may be needed. Those not in a condition for immediate removal to hospital, or cannot benefit from hospital treatment, will be taken to the Holding Unit where they will be made as comfortable as possible.[70]

Visualising the idea that seriously injured people could not be hospitalised was radically shocking and with the association of holding units becoming conscience saving dying spaces not particularly the best of images to promote for gaining more nursing volunteers. Predictably, recruiting campaigns buried war ever deeper with a preference for presenting what a trained first aider could do to help in accidents in the home. War as a themed message had become an under the counter affair to be sold only to those interested in a more bellicose vision of the NHSR. Expunging nuclear reality undoubtedly possessed advantages as it turned the NHSR into a more palatable marketing proposition.[71] In 1962, for example, *Woman* magazine, with a circulation of three million, included an article about the Reserve in its hobbies supplement.[72] Another publicity coupe came when the Executive Committee of the National Federation of Women's Institutes agreed all their affiliated Institutes could participate in civil defence. In the past, the general policy of the National Federation had been against Women's Institutes becoming involved in such activities.

Following discussions with the Home Office, however, the National Federation accepted members of the Institute should be encouraged to join the National Hospital Service Reserve with the decree that an Institute may take steps to enable their members to become better informed on how to look after themselves and their children in the event of an emergency.[73]

Driven by this desire to dilute the nuclear war aspect as a means of encouraging recruitment, a real thorn in the side of the Ministry of Health became the Minister's Challenge Cup Competition. The event had been suspended in 1958 and then restarted in 1959 at the Royal Albert Hall.[74] With the Mobile First Aid Unit replaced by the Forward Medical Aid Unit a new competition plan was necessary to devise. The change could not have been a more prickly issue for the Ministry of Health. It held out the prospect of having to confirm publicly a major alteration from the hospital support always promised to the seriously injured to a policy of sorting, a concept completely alien to the British public. The 1960 competition did not take place and the Ministry would have preferred its completed closure. Typical of the situation, the South East Metropolitan Hospital Board complained several hospital groups possessed equipment, trained nurses and NHSR auxiliaries, but still had been unable to secure the services of general medical or even dental practitioners to lead and train the units. The Bromley Hospital Management Committee in Kent expressed the point in the following terms:

> We have explained from time to time that medical officers are needed to train these units and none have been forthcoming for some years although about 20 doctors have been approached. We cannot see the position altering unless we are able to get some public spirited doctors with sufficient time to spare to take on these units or until some financial inducement can be offered: or alternatively, until compulsion can be brought to bear by means of tying in the duties of training mobile first aid units with some of the more junior medical appointments.[75]

Revealing the completely disjointed nature of the NHSR, some regions were strongly of the opinion the competition should continue as a morale boosting exercise, whilst others felt it to be a distraction and a complete waste of time. Although the Ministry acquiesced to keeping the competition, a critical change appeared to the format and instead of being a field-based event its focus turned towards examining hospital procedures within an acute ward. Conveniently, this circumvented the issue of medical problems in the nuclear frontline. It also meant new training systems did not have to be devised that would risk exposing the NHSR as a weak link in the medical chain.[76] To quell any further discontent, the Ministry of Health also employed its signature tactic of suggesting if Regional Hospital Boards wished to conduct their own exercises and experiments they were free to do so.

If anything, the fears the Ministry of Health about the abilities of the NHSR to cope with much more than basic first aid appeared correct as a result of the action taken by Birmingham Regional Hospital Board. They went along with the Ministry's idea and undertook an experimental FMAU competition on Sunday, 8 November 1964 at St Matthew's Hospital, Burntwood, near Lichfield. Awaiting the four competing teams, another more unpleasant ingredient appeared in order to test their nuclear skills with the menacing name of 'relative overload'. This involved an excessive number of tasks in a short period of time that included sorting procedures, extended first aid, nursing tasks, recognition and use of equipment, teamwork and the discipline of the team members, as well as the organising ability of the team leader. Four casualties were involved with wounds ranging from minor injuries to serious complications. Furthermore, one of their number was to exhibit signs of psychological trauma and disrupt the team, with marks then deducted for any distraction leading to incomplete work. The results of the exercise made for precisely the kind of discomforting conclusions the Ministry wanted to hide:

> Although the casualties were realistic and the briefing made clear the extent of the injuries (e.g. arterial haemorrhage) the reactions of the teams were not satisfactory. It appeared that their knowledge was inadequate not only of major conditions (e.g. pneumothorax) but also of simple procedures (e.g. taking a blood pressure measurement, handling oxygen equipment). The teams which competed would normally be considered above average. Their apparent ignorance was thought to be due to the difficult conditions imposed by the rules of the competition. A more leisurely test would no doubt have produced more impressive results. It is considered that this is further evidence of the 'relative overload' principle.[77]

Birmingham's main deduction over the experiment further illustrated the impossibility of tackling the nuclear medical problem through the medium of the NHSR and the overall level of medical competence it possessed. Their report stated: 'The results of this exercise are an emphatic reminder that FMAU nursing duties require a depth and range of knowledge which cannot readily be obtained by personnel who are not undergoing full-time nursing training'.[78] Beset by a whole array of problems it may have seemed odd the organisation managed to exist at all. The fact remained that the NHSR fitted in precisely with the Government standard of achieving visibility at least cost. Many of its overheads were absorbed by the NHS and cost £200,000 p.a., against the £8 million or so to keep the rest of the civil defence services in place.[79] As a national asset its only danger, ironically, seemed to originate in the discretionary arrangements over membership afforded to the voluntary aid societies and these had to be addressed!

A review, ostensibly to strengthen the hospital side of things, was announced by the Ministry of Health which innocently claimed its introduction being necessary 'after fifteen years of experience' with the main focus being on the relationship between the NHSR and the voluntary societies. Given the history, the exercise actually raised a certain inevitability about the outcome. On 10 January 1967, Regional Hospital Boards received a summons to hear the result of the assessment and the Ministry of Health did not disappoint them. It announced its preferred option was to terminate the enrolment and training arrangements of the auxiliary nurses by the voluntary societies and that these aspects would be left entirely in the hands of hospitals. Minutes of the meeting record the hospital representatives being 'unanimous' in their support for this, a position essentially reflecting their long-held view the voluntary societies had too much influence which hindered attempts to bolster the NHSR support for hospitals.[80]

Armed with such a complete empowerment for change, the Ministry of Health summoned the voluntary societies to a meeting in January 1967 that possessed a distinct air of a carefully orchestrated kangaroo court. On the Ministry side sat three male officials representing the civil division and a female nursing officer. From the St John's Brigade they included, Superintendent-in-Chief Marjorie Pratt, Countess of Brecknock and the British Red Cross contingent were led by their Vice-Chairman, Dame Anne Bryans. It was obvious there was to be no surrender to the senior grandees present and three quotes illustrate the charges they collectively faced which amounted to systemic sabotage, inappropriate administration, as well as creating a general state of irreconcilable difficulties:

> The national headquarters of the Societies readily co-operated in ironing out local difficulties which were brought to their attention, but the Ministry's

> officers in their visits to local competitions and meetings had been made aware of many small difficulties which were inherent in the system of divided responsibility and which for various reasons were not brought to the attention of the Ministry or the Societies.[81]
>
> The NHSR is a hospital reserve and the hospital should be the focal point of activity: under the present arrangements the association with a hospital for which many members join the Reserve is usually absent for most of the first year of service, when the member is training with the Voluntary Aid Societies; the Reserve loses members in this period.[82]
>
> The system of divided responsibilities has inherent weaknesses and in the case of the NHSR inevitably breed problems in local organisation, communications and personalities which cannot satisfactorily be cured by liaison machinery. It would be advantageous for the hospital service if the basic training of its Reserve members were more closely directed to the needs of the hospital than can be achieved through the present first aid and home nursing syllabuses.[83]

Despite mounting a staunch defence, the societies met a rehearsed rebuttal of exceptional harshness. Mercilessly, the fatal blow levelled at them came in a statistical line that the auxiliary membership of the NHSR included 26,000 who belonged to the societies, but only 7,500 had secured any kind of hospital experience during the previous year. The Ministry took this lack of involvement in hospitals to kill off the relationship. In a statement, which reached the pinnacle of hypocrisy, it expressed a preference for the NHSR to consist of those prepared to participate in hospitals and the societies stood accused of making little contribution towards that objective.[84] Such views exhibited signs of selective amnesia, given the terms and conditions agreed were in place simply to bulk up the recruitment stats. At a stroke, the arrangements appeared to count for nothing. In the new scheme of things, the Ministry of Health decreed nursing auxiliaries would be enrolled and trained by hospitals and totally severed their administrative and management links with the societies.

No external hint of this catastrophic event surfaced publicly. Amendments to the NHSR training manual continued as if nothing had happened, though the timing of the deconstruction of the NHSR turned out to be the final irony. Shortly after the axe had come down on the voluntary aid societies, the axe then descended on the NHSR and the other civil defence organisations so the opportunity to fulfil the grand plan disappeared. Whilst the endgame possessed no further historical impact, it provided an exceptional insight into attitudes, relationships and sheer scale of political manipulation that beset the articulation of the nuclear nursing resource. The ruthless dispatch of the societies exemplifies the brazen audacity of the Ministry in the degree to which they had been used, a point shown up when the minutes recorded: 'They also sought confirmation that the object of the Reserve was still to supplement hospital staff in wartime, as publicity leaflets referred to peacetime help given by the Reserve'.[85] In every sense, the question about what the Reserve was for and raised after nearly twenty years of its existence provides an extraordinary verbal monument to the whole affair. The Ministry of Health had become the 'Ministry of Stealth' in its secret mission to nurse numbers and through that to maintain the idealised view of nurses and doctors still bringing the compassion of the NHS to the nuclear battleground.

Chapter 8

ALTERNATIVE MEDECINE

Until the end of the 1950s, the secret remit of 'the nuclear health service' was simply to project the promise of mass compassion as a mythological statement to protect the British bomb. It meant Whitehall juggled with two nuclear realities. One involved the construction of an environment conducive to maintaining the logical appearance of the facade. The other arose from the military assessments that were increasingly showing destruction completely off the scale of human comprehension. On the other hand, during the 1960s the legacy of running with such a policy began to trouble the government. The Berlin Crisis and the Cuban Missile Crisis were blunt reminders of the possibility of war. Against that background the continuation of the medical myth was all very well to promote as a psychological war game, but did nothing to answer the question rising up the nuclear agenda how the survival of the state itself ought to be organised given the conditions that threatened to destroy much of it both physically and as a governable entity.

The government possessed a hospital evacuation and casualty sorting strategy where the administrative side had progressed well, but with no way of distributing surgeons and hospital doctors within it.[1] Medical Officers of Health had become an integral, not to mention, indispensable link in the local authority civil defence chain. Moreover, their professional organisations were sympathetic towards being involved in any public health matters related to the post attack environment. Completely juxtaposed to that position, the BMA acting on behalf of the general practitioners, continued sitting on their political fence about the inclusion of doctors into any kind of medical command structure. Altogether the call up and nuclear management of the medical profession remained ineffectual with the potential of becoming politically humiliating, if not disastrous. Something had to be done to bring closure to the situation whether by fair means or foul; alternatives that would have a profound influence on the final shape and form of 'the nuclear health service'.

Critical Conditions

The legacy of the negotiations between the Ministry of Health and the

British Medical Association amounted to little more than a reconstituted version of the Second World War protocols designed for calling up medical recruits for National Service. The very factors endearing it to the medical profession as a self-disciplinary system with its maze of committees only offered a cumbersome machine compared to the instant mobilisation of a National Medical Corps originally intended. Yet it became an extraordinarily important vehicle in the military scheme of things and by the time National Service ended, the process had over the twenty-one years of its existence recruited over 27,000 doctors to the three Services and dealt with thousands of applications for deferment.[2]

The position in respect of dentists was not dissimilar. Agreement in getting them signed up to a comparable structure took an interminably long time and only in August 1955 did formal protocols under the euphemistic title of 'Control of Dental Manpower' reach the form of a finalised Skeleton Plan. With a new register planned, it followed the BMA system ending up as no more than a network of self-control to cover the screening of dentists and dental technicians for National Service. The only direct benefit to accrue as far as the nuclear connection was concerned appeared during October 1955. At that time the Ministry of Health advised all hospital Senior Administrative Medical Officers the British Dental Association had given an assurance every endeavour would be made for their members to support the Mobile First Aid Units. A letter affirmed this in very positive terms: 'The Association have accordingly undertaken to help Regional Hospital Boards to get in touch with practitioners who would be willing to lead units in wartime and, no less important, to assist in the training of units in peacetime'.[3]

After years of painful wrangling, the Ministry of Health were really beneficiaries of only a complex web of administrative procedures to deal with National Service. On the other hand there were still signs inside the BMA that the nuclear door might still be possible to open. At one level, the organisation actually seemed remarkably amenable to the prospect of doctors being involved in patching up the nation after an attack by hydrogen bombs. A report prepared by the Association's Medical Manpower Evidence (Steering) Committee, passed on to the Willink Committee then considering the future provision of doctors, emphasises the point with some clarity. For the purposes of the Cold War, which at the time still remained underwritten by National Service, the committee noted it would need at least 1,500 students a year to maintain the 800 to 900 or so National Service doctors required by the Armed Forces. It stressed this should be borne in mind if any reduction in their numbers were to be contemplated. Referring to the possibility of a 'warm' war, they believed that was possible to cover by the government recalling medical reservists as had happened in the Korean War without any appreciable effect upon the National Health Service.[4]

Nor did the committee seem at all concerned by doctors becoming involved in a full scale nuclear exchange, which it termed as a 'hot' war. Despite cataloguing some of the horrific conditions that might come in for medical attention the report, somewhat bizarrely, pointed to the risk of not enough doctors being available for nuclear war because of medical recruitment policy, rather than through the event itself:

> It must therefore be assumed that nuclear warfare will involve a greatly increased requirement for doctors. The Committee is not in a position to estimate what surplus of doctors would be required in nuclear warfare. The initial needs of the Services in war are not likely to be large and could probably be met without undue dislocation of the civilian medical service. The subsequent needs of the Services depend entirely on the nature of the warfare, and any forecast must necessarily be blind. If, however, the Departmental Committee should decide to recommend a reduction in the annual out-turn from the medical schools, the number of doctors available might not prove adequate in time of nuclear war.[5]

Still in this cooperative frame of mind, the committee also looked at the flip side of the problem and the difficulty of ensuring enough trained personnel were available without creating a surplus of doctors who could not be absorbed into medical practice during peace. Far from being obstructive or defeatist, it put forward radical plans suggesting some of the 7,000 fully or partially retired doctors could plug the gap in numbers thereby circumventing the problem of diluting the profession, whilst maintaining a reserve. Another possibility the committee raised involved a highly provocative gender based idea on the assumption that because medical women would marry and some retire permanently, whilst others might continue in part-time work, medical schools could accept a larger number of women and proportionately fewer men. If an emergency did occur, the theory went, such arrangements could provide a potential resource for the Forces. Alternatively, if the government were reluctant to apply conscription to married women, they might take over a greater share of the civilian duties to release more men for active service. In order to protect such an investment, the package even came with the idea that state grants for the medical education of women should be subject to a condition they complete their two pre-registration posts and become fully registered practitioners.[6]

Encouraging signs of possible nuclear participation were also reinforced by the involvement of the BMA in compiling the Central Emergency Register. On 8 July 1953, the Association announced the first analysis was ready. By that time, the register had reached a stage of being 83% complete and frozen on 31 December 1953 to allow the raw data to go through the sifting and logging process. The record of the event states seventy-five staff of the BMA took part who worked throughout Saturday 2 January and for half of Saturday 9 January 1954. Covering both England, Wales and Scotland, it subdivided a total of 58,572 women and men doctors and surgeons into their respective areas of practice, age, qualifications, and mobility and included those who had retired.[7] Equipped with this information, the Ministry of Health started again to try to crack the mobilisation and deployment problem. Another Skeleton Plan – the third – began its journey in the hope the committee structure, combined with the register would finally provide the right ingredients to achieve an agreeable outcome, especially given that the medical profession had accepted both elements.

For a second time Russell-Smith faced Dr Solomon Wand over the negotiation table to begin discussions; on this occasion, to meet the hydrogen bomb age. Again, the results soon descended into a bureaucratic ordeal and had Wand's fingerprints all over the terms demanded. Once more he looked on the whole process as another union affair to safeguard his profession against whatever nastiness the state might think up, which could lead to the complete control of the medical profession in peace, let alone war. The nuclear terms Wand sought, and indeed achieved for his membership, reflected that obsession. Medical practitioners in evacuation areas and due to be posted into reception areas were to be given a preference where they would like to go to on the basis they 'be allowed to follow their own patients'. Families of doctors would be treated in the same way as the general population and the usual caveats about direction gave assurances regarding compulsion to ensure its meaning was watered down to insignificance. Controls were to be no more stringent than applied to others, only to be introduced as a last resort, and finally, undertaken in 'the closest consultation' with the appropriate medical recruitment committee. Other guarantees included the possibility of reintroducing the Protection of Practices scheme, agreed at the time of the Suez Crisis, to make up any financial loss suffered by surgeries whose doctors had been called up and to apply this for as long as possible. The dread of state control also came into the equation with the demand, 'a firm undertaking should be given that a salaried general practitioner service would not be introduced at the end of the war'.[8] Neither did the question of 'nuclear' pay escape the process and a general statement agreed with the Treasury designed specifically to mollify Wand.[9]

Agreement over the nuclear terms of employment may have seemed to reach some kind of closure, but it still left the question of which branch of medical profession should act as medical directors to ensure personnel were in place in the pre-attack phase and facilitate any post-attack movements to areas of greatest need. In theory, the answer stared the Ministry of Health in the face. The Medical Officer of Health had to be the logical choice for the appointment, particularly since local authorities possessed established civil defence networks to conduct that task. Straightforward as such a step may have appeared on the surface, underneath it carried the heaviest of historical baggage possible to imagine in view of the recent past. Especially pertinent to the situation were the battles by GPs to prevent local authorities gaining ascendancy in the NHS through their local health centres. Certainly, the sheer trepidation that gripped the Ministry of Health about taking this route is evident from Russell-Smith's aside. She voiced her reservations to Sir Frederick Armer: 'It will be necessary to agree with the BMA in peacetime on the proposal to be used in war-time for the transfer of general practitioners and it will in my view be most difficult to persuade them to agree to proposals which will appear to them to be giving the Medical Officer of Health of an area the right to order about the general practitioners in it.'[10] That feeling of insecurity displayed shows the sense of trepidation about dislodging the BMA from its established comfort zones. More incredible is that such fears surfaced in a situation where the BMA held virtually no bargaining counters in the form of mechanisms to move medical resources to where they were required. In this particular argument about handling reinforcements, the BMA were in a tight corner since it operated as a resource supplier to the civil defence system and possessed none of its operational equipment or networks that included bunkers, radios, radiation monitors and so on, all the operational trappings necessary to instigate changes in the game plan.

For all that, the circumstances dictated something had to give if the means of securing movement controls in the post attack situation were to be established. Control of medical manpower had reached a watershed. The Ministry of Health suggested a new operational directive in the Skeleton Plan that took a step towards recognising the inevitable operational realities. However, in order to placate Wand by keeping general practitioners fully in the communication loop a convoluted approach to the issue was proposed on the following principles:

> In each local area requests for help will be channelled through the Medical Officer of Health of

the county or county borough. If arrangements are made for him to be in close contact with a representative of the hospitals situated in the area (a Hospital Area Officer) and with a representative of the Local Medical Committee covering the general practitioners in the area probably in most cases the Chairman, machinery would exist by which the doctors to be sent to the area needing help would be picked out and given all the necessary detailed instructions.[11]

Achieving this high level of coordinated action meant every person involved in the medical control structure was to possess a local copy of the emergency register. Best practice suggested the document would be the object of constant updating to keep a track of doctors in the area and facilitate their dispatch to sectors of urgent need. When Dr Solomon Wand considered the proposal, his reactions clearly showed complete disdain for placing the Medical Officer of Health at the hub of the arrangements simply on the grounds he owned the office and the staff available for handling the requests. However, being the consummate union negotiator, Wand must have also realised the futility of pushing for more on this issue and in protecting the benefits secured, he agreed the historically significant principle that the Medical Officer of Health should become 'the' medical supremo and have control over general practitioners.[12]

The outcome may have represented a glimmer of hope towards reaching a conclusion over the control issue, but reality had a nasty way of intervening and the terms were overtaken by a new strategic appreciation whereby mobilisation plans needed to become operational in two or three days let alone seven. Attention to the minutiae of employment detail Wand had demanded was part of a world that had ended abruptly. London now described the Skeleton Plan Wand had turned into another domestic contract of self-protection as 'hopelessly complicated'.[13] Edinburgh concurred, commenting 'the elaborate scheme worked out over the years does not now meet the situation and that quicker procedure is required'.[14] With those essential truisms, any chance of the third Skeleton Plan being finalised came to a sudden and unceremonious end.

The closure of the initiative on the basis that a 'quicker procedure' was required appeared to consign any mobilisation formula into the realms of impossibility. There seemed no way of breaking the intransigence of the BMA on the issue and as London remarked in desperation the Association was 'wedded to the profession making its own allocation.'[15] A number of possibilities to bypass the labyrinthine medical committee system for allocating doctors had already been discarded. The Ministry of Health momentarily even thought about attempting to establish a National Medical Corps by using a different name, the Emergency Medical Corps.[16] One more precarious idea to surface out of the sea of anxiety swirling around the Ministry corridors included the possibility of the National Medical Manpower Committee encouraging the Forces to call doctors to their fullest requirements. Placed under military discipline, so the theory went, there would be no problem sending doctors under orders to any area of the country. Nonetheless, the somewhat dubious nature of that kind of approach was recognised in so far as such a move would not only require government approval, but the Commanders-in-Chief might find it odd to have the casualty needs of civilians included as part of their responsibilities.[17]

The trouble was that not just the medical profession were being elusive. The Ministry of Health had virtually excluded general practitioners from 'the nuclear health service' altogether as individuals and showed no real enthusiasm to remedy that omission on a seriously grand scale as evidenced by its subsequent actions. Dr Ernest Claxton, Assistant Secretary of the BMA, started a campaign to persuade the Government to publish a booklet especially for general practitioners. The clamour for information also reached the British Medical Association Annual Representative Meeting, which as a national debating forum on medical matters resolved during its 1956 session the following demand:

> That in view of the fact that any future war is likely to start with little warning it is essential that members of the medical profession should understand the medical implications of modern weapons. This meeting therefore believes that the Government should arrange courses in these subjects which may be attended by any interested practitioner.[18]

With all civil defence expenditure tightly controlled by the Treasury, the Ministry of Health tried the cheap-option approach to the problem. Between 1950 and 1951 a thousand hospital radiologists had attended a course on the atom bomb at the Alverstoke Naval College. Subsequent attempts were made to enlist them to lecture about the radiological problems associated with the hydrogen bomb, on the grounds the medical principles were the same. Some Regional Hospital Boards were more successful than others in arranging lectures, but the majority view veered towards incredulity such a scheme could be started without the radiologists themselves being updated about the more complex issues the new weapon posed.[19] Using every delaying tactic possible the Ministry of Health held out for four years against a barrage of stiff reminders sent by the BMA before finally acceding to a course for general practitioners being laid on at the Sunningdale Staff College itself about the wider issue of casualty arrangements in place. What then actually caused the change of heart to do something resulted because of the mounting embarrassment the silence was causing the Staff College when lectures on medical civil defence were given. With the nuclear hospital plans prepared, the casualty collection plan in place and the Forward Medical Aid Unit also established, the missing link stubbornly remained the general practitioner.[20]

Matters had even deteriorated to a point where General Matthews, the commandant of Sunningdale, found it necessary to notify the Ministry of Health that the absence of any official guidance about the place of non-hospital doctors had become a source of severe awkwardness. Staff College lecturers were floundering when facing questions on the role of doctors, the General's questions revealing the complete operational inertia that had gripped the system:

> For Instance, I understand it is almost impossible to get the General Practitioner to come forward and train with FMAU and what is more there seems to be little direction at the moment as to where the General Practitioner is to be in the event of a crisis. Does he stay with his attenuated population or does he move? Does he work with the FMAU?[21]

Forced by the growing sense of dysfunction in nuclear healthcare arrangements, the Ministry agreed a course should be run and arranged for representatives of the British Medical Association to attend on 9 and 10 July 1960. As it was, any hopes of a 'big bang' approach to the issue of medical practitioners were shattered when the course notes hinted to those attending they were likely to be the first and last beneficiaries of such an event:

> This course would be intended to serve as a pilot course for representatives from British Medical Association Branches and Regional Hospital Boards who would later arrange courses on similar lines throughout the country to cover all general practitioners. The primary objective of such courses is to study civil defence, in order to stimulate general medical practitioners to take an interest in

civil defence and to volunteer for training with hospitals and Forward Medical Aid Units, but some instruction in the peacetime hazards of radiation will also be included.[22]

Only seventy-five places were allocated to the BMA on a once-and-for-all basis, and twenty to Regional Hospital Boards, the intention being that from this apostolic laying on of hands at Sunningdale a great wave of nuclear indoctrination would spread across the country.[23] Really, the event was nothing more than a ploy to calm things down. 'The nuclear health service' continued to exist as an array of organisational contradictions. Doctors were being encouraged individually to learn more about the casualty plan and urged to act as instructors in a volunteer capacity, but not explicitly informed about their role, although implicitly this had become apparent. Even by December of that year, when the third Skeleton plan had been torn up because of its inherent bureaucratic complexity, the Ministry of Health refused to come clean officially about the redirection of doctors to hospitals. One Regional Hospital Board lost patience and simply took matters into its own hands advising Local Medical Committees in writing that general practitioners would be called upon to support the vastly expanded hospital system, as well as the Forward Medical Aid Units at the nuclear frontline.[24]

With the embarrassments mounting, the Ministry of Health made a confession of sorts and in a letter advised the BMA of what lay in store for general practitioners, albeit in somewhat oblique terms:

> One cannot envisage such an expansion of the hospital service without the help of general practitioners and this has been generally understood. Hospital duties would include work in emergency and auxiliary hospitals or with Forward Medical Aid Units but general practitioners would also be needed to continue to provide medical care in the community and for the homeless. We cannot, however, as yet say what the precise arrangements would be for the allocation of doctors to particular services and in preparing any such plans we should of course consult you at an early stage.[25]

For all its obliqueness, this outline of intent delivered in 1961, simply had never combined with the hospital plan officially and excuses always found to delay its formal unveiling. Either evacuation or dispersal plans were changing; the mechanics of redeploying general practitioners still required working out, or the basis of paying practitioners in their new employment remained outstanding. When the BMA goaded the Government for greater inclusion into the civil defence regime, the Ministry held their ground with the Sunningdale principle of indirect approaches by doctors being the preferred method of dissemination, a fact revealed in an internal Ministry note exchanged between officials on the matter:

> It may be argued that this does not represent progress of a sufficiently rapid or systematic nature, but in general I feel that it is in accordance with the general government policy of gradual dissemination of information about nuclear warfare as exemplified in our other fields of education, e.g. Medical Officers of Health, Public Health Inspectors, Nursing Officers, Ambulance Officers etc.[26]

Admitting to the failure to bring in the general practitioners into the hospital plan along with the disparate system of communication on nuclear information says much about the medical facade and its operational bankruptcy. Everything had degenerated into a drip-fed and random process accompanied by a cat-and-mouse game played out principally by the BMA and the Ministry of Health. Having said that, it also reveals an essential feature of the illusion whereby organisational detail and nuclear information came in for manipulation to create and sustain a false sense of cohesion. Unfortunately, it also left the awkward question hanging in the air about whether any kind of reality could ever be breathed into the unrealities, without destroying the mythology they supported.

Bloody Doctors

Fortuitously, just as the injection of any kind of operational structure seemed an impossible endeavour, something occurred in 1960 that brought a new dimension to the situation. Due to the changing impact between the atom bomb and hydrogen bomb on military strategy, plus a reduced commitment to policing a diminishing empire, the Services had found it difficult to settle on the number of medical professionals they would call up. Resulting from that, a continuous stream of uncertainties had always hung over the hospital and casualty plan. But once new military strategies were eventually established that also involved the end of National Service, the outcome favoured civil defence as the Services reduced their potential call on civilian doctors and surgeons. The situation altered dramatically and though the possibility of 8,000 'specialists' had at one time come into the planning frame as the figure the military might conscript, the final requirement came down to just 1,500. Representing a welcome reversal of fortunes, it spurred on the Ministry of Health to bring closure to the issue of mobilising and deploying the medical profession that had existed as an intractable thorn in their side for so long.[27]

Along with that new assessment, a potential solution came about because of studies begun in Scotland during 1961 to get the doctors quickly into place if all else failed. Possessing a smaller medical organisation run through just 25 Executive Councils, against 138 in England and Wales, a simple method had been devised, but its principles seemed to offer the means of creating a national strategy. The first thing the Scottish model discarded was the contractual approach relating to the weighty baggage of doctors and surgeons already in the hospital service. Since civil defence hierarchies already existed throughout the hospital organisation, they could manage their own resources. In order to speed up the general practitioner side of mobilisation two basic approaches were proposed. Firstly, a standard doctor/patient ratio for general practitioner work based on 1 doctor to 10,000 patients was to be applied both to evacuation (target) and reception areas and the balance left for distribution amongst the hospital services. (Sunderland, Orkney, Shetland and the Outer Isle were to be omitted) On the dental side, a ratio of 1 dentist per 20,000 of the population was imposed on a similar basis to maintain essential dental services, the rest also transferred to other duties in hospitals e.g. in minor surgery or anaesthetics. As to the second element, this was about putting faces to the numeric based distribution plan. The most effective route to fast selection seemed achievable through small teams being formed consisting of people chosen from the established Local Medical Committees who would represent local general practices and the hospital services. Working together, the Scots felt, these could decide which practitioners should go or stay and inform them directly of their decisions. Also by relying on local knowledge the feeling prevailed it would provide the means of better management of married women doctors, retired doctors, those in private practice, as well as trying to identify persons with military obligations. Finally, a sweep of any remaining doctors would take place through a broadcast asking them to report to their nearest Executive Council offices immediately.[28]

The Ministry of Health decided to adopt the philosophy of the Scottish method, especially its simplicity, and began to turn it into a national strategy that could be set in place during peace so it was ready to activate in the event of a national emergency. Work on assessing how the size of the medical cake and its division between England, Wales and Scotland concluded at the beginning of 1962. The exercise established the number of doctors engaged in the peacetime hospital service throughout England

and Wales amounted to about 20,500 and 3,100 in Scotland, excluding general practitioners. Nuclear preparedness according to the plan then in place required at the very least 33,000 doctors (excluding last year medical students).[29] A standard formula was, therefore, set to make up the difference. This required every Executive Area, in whatever designation (reception or dispersal) to contribute 10% of practitioners under contract. Areas classified, as 'dispersal areas' (namely the target areas) were then to add a further 65% doctors on their membership lists. Prescribed exceptions included doctors involved in hospital work, teaching, medical research, full-time members of the staff of local authorities and those still having a commitment for immediate recall to the Armed Forces. Regard to their geographic spread was desirable if circumstances allowed, but those volunteering their services who were in reception areas would be accepted into the hospital system with the possibility they could state a preference as to where they might be sent. Finally, any women doctors with children under the age of 18 would be entitled to be moved as 'dispersees' and exempted from transfer to the hospital service.[30]

On completion of the calculations, Scotland found that having applied the 75% rule their main target areas, Edinburgh and Glasgow had too little home cover that led to a revised percentage applied. The process across the country finally resulted in 700 out of 2,800 general practitioners in Scotland and 9,000 out of 21,000 in England and Wales being allocated to the hospital service.[31] It left potential support in target areas to nothing more than a symbolic presence. Ideally the Health Departments would have wished even more medical resources to be withdrawn, but had felt that public opinion would not accept any greater dilution.[32] So with that, an allocation of registered medical practitioners appeared for planning purposes which settled on a division in the following way:

Armed Services	1,500
Hospital Service	33,000
General Practice	15,450
Local Authority	2,500

The breakdown represented the final mathematics that the National Medical Committee were to agree as a strategic objective for the proposed nuclear mobilisation plan.[33] It also came with two provisos, the first being that when hospital work tapered off an increasing proportion of general practitioners would be allowed to return to general practice. In England and Wales those general practitioners working in reception areas were to remain, subject only to their recall to the Services.[34]

Next, the process had to grapple with the more stubborn difficulty of the actual choice of general practitioners, and what arrangements were needed to ensure resources could be moved to areas of greatest need. At this point, the Ministry of Health suffered a moment of deep introspection about divulging the plans to the Central Medical Recruitment Committees given many general practitioners were members. Exhibiting anxieties caused by previous encounters over the negotiating table, the Ministry felt such a move risked the profession once again becoming totally obsessive about control and would consider the approach as a signal that 'they have a prescriptive right to be consulted about the manner in which medical manpower should be deployed in time of war'.[35] Sheer practicality won in the end and the Central Medical Recruitment Committee approached to turn the mobilisation framework into an operational reality.

After giving the matter due consideration the CMRC agreed, but had no illusions about how problematic this could be. The committee cautioned, 'the selection of general practitioners for allocation to the hospital service in wartime will be a very onerous, difficult and perhaps even invidious task'.[36] Inconveniently, the advice went further, with a caveat raised that if the plan was to stand any chance of being rolled out the selection process needed to adopt complete transparency with doctors fully involved and consulted by their Local Medical Committees. Any political wriggle room also disappeared when the National Medical Manpower Committee strongly endorsed the recommendations as the right way forward. Also, because there were 'political implications' of telling so many doctors of their wartime assignment, it did mean sounding-out Ministers responsible for civil defence planning since the exercise would require the general practice side to become involved in civil defence courses and associated medical support issues.[37]

'Transparency' may have added the aura of a participative exercise, but it did not provide complete comfort for the politicians. Whilst approval was given to the action and the Minister of Health invited to consult the Home Secretary, the question remained as how Parliament should be informed of the arrangement. As to whether the announcement was to come through 'an Adjournment debate or by other means' provided a moment of nervous apprehension about the reaction in the House of Commons.[38] In spite of all the reassuring utterances on the matter, the safety and seclusion of 'other means' was adopted, rather than risking a full debate. Therefore, one of the most important announcements affecting the National Health Service was delivered on 23 March 1964, the Minister of Health replying to a written Parliamentary question specifically prepared for the purpose. Deftly scripted, to keep the information to the very minimum, he restated the National Medical Manpower Committee had recommended the transfer of considerable numbers of doctors who required removal from general practice to the hospital service if wartime needs were to be met. In order to achieve this, the Minister also made the announcement the process would begin through the existing machinery and doctors consulted, with those selected informed where they should report in the event of a national emergency. A neat finishing flourish came with a disarming statement of implied consensus that, 'My right. Hon. Friend and I have accepted this advice as being in accordance with the Government's policy of preparedness in home defence planning, and we now propose to consult the medical profession with a view to carrying it into effect'.[39]

With the Parliamentary announcement out of the way, a new NHS memorandum embodying the principles of medical participation in nuclear medicine started to be drawn up and traded in the old heading of 'control of medical manpower in war' for the more user friendly title of 'Allocation and utilisation of medical manpower for the civilian health services in war.' (Appendix 5) This remarkable document distilled nearly fourteen years of discussion into just three pages. It was a masterpiece of moral contortion by putting into an organisational format the flirtation the BMA had always had in professing interest about becoming the medical saviours of the nation; explained why the NHS contracts could no longer subsist, but offered an alternative to enable them to conduct their nuclear duty. Importantly, the arrangements were based on voluntary cooperation and still allowed general practitioners all their cherished medical committees to make the allocations. Even the usual platitudes reappeared about remuneration and how this or that might be done. A rational explanation of why the general practitioner could not undertake the civil defence control function, clearly designed to defuse situation, featured in the calming measures. Nevertheless, the bottom line of the protocols stated with unambiguity: 'Local health authorities should have responsibility for organising general practitioner services to cover the period following attack and that general practitioners should be in contract with and remunerated by them'.[40]

The Ministry of Health sent this paper to the BMA, which its Committee on the Control of Medical Manpower in War then considered on 7 May 1964.[41] A deputation from the BMA met representatives of the Ministry on 22 May 1964, the minutes recording: 'Explanations were given by the Ministry on all points raised with agreement reached the draft plan should be submitted to the General Medical Services Committee, the Joint Consultants Committee and the Public Health Committee for their comments'. All three committees passed the memorandum, the only substantive observation made by the consultants who agreed, but on condition the suspension of teaching of medical students in the event of war would be introduced only as a short-term measure. The Public Health Committee reflected on a more practical point critical to the whole plan. It hoped that the placement of general practitioners under the control of the

Medical Officer of Health would be completed in a spirit of full cooperation. On their part the Ministry of Health requested the agreement should, for the time being, be regarded as confidential and the BMA was not to publicize it in the medical press. Nothing could have been clearer and unambiguous.[42]

So very real did the prospect seem of a resolution to the control of medical manpower problem the inevitable detractors and doubters began to appear. London County Council made representations that the proposed transfer of general practitioners would deprive the population in their area of adequate medical facilities during the precautionary period. With the scheme involving some 75% of doctors being removed immediately out of target areas in England and Wales, the Home Office caustically considered it to be nothing more than a dispersal scheme for doctors. The Ministry of Health even had to justify the plan by arguing such doctors would be transferred to hospitals which would serve the areas after an attack from which they had come.[43] For certain, by the end of December 1964, everything pointed to the problem of the mobilisation and deployment of doctors being settled at last. As part of that positive movement detailed schedules were prepared showing the quotas proposed for each Executive Council throughout the country. South of the border, 9,000 doctors were formally to be drafted and 700 in Scotland, with Edinburgh and Glasgow contributing the major share.[44] The feeling that the nuclear control issue was on the very brink of being settled is very much evident in a letter sent to the Secretary of the Central Medical Recruitment Committee for England and Wales at BMA House by the Ministry of Health. This confirmed the work of selection should begin with a draft statement agreed and held in readiness for insertion in the medical press.[45] Draft letters to the Local Medical Committees and practitioners were also ready to go into print.[46] Scotland went ahead of their partners holding a meeting at the BMA Regional Office in Glasgow with representatives of their medical committees and executive councils, as well as Medical Officers of Health, where a great deal of fine tuning to the Scottish plan took place.[47]

Because of just such frenetic activity, the result was both shocking as it was unexpected. At the very last moment a loss of nerve occurred, but not by the Scottish Department of Health nor the Ministry of Health. The Central Medical Recruitment Committee for England and Wales itself, suffered a deep anxiety attack and decreed no further selection arrangements were to be undertaken until, as they put it 'a better climate in the practitioner field' had arrived.[48] With that signal, the entire process ground to a painful halt and the Scottish Central Medical Recruitment Committee also confirmed its intention to put everything on hold until 'the climate' changed.[49] Behind the scenes a secret advice emerged from the hiatus, prepared for the private information of Staff College officials as to why the plan had suddenly hit the buffers.[50] Not only did the proposed mobilisation and deployment contract contain the contentious clause that doctors outside the hospital service would come under local authority control, throwing it to the general practitioners could not have come at a worse time.[51] Indeed, the Sunningdale note explains clearly why the retreat had been sounded. In no uncertain terms it warned about the politically explosive mixture 'the contract' and 'the climate' could become:

> Currently general practitioners have worked themselves into a somewhat belligerent mood on the question of remuneration and terms and conditions of service. The Minister would not wish to give the more militant members of the profession the opportunity of using this scheme as a bargaining counter in negotiations on terms and conditions of service.[51]

The pages of the committee book of the British Medical Association recording the events confirm why the Ministry of Health found the situation so troublesome. General practitioners had indeed worked themselves into a seething mass of discontent with a long list of grievances brandished in front of the Government. These were contained in a paper titled 'Objections to the Present System' which reflected in no uncertain terms the deep seated concerns about their place in the National Health Service. The General Medical Council felt that they had lost ground to Area Health Authorities and exclaimed in disgust 'a great profession has been divided'. Just about everything within their ambit came in for criticism with an overriding fusillade of displeasure: 'The Hospital Service has undoubtedly attracted political and financial support, albeit necessary, but to the detriment of the General Practitioner Services'.[52] Added to the list came a measured tirade hurled against the Public Health Services and the way their Maternity Services and even the Ambulance Service were preventing general practice to flourish as a multipurpose team. This stemmed from a situation where the general practitioner was employed under contract with his or her Executive Council, but a different authority provided the health visitor and home nurse. More than that the sense prevailed the profession had been overshadowed in other areas, the depth of disgruntlement being voiced in the overall statement: 'General Practitioners have witnessed the great empire-building in the hospital field at the expense of General Medical Practice where there has been little or no capital expenditure since 1948 by the State'.[53]

Dissatisfaction over the direction of general practice also merged with the question of pay aggravated by its links to 'the pool' and the highly complicated calculations the arrangements involved. Since 1961, a bitter dispute had blown up and although a review body was supposed to have settled the matter in 1963, its recommendations did nothing more than create further resentment with the conclusion it had caused final disillusion with the pool system. The *GMS Voice*, the equivalent of a trade union news sheet, fanned the flames of discontent by confirming that the arrangements could no longer be accepted because they were not geared to workload and responsibility. Doctors felt trapped by a vicious circle whereby the family practitioner had to care for more patients with the growth of population and yet the conditions of service were leading young doctors to avoid general practice that made the position worse. General practice, according to the union story, appeared to be in a spiral of decline increasingly funded by the goodwill of doctors through working longer hours or financing improvements to practices themselves. Finally, the protest note came wrapped up in the overall conclusion, 'the real issue is the fact that general practitioners can no longer have any confidence in their terms of contract under the National Health Service'.[54]

Exactly what brought the Central Medical Recruitment Committee to make their decision to curtail the mobilisation plans against this exceptionally difficult climate does not survive. Anyhow, little imagination is required to appreciate the circumstances in 1965 for persuading individual general practitioners to accept a nuclear contract and come under the control of Medical Officers of Health were not auspicious. Always a sign of being serious, The British Medical Guild, the BMA's weapon of last resort, had again been primed in order to circumvent the legal position of the British Medical Association not being able to organise and finance any action against the NHS itself. It advised all general practitioners to prepare letters of resignation from the National Health Service and deposit them with the Guild so they were ready for dispatch in the event of an unsatisfactory settlement. So not only had the dispute raged about pay, it also raised the desire for a fundamental change of attitude by the Government to general practice involving greater investment and rationalisation, but still with old battle cry voiced about minimum interference by the state.[55]

Neither did that particular crusade exist as a solo effort. The British Medical Association minutes also reveal the consultants and specialists were indulging in a war dance of their own. They claimed hospitals were the real losers that had suffered through a lack of money, buildings, and equipment and only their goodwill had bridged the increased demands placed on the system. Moreover, the consultants and specialists argued it was they who had been forced to tolerate 'unsatisfactory conditions and to overcome shortages by exertion beyond the call of duty'. The rationale of their committee for more investment in the NHS came in rhetoric that bluntly revealed how things seemed on that side of the medical fence:

> The public is almost totally uninformed about the finances of the hospital service. The hospitals cost the nation over £600m. a year (or £12 a head). Of this sum, about £100m. comes from the 'weekly stamp' and most of the balance from taxation. At the same time, the nation spends £2,500m. a year (£50 a head) on alcohol and tobacco, and £900m. a year on gambling. After 17 years of the National Health Service, it has become all too clear that fiscal and political, rather than medical considerations determine how much money is available for the hospitals. The nation must now face the fact that the concept of 'free' health care financed through general Exchequer funds has failed to provide a modern, advancing comprehensive hospital service. If there is to be such a service then some way must be found of liberating the hospital finances from the political and other pressures to which it is meantime subject, or else other sources of income must be made available to the hospital authorities.[56]

Despite the emotive medical politics, Scotland's reaction to the contractual disaster, at least publicly, amounted to one of diplomatic disappointment since the country had received a good reception from all the medical committees and no hostility at the official level. Internally, General Richardson exploded with incandescent fury. He vented his feelings in a file note, angrily stating 'What a BLOODY lot we doctors are', the word 'BLOODY' capitalised and appropriately highlighted in red ink.[57] Expressing a personal opinion to a colleague at the Scottish BMA, Richardson maintained the approach to practitioners was too cautious, 'too like a cat on thin ice'. The way the general saw things appeared in a summary that highlighted the dilemma of the moment between the medical profession accepting its role as a humanitarian part of civil defence, but without the political connotations of support for nuclear war and weapons:

> Doctors being the guardians of public morale ought to know the facts as opposed to the fictions of nuclear war, and should be able to play a part in

> educating the community in what one might call 'survival under nuclear attack'. I have been told that many of them are more interested in C.N.D. than in C.D. and would resent being asked to play any part in planning for war. Assuming that the motives of C.N.D. are basically humanitarian it is no doubt right and proper that many doctors should feel inclined to support some of its aims, but this should hardly make them deaf to our explanation that every minute spent in C.D. training is in preparation to mitigate a possible catastrophe, and to ensure that something can be done to help survivors and to ensure the future of the race.[58]

Not much altered after the collapse of the nuclear contract. As late as 1967 the Ministry of Health continued to be fearful of the reaction of the medical profession. Some attempts were made to salvage the mobilisation scheme, as agreed in principle by the BMA, but the essential momentum had been lost. In a sense, the only external evidence to come out of nearly twenty years of deliberations became a fitting symbol to the whole mobilisation fiasco. This existed in the apparatus of the National Medical Manpower and Recruitment Committees that endured until disbanded in 1978, an extraordinary mechanism which had allowed the illusion of mass compassion to survive by being there, but not being part of it. Yet at the time the question still obstinately remained exactly how the 'BLOODY' doctors could ever be integrated into a nuclear war plan.

Bitter Pills

During the 1960s the external development of 'the nuclear health service' had steadily progressed towards a complete working strategy. However, with the inexorable development of weapons and the possibility that the country might not just take ten hydrogen bomb strikes, but hundreds, brought a new dimension to the problem of nuclear survival. The realisation within government increasingly narrowed to the view that the real battle was not going to be a matter of managing mass compassion, but in reality mass abandonment. Patching up some survivors, albeit with ever decreasing resources, still held propaganda value to keep the image of the caring state in front of the public, but secretly the position needed to be faced that any remnants of resources left would have to be applied towards saving the future of the state itself. This presented the critical challenge of keeping hidden the social violence and raw power of government machinery such a policy would represent.

So just as the symbolic value of the hospital plan and the casualty chain appeared to be most complete, the realities of its fragility were becoming apparent in Whitehall. Covert arrangements prepared for a crisis over Berlin provided a premonition showing just how ideologically brittle the iconic symbols of care such as the Ambulance and First Aid Section had become. Draft letters to Regional Hospital Boards admitted the previously idealistic instructions involving the integration of the section with peacetime ambulances and the organisation of mobile columns at operational bases, were no longer tenable. Really, the letters represented a final and brave attempt at some kind of salvage operation to save some of the protocols that had been the object of indoctrination for years. Any arrangements would depend on circumstances, the likelihood being there would not be enough time even to distribute any stretcher fittings to convert the vehicles to carry four casualties. Instead of the injured being treated with due dignity promised by civil defence exercises, instructions indicated they would have to be unceremoniously pitched onto the floor of the ambulances or any other vehicles requisitioned. For all the signs of hopeless endeavour, some particles of optimism did still manage to surface. Members of the Ambulance and First Aid Section were to remain in their homes and after an attack lend themselves towards treating the lightly injured in their local area, as well as preparing the more seriously injured for transport to Forward Medical Aid Units when the ambulances arrived.[59]

It was to be the last grain of hope. NATO EXERCISE FALLEX 62 arranged to test national reactions through the network of government bunkers, officially known as Regional Seats of Government, set out a new and indescribably horrific scenario likely to result from a nuclear war. The bomb plot involved about 200 megatons aimed at missile sites and airfields, plus megaton bursts on sixteen or seventeen cities, all in a matter of just a few hours. Estimates suggested about ten million people might die immediately, and three million seriously injured. Horrific calculations assumed a dispersal scheme had been put in place otherwise the casualties would be even higher. The post attack aftermath pictured added to the awfulness, between ten and fifteen million deaths expected within twelve months. It left the prospect of some thirty-five million people surviving and huddling into grossly overcrowded buildings still standing, with little food or water and no public utilities. They would also witness people drop dead in the street, as the irradiated victims suffered the final ravages of radiation sickness.[60] Politically embarrassing, this dreadful scenario fell into the hands of the Campaign for Nuclear Disarmament and disclosed with elation at the organisation's annual Aldermaston march, completely justifying their prophecy of social disaster.[61] Ironically, inside the Home Office, the truth was equally causing a high degree of gloom.

Theoretical ideals of forces coming in from prepared positions outside a smitten area appeared no longer defensible, or as officialdom now frankly put it: 'The truth is that the feasibility and the correctness of this early action have been overtaken by the changes in the scale of attack. With fallout on a wider scale and overlapping plumes causing increased radiation intensities, many services could no longer be mobilised for some considerable time'.[62]

The whole system was effectively falling into a state of paralysis, which soon became more visible. Compared to the comparatively slow-moving Berlin Crisis that culminated in the building of the Berlin Wall, the Cuban Missile Crisis of 1962 showed the facade could not respond to fast moving events with the result the organisation remained embarrassingly impotent. It exposed civil defence more publicly as a possible irrelevance causing the worst ever crisis for civic confidence, particularly as the control arrangements then in place simply were just a facade. *The Economist,* in an article titled 'How much Shelter' argued not for scrapping civil defence, but completely overhauling it as a deployable force. As it pointed out, its critics had made much out of the episode: 'A lot of people, reportedly including many neutralists and nuclear disarmers, buzzed their local town halls and police stations in Cuba week to find out what arrangements had been made for their personal survival, and were chagrined to learn that the answer was precisely nothing'. Damaging rumours even suggested the inactivity had resulted from a purposely engineered ploy to protect civil defence inadequacies becoming openly apparent and falling to scrutiny by the Campaign for Nuclear Disarmament.[63]

From these reality positions emerged a reality plan, of sorts, on the basis the changes would have 'tremendous advantages' in holding community morale. An important circular, dated 19 August 1964, covering the nuclear situation through somewhat less optimistic eyes warned the information given was not to be communicated to the Press indirectly or directly, nor to any person not authorised to receive it. Headed 'Mobilisation and Deployment for Operations' the instructions represented the combination of the Berlin/Cuba experiences and the conditions of FALLEX 62. If there was preparation time, Ambulance and First Aid crews were to report to their local depots and help installing stretcher racks into requisitioned vehicles before returning to their homes armed with a medical kit to establish a first aid organisation in their local area with help from local wardens. Reduced to a few pitiful rituals, they remained the only simplistic advice possible in view of the overwhelming nature of the radiation hazard anticipated. Forward Medical Aid Units could be trapped at their hospitals by fallout and ambulance teams might not be able to become operative for the same reason.[64] Even the most basic assumption, acted out for several years, that these two elements would combine into an efficient lifesaving chain evaporated. The terminology now changed to the use of *ad hoc* moves which involved nurses and doctors sent out 'as and when' circumstances allowed to provide whatever support was possible to give.[65]

The anticipated breakdown of the medical arrangements also mirrored a much wider concern about the collapse of society generally. Berlin and Cuba accelerated the need for the state to take powers to keep some kind of social structure intact. Way back in 1956 ministerial departments had received an invitation to submit to the War Legislation Committee a statement of their existing powers and any new requirements they considered might aid the process of raising something out of the ashes of civilised society. What emerged as a result of that exercise was a radically new enabling act called the *Draft Emergency Powers (Defence) Bill, July 1958*. The idea behind it was to allow the introduction of a raft of Regulations, which would be necessary to put in place before a nuclear war and the first three months after the attack. In truth, the socio-political monster this represented becomes clear when the Home Secretary, Rab Butler, wrote to the Prime Minister on the 7 February 1959 advising him it would be a mistake to try and put the powers proposed onto the statute book during peace.[66] That moment saw 'nuclear law' being ring fenced as totally unsuitable for scrutiny under normal parliamentary procedures. As Sir Norman Brook, still chairman of the Defence Transition Committee, reported to Ministers, any attempt made under democratic conditions to introduce such legislation would leave the final version 'so emasculated, by limitations and provisos of various kinds, as to render it inadequate for the purposes for which it was designed'. All necessary Bills and Regulations had in the future to be prepared secretly and held in readiness for ratification during the last moments of peace by Orders in Council or Royal Proclamation.[67]

Essentially the *Emergency Powers (Defence) Bill* provided the final bulwark for the secret state to protect itself against total annihilation. A new dark age of planning began for the virtual demise of individual freedom, far beyond anything adopted in the last war. Applied to the medical practice side, the draft regulations had far reaching consequences. It was possible to wipe the entire slate of existing legislation relating to the National Health Service and start again in every sphere of hospital administration, general medical, dental, pharmaceutical and ophthalmic services and the Public Health Laboratory Service. Powers were prepared to dismantle one Regional Hospital Board area and vest its management with another. At lower levels, the same principles could apply with the powers of management committees and hospital boards transferred in whatever ways circumstances demanded.[68]

Within that dismantling process, perhaps the most breathtaking and unthinkable prerogative came in the power of government to dissolve the Executive Councils of the general medical and dental services, pharmaceutical services and ophthalmic services. It was, of course, a move towards the final destruction of the machinery representing the independent governance of those medical areas, so diligently respected in the past. As to remuneration, this remained in its simplest form being settled by possibly 'a fixed salary or otherwise'.[69] Many directives recognised the departures likely to occur from the normal practices of the pre attack world. Under draft Regulation 18, persons authorised to dispense or supply medicines on a prescription were entitled to substitute an appropriate alternative 'ingredient' for a scarce substance, but were required to take reasonably practicable steps to notify the person prescribing. Draft Regulation 21 enabled the Minister to suspend or modify provisions relating to the notification of infectious diseases, food poisoning, as well as the prevention and treatment of infectious diseases. Signalling the likely impossibility of the situation new rules also provided a catchall position: 'When the health services are being put on a war footing it would not be practicable for all these provisions to continue to be observed, and the Regulation enables the Minister by order to substitute others more appropriate to the circumstances'.[70]

Private hospitals were to be nationalised in all but name with Regional Hospital Boards able to give directions about the management and use of such hospitals for the care of the sick and as maternity units. The provisions of the *Mental Health Act 1959* relating to the care and treatment of the mentally disordered, as well as the legal obligations to make provision for those purposes, all dropped out of the medical system. Provisionally and temporarily registered doctors, last year medical students working under supervision and dentists working in hospitals were all empowered to undertake anything a fully registered medical practitioner could do. The appropriate Minister could also allow the employment of unregistered persons with Commonwealth or foreign qualifications as medical practitioners in hospitals or institutions. Certain classes of nurse received legal powers to practise midwifery, notwithstanding the provisions of the *Midwives Act and Midwives Rules*. A more ominous proclamation of intent came under the heading of 'control of professional employment'. No longer did the assignment of duties come as a debatable option over a negotiating table, but the blunt instrument of state control would cut across individual freedoms without an ounce of compromise. Medical practitioners and dentists were resources that would come under the direction of government officials, or those delegated by them, 'to any employment' where a medical background would be of use. Similar conditions applied to every other branch of the profession as well as persons being trained who all could be ordered to carry out work in their discipline, although not formally qualified.[71]

With the threshold crossed where democratic processes no longer held any relevance, the move dragged in an entire system of nuclear law that would underwrite the relationship of citizen and the state in a new and unimaginably brutal form. The *Emergency Powers (Defence) Bill* allowed individual Ministers to delegate specific powers to Regional Commissioners enabling them, either directly or by delegation, to legally exercise the appropriate functions of the state if communications were broken between the Government bunker and the Regional Seats of Government. In war, ten such commissioners of Cabinet Minister status would exercise virtually sovereign powers which would aim at gleaning any resources towards the survival of their fiefdoms. The gist of how their power would be unleashed appeared in their manual of governance:

> The combined effect of the widespread casualties; of the devastation of food and water supplies, buildings and communications; and of the hazard of fallout; would be the sudden disappearance of our present relatively safe and comfortable way of life. Survivors would have to accept an extremely primitive standard of living for some considerable time; and in these circumstances the enforcement of law and order would assume an even greater importance than it now possesses as a pre-requisite to the maintenance of public morale. It would be imperative, therefore, for justice to be swift, summary and effective; and these considerations dictate a need for simplicity and, above all, flexibility in the machinery of justice.[72]

Survival, in effect, was to depend on a new ruthless relationship between the leadership of those in authority and an unquestioning obedience from survivors. That presumption necessitated comprehensive powers which the *Defence (Public Security) Regulations* obliged by creating a number of new wartime offences including, misleading acts, misrepresentation, seducing persons from duty and causing disaffection. Critical to the new medical rules, disobedience or neglect to comply with <u>any</u> provision of the Defence Regulations would be an offence automatically attracting a verdict of guilt without a grain of mitigation taken into account.[73]

What then turned everything into an abject regime of institutionalised barbarity came in the *Draft Emergency Powers (Defence Bill)* introduced in December 1964. Set against a post attack world where necessity demanded the release of most prisoners, a new system of punishment had to be accommodated. Ironically, at a time when Parliament felt it was no longer appropriate to continue with capital and corporal punishment in peace, these methods were introduced with unimaginable ferocity to deal with the expected breakdown of post attack society. Whilst a generous interpretation of the results might be defensible on the grounds of recognising nuclear reality, a more cynical conclusion could be that the new representation of the rule of law was nothing more than a move to legalise mob violence.[74] Reconsidering the problems of social breakdown, drafting instructions directed: 'The emphasis of the Regulations should therefore be on making the process of criminal trial as short and simple as possible and in removing restrictions on the court's powers, rather than on safeguarding the rights of the individual.'[75]

The future foundation of the purpose of law thus embraced a new recognition: 'A state of anarchy would soon ensue unless the community could exercise restraint over those of its members who would otherwise take advantage of circumstances to inflict grievous hurt on the state or on their fellow survivors.' Linking law to community morale, in effect, produced a new prescriptive nuclear morality. Apart from capital offences, the circumstances of an offence would determine its severity rather than any intrinsic 'wrongness'. Depending on the conditions in which they were committed, minor violations such as stealing a bottle of aspirin could become grave threats, whereas other transgressions, regarded as serious during peace, might justifiably be ignored. As a safeguard to ensure that only 'appropriate offences' were heard, emergency courts had the right to refuse to hear or determine any case brought before it.[76] The extent of the viciousness enshrined in the nuclear legal system especially showed its teeth in a drafting discussion over the question whether the death penalty should be used against children and though seriously disliked was not entirely ruled out:

> Need we, even in these conditions, contemplate the death penalty for children? I suggest that the sentence might read 'A formal lower age limit for the penalty should perhaps be avoided, but administrative guidance to the courts would no doubt emphasise that its use against young offenders should be wholly exceptional and very much a last resort.'[77]

When Lord Stoneham, then an Under Secretary at the Home Office, advised the Home Secretary Sir Frank Soskice about the matters of 'utmost gravity' as to how the law of the land was to be administered during the early days after a nuclear strike, his presumption proved to be no exaggeration. In the new scheme of things, swiftness and potency mattered most. Procedure, rules of evidence and rights of audience would be at the whim of the judge; no decision was to be invalidated by an alleged defect in procedure and no appeals, nor provision for defending counsel or legal aid provided for.[78] Sentencing under regional control meant death would be meted out in the most perfunctory terms, as the situation demanded. With cold exactness Clause 8(3) of the new *Defence (Administration of Justice) (England) Regulations* turned the punishment side of the equation into a working proposition on the following terms: 'Where in the opinion of the court, by reason of the nature of the offence or in the circumstances for the time being existing, and having regard to the attainment of any of the authorised purposes no other form of punishment is appropriate.'[79] Methods of punishment were not likely to have the same peacetime alternatives. Imprisonment or even forced labour raised the prospect of being fed and looked after which might be regarded as a privilege rather than a punishment, a situation that left the choice between the death penalty and flogging. As the Secretary of the War Planning Committee succinctly put it, 'in the traditional philosophy of punishment, deterrence, retribution and reformation, the last had no further purpose'.[80]

The administration of this nuclear law was to be through any legal adjudicator still surviving which could mean anyone from a lay magistrates to a high court judge. They were all to be given the power to pass down the death penalty in a nationwide network of single tier courts with a single judge. The argument went this organisational simplicity was essential to appease community feelings and only judicial force acceptable to the public would suffice to restrain the heightened mood likely to exist. This meant giving emergency courts powers based on the most difficult times. It would then be for the Regional Commissioners to modify those powers by gradually restricting the penalties available and the procedural aspects as the situation became more normal.[81] Flexibility equally applied to penalties and emergency courts could make any order or impose any punishment authorised. No less flexible, corporal or capital punishment was possible to apply to any offence when the conditions were at their worst. Sentence of death would likely be by shooting since skilled hangmen, the preferred method of state killing at the time, would not be readily available, nor the equipment. Responsibility for securing the carrying out of the sentence rested with the court and the place of execution likely to come down to mere practicality. If under 'prison' guard convenience suggested that executions be undertaken within the confines of that area, or if under police custody, then it would be expected that the police themselves would complete the job by a firing squad and as quickly as possible.[82]

Unpalatable as these new rules were they continued to form the basis under which real 'the nuclear health service' would have to operate. After years of being hidden, Strath's warning of the need to recognise the consequences of social breakdown now had a place in the secret nuclear constitution. With the inevitable rationing of highly desirable medical resources, the consequences of such constraints to protect them from the desperate were profound and unimaginably different to the ethics of normal society. Coupled with the policy to focus medicine on those of value to the reconstruction of post attack Britain, the potential for a toxic barbarity was enshrined into these hidden powers. It meant that the smallest transgression could attract the death penalty, the judgement made against the fragility of mob opinion and passed down by any lay magistrate who might still be available. A crucial stage had arisen as to whether the facade could finally cope with the ever more coercive side of government being folded into the civic domain so that externally a more acceptable model of post nuclear attack conditions remained in place. From the medical side, it meant the ultimate test of hiding a draconian reality plan behind the benign image of a 'nuclear health service' in which general practitioners were never likely to become a fully integrated part of its structure.

Chapter 9

WHICH DOCTORS

Although embedded as a fundamental expression of the secret state, the creation of the emergency regulations did provide the conditions for a final test of government resolve either to stick with the facade or come clean with the public about the realities it was hiding. A third Home Defence Review started by the Conservatives, but concluded by the new Labour Government in 1965 began to consider the question against the possibility of some ideological rethink on the civil defence issue. The odds against the hitherto reassuring charade holding appeared to shorten further when Labour promised high priority to public expenditure described as having 'social and economic' value to put right the parlous state of the economy at the time.[1] Politically, the circumstances provided an incredibly important historical crossroads moment. However, the choice of directions now faced new problems in view of the repressive nature of the Defence Regulations. Especially problematic to the continuance of the facade was the question as to which sector of the medical profession could be trusted to encompass the comfort of civil defence in the old sense on the one hand. On the other, it would need to underwrite an insurance policy by accepting a leadership role in the fight for survival if the worst did happen, with all its attendant ferocity prepared to go constitutionally correct.

Local Anaesthetic

Unexpectedly, the idea of a new approach to the issue of civil defence surfaced through the chairman of the Home Defence Review committee. Sir Phillip Allen, Permanent Under-Secretary of State at the Home Office, no longer felt the Bishop doctrine of civil defence linked to deterrence policy realistically held any further validity. According to Allen, the only issue outstanding was somehow satisfying the needs of survivors, which he explained with a dose of pragmatism:

> Civil Defence Corps Ambulance and First Aid Sections have about 38,000 members. This would be a mere drop in the ocean. If we are serious about this, simple first aid ought to become

compulsory in the fourth and fifth forms of every secondary school in the country. This would give an annual output of thousands of trained people with a basic knowledge that is useful in peace as well as in war. I understand that in the past the Ministry of Education has refused to consider the introduction of such courses. They should be told to think again. It is of course a waste of time and money to provide ambulance vehicles. If an emergency comes we can take over the millions of vehicles we need. After a nuclear attack or even before it sick and injured people will not worry whether they are in a purpose-built ambulance, a private car or a coal lorry so long as they are being taken care of. The problem will not be a shortage of vehicles; it is more likely to be a shortage of fuel.[2]

Allen thus offered an alternative method to instil public confidence through greater transparency, by what he called stripping away 'the secrecy' of the United Kingdom's preparations. This meant the Defence Regulations prepared to deal with the direction of labour of just about every survivor would go public, so everyone could learn about what lay in store. In this way, he argued, the pretence of a trained volunteer force could finally end. Unsurprisingly, the response to the suggested greater dissemination of public information and the stress for self-help proposed by Allen exposed the deep political anxieties still haunting Whitehall. It was felt that to acknowledge the risk of nuclear attack, coupled with a reduction in civil defence expenditure, would be politically impossible. Moreover, wider disclosure to members of the public of the secret rules and their possible assignments to wartime tasks sent a shiver through the corridors of power with the consummate reaction, 'indeed some are so stringent that their publication might cause unnecessary controversy.'[3]

Given a choice, faith in the comfortable symbolism of civil defence stubbornly persisted. Against a changing world background to the civil defence debate, new anxieties suddenly appeared. Whilst political thinking ran along the lines that the superpowers would be more vigilant after the Cuban Missile Crisis over a possible confrontation, the explosion of a nuclear device by the Chinese added a fresh uncertainty. Prime Minister Harold Wilson had become personally committed to the idea of keeping a highly trained nucleus of Corps members and the outcome reflected the Government's determination to maintain the facade behind that philosophy. The Home Secretary, writing to Allen agreed many aspects of the Civil Defence Corps needed rethinking, but considered the retention of the warden organisation vital to maintain the essential link between the council and the public. Nor was the disclosure of the enormity of the real task of civil defence preparations considered wise. When put to the final test, the political preference still existed for the truth to be concealed behind a mythological perception based more on historic sentimentality rather than reality.[4]

The price of that sentiment did not come cheaply. With substantial local and national overheads to retain, even a cut of Civil Defence Corps numbers from 152,000 to 87,000, representing the lowest figure at which a viable force could operate, achieved only a comparatively small reduction from the yearly spend of £8.25 million to £7.5 million. Felt to give the biggest contribution to the facade, as well as attract the most public confidence, the reduced Civil Defence Corps turned its focus on the control function undertaken through the Headquarters and Warden Section run by local authorities. Other functions, including welfare, ambulance work and heavy rescue were to be given over to local authorities and their staff, as well as being distributed amongst voluntary bodies. The general public would be mustered into first aid or rescue parties.[5] Altogether this package allowed Labour Home Secretary Roy Jenkins to proclaim to the country that their nuclear future had been secured, though with less money.[6] It still just about purchased the means to reiterate the old mantra of reassurance when he advised Parliament: 'The Government believe that by carrying the measures I have indicated they will retain on the most economical basis a pattern of civil defence preparations which, if there were a nuclear attack on this country, would enable many millions of lives to be saved'.[7]

Translating all that into an action plan meant Whitehall had to find leaders who would wholeheartedly embrace the secretly-acknowledged nuclear reality, but through which the powers described were possible to defuse in peacetime. The Government did not have to look very far. Civic pride and the desire for control already existed in the constitutional framework of the country. Civil defence had evolved through a unique relationship between local and national government with self-interest politics supporting the new 'Home Front' in ways not always open to public scrutiny. Those politics were bound up in the complexities of domain power that now reached their natural zenith in a transition that had changed the strategic role of civil defence from its traditional form of immediate rescue to long term survival. In the Cold War struggle against communist totalitarianism, the idealised picture of democratic structures remaining under civic rather than military or police control presented a perfect allegory for government that the Ministry of Housing and Local Government offered as the final throw of the political dice:

> The local authority peacetime structure in this country covers a vast network of organisation built up over the years. It employs a million people (including school teachers) with tremendous experience in all matters concerning our daily existence. Without this organisation survival and restoration after a nuclear attack would be unthinkable. Until recently little thought has been given to the part local authorities would have to play in the survival phase. It is recognised that this would in fact be their major role and that the organisation must be preserved and rebuilt to full strength as soon as possible after attack.[8]

Accepted as the way forward and aptly named after the mythical two-faced god, STUDY JANUS 63, held between government departments and nationalised industries at Sunningdale began to turn the philosophy into an operating system. On the medical side, the hospital still remained as a default position in caring for the injured.[9] At the same time secret concerns were expressed: 'The most urgent tasks would lie with the public health service and its ability to control probable future epidemics and deal with public hygiene in the absence of mains water and sanitation'. Any surviving general practitioners, the thinking went, would under such conditions need to be organised and controlled by the local authorities.[10] With hospitals depleted of drugs and medical equipment, as well as a highly diluted staff, there was an inevitability now being recognised that the emphasis would fall on the greater medical battle having to be fought outside the traditional areas of care.

The idea of a reverse flow even entered the debate during that study whereby nurses, nursing auxiliaries, works and maintenance staff would need to be organised into flying squads able to assist in the treatment of epidemics, select patients for admission to hospital and deal with obstetric emergencies, the whole grizzly picture painted in a few words:

> Special arrangements will have to be made for caring for those suffering from and, dying from, radiation sickness in the next few months. The burial of the dead killed by the immediate effects of the bombs may not be such an enormous task as many of them will be under the rubble and it may be simpler just to seal off the heavily damaged area. But thousands will have to be buried. And many

> more thousands have still to die. We may indeed return to the death-carts of the Great Plague.[11]

In the shadow of that kind of thinking about the charred and unpleasant Jerusalem in prospect, civil defence was reorganised entirely on administrative county and county boroughs by a nuclear charter giving dictatorial powers to local governance:

> Supreme authority at a local authority level of control should be vested in a single controller or commissioner. He might be supported by a small advisory committee but should be free to accept or reject their advice as he saw fit. He would derive his powers direct from the Regional Commissioner.[12]

Raising the stakes to the realm of 'supreme authority' meant the powers and responsibilities of an emergency committee of the council in war could be unlimited. The list involved requisitioning, rationing, control of food stocks, issue of money tokens and many other means of re-establishing the basics of civilised life to enable the nation to survive. Even in peace, such plans carried immense status implications and characteristically the County Councils Association and Association of Municipal Corporations picked on the term 'a small advisory committee', that inferred officers of the council could be given the same controlling status as elected representatives. Refusing to compromise, a deep and final irony occurred that 'control' in nuclear war eventually entered into local war books as a wholly democratised process. Emergency legislation would provide for the delegation of local and national powers to a small emergency committee of elected members and vest them with responsibility for preserving a framework of administration. Through that structure, they could utilise the resources still available in the community, maintain law and order and generally navigate their area towards a more normal life. Whilst circumstances might arise where a controller, usually the town clerk or chief constable, would have no alternative to act on his own initiative, he still needed to account to the emergency committee for any activities undertaken in relation to local government functions as soon as practicable, a signal undoubtedly designed to imprint local democracy in some retrospective way.[13]

With those principles embedded into local constitutions, towns and cities across Great Britain embraced the most complete form of civic garrisoning ever undertaken, mostly in basements of town halls. All chief officers of councils, which included the Medical Officers of Health, were to prepare detailed plans for the operation of their departments in war. *The Civil Defence (Public Protection) Regulations 1967* set out an explicit duty to train council staffs in the control system emphasising this to be the most important of the functional areas contributing to national survival that could not be left to chance. Reflecting the theme of employee participation, even the term 'warden' disappeared with more modern terminology referring to 'the mobilisation of community resources' and responsibility placed on 'control officers'.[14] Local government took on a new meaning. Even though in the local setting the civic structure would turn into a network of mini national governments housed not in separate bunkers as in the atomic era, or way outside the city boundaries, but in the heart of their civic centres to provide for twenty-four hour cover and rapid activation.

In order to hardwire this philosophy into an operational reality a programme of adapting town halls prescribed standards of radioactive protection, including air filtration, self-sufficiency in water, food, and power generation for twenty-one days. One hundred and forty-seven of the three hundred local authority controls planned before January 1968, were built or in the process of being built. If an emergency had occurred those councils not possessing such 'bunkers' had to rely on just their existing offices with all the attendant risks of fallout, failure of power supplies and without special communications.[15] The phalanx of officialdom placed in bunkered accommodation to clear up the nuclear aftermath thus involved a formidable array of anticipatory administrators. Local authority staff would be allocated places, along with representatives from the Whitehall Ministries, Police, Armed Services, Fire Authorities, Public Utilities, Petroleum Industry and the Hospital Boards.[16] Naturally, the Medical Officer of Health had his slot to provide the critical link between local government and the hospitals, as well as the key figure in the new survival regime.

Quite remarkably, despite all this attention to detail, the complete absence of thousands of general practitioners in the medical arrangements continued. Their position simply rested on sweeping pronouncements that hospitals would receive allocations of doctors and preparations required to receive their help at the appropriate time. Assurances given to the Regional Hospital Boards over the entire issue of control remained a curious mixture of democratic intent and having to fall back on the circumstances of the time:

> The position was that the last government had accepted that arrangements for selecting and issuing mobilisation instructions to general practitioners should be made in peace-time. The timing of the

operation could only be settled by government and the profession jointly and, as it involved a planned reorganisation of general medical services in war-time following the withdrawal of more than one third of general practitioners from their present jobs, it was obvious that a new pattern would have to be worked out. That pattern would depend, among other factors, on the views of the profession, the position and war-time responsibilities of local authorities in the civil defence control chain, the place of executive councils in war, and the extent to which government might take powers to direct manpower. Whatever the timing and the pattern it was clear that a reorganised general medical service would have to fit into the overall pattern of war-time government and control.[17]

Compared with the somewhat cloudy picture of general practice in nuclear tactics, the position of the Medical Officer of Health came into much sharper focus. With the shift of the medical battle to outside the confines of the hospital, the Scottish Health Department started compiling a more detailed assessment of MOH duties to inject greater realism. Called the *War-Time Responsibilities of Local Health Authorities* it aimed to put as much nuclear nastiness under the medical officer's jurisdiction as possible. Although civil defence ended before it could be issued, the document does extend the view of the operational regime being constructed. Apart from codifying all the public health issues which had been recognised in the past, other problems never considered before were included. The peacetime responsibility of local health authorities for mental illness was to continue in wartime, but a new and sinister concept began to find favour related to the handling of individuals showing mental illness caused by the nuclear attack. With the dangerous prospect of stupor, hyperactivity or severe physical prostration by those affected disturbing public morale the issue now came in for attention. During peacetime some of these conditions were treatable by psychiatric drugs, but in nuclear war such valuable resources would be reserved for surgical and medical needs. A further extension of 'home nursing' thus offered the means of introducing a system of 'ghetto isolation', a summary measure to prevent a demoralising effect on the rest of the survivors, even if that required removal from their homes.[18] Essentially a process of collectivisation and segregation was to protect any speck of normality that might have survived. Attractive as that route seemed, the medical consequences of dealing with only selected casualties prescribed under the sorting rules also raised the additional problem of many survivors left with horrendous disabilities. No real answer appeared as an overlay to that aspect, other than it would quite simply and naturally become another issue for the MOH to manage.[19]

Although the Government had lost its nerve over the issue of formalising the mobilisation of the medical profession, the Scottish draft manual also confirmed the operational principle that Medical Officers of Health and some of their staff would have authority delegated to them to organise local health medical services and set this out in the following way:

> The services would have to be organised by a body in possession of information about damage, casualties and fallout and with access to civil defence communications. The Medical Officer of Health as medical adviser to the group or area civil defence commissioner would have access to this information. Provisional agreement has accordingly been reached with the local authority associations, the British Medical Associations and the Association of Executive Councils that the responsibility for organising (the) general practitioner service to cover the period following attack. It is envisaged that similar arrangements would be applied with regard to dental, pharmaceutical and optical services but consultations with representatives of these professions about the possible role which they might play in war have not yet taken place. Further guidance on this subject and on the organisation of general practitioner services will be provided in due course.[20]

Vitally, this snapshot provides an insight of just how other sectors of the profession remained isolated from 'the nuclear health service' and even by the close of 1966 had no formal operational connection with it. Indeed, the only area of the medical profession where a professional body and its membership appeared to work in complete nuclear harmony was in the network of Medical Officers of Health. Across the country, they had attended courses at Taymouth Castle in Scotland and south of the border the picture was no less purposeful. Several hundred Medical Officers of Health passed through the Staff College at Sunningdale in an intensive indoctrination process begun as far back as 1960, with a special course also arranged for Public Health Inspectors at the Army School of Health, Mytchett, near Aldershot. Records show many on the local health authority side had even attended Sunningdale more than once contrasting sharply to the meagre 75 places afforded to general practitioners on a once and for all basis.[21]

During 1963 the Medical Officers of Health at Taymouth, recorded concerns that adds further evidence about the difference between the willingness of the MOHs to become involved in medical civil defence, compared to the position of general practitioners. Attendees felt that they should be given explicit powers of direction to deploy their doctor colleagues in general practice. Moreover, they expressed fears that doctors having had no training in their allotted post in FMAUs could become a hindrance. But as a significant body of Scottish attitude, the most important point came with their collective view, 'the balance of opinion was in favour of the medical adviser to the Controller taking responsibility for the general medical service in his area'. Accordingly, it was suggested the Health Department should take the early opportunity of raising the matter with the BMA.[22]

That desire to acquire the leadership role over general practitioners materialised two years later, but through a completely different channel given that the 1965 mobilisation agreement had not been formally completed. Instead, their job description appeared in the framework of NATO EXERCISE CIVLOG 65, designed to test home defence preparedness across a wide area of resource planning by Whitehall Departments. This assumed an attack by eighty eight nuclear weapons and a script to match for national survival which sent out a message of considerable importance regarding the medical aspects. It defined the Medical Officer of Health as a leader of the medical effort in three significant ways. Firstly, it ensured the post itself always stayed outside the melange of destruction and did not become a victim of annihilation. Secondly, the investment of years of indoctrination was realised through resourcefulness and ingenuity applied to the crisis in the likely absence of much else. Finally, the primacy of the role appeared through a staged progression of events that supported the MOH as a logical leader and potentially becoming a national treasure once more.

Many realities of the hospital evacuation plan occurred in ways that never surfaced publicly. Far from being the kind of precision planning outcome envisioned in civil defence exercises, the post attack picture descended into a catalogue of hopeless catastrophes. It was concluded that at the time of the attack hospitals had only managed to form 400 Forward Medical Aid Units, but this strained nursing resources greatly with little added through the National Hospital Service Reserve. Crucially, the exercise assumed the mobilisation of medical manpower also failed to reach what was required, even though the Minister of Health exercised powers under the Defence Regulations to relax the qualifications of medical practitioners. Another potentially debilitating threat to the hospital service was also depicted through a chronic shortage of maintenance and domestic staffs, many of whom refused to move with their hospitals. As a result, the conclusion of the narrative was that the hospital services throughout the country were grossly overburdened, with the number of beds available substantially reduced by blast damage and high intensity radiation.[23]

At 30 days CIVLOG depicted an overloaded system with understaffed hospitals using crude facilities, any staff left more often than not suffering either exhaustion or radiation sickness. Attempts, it was said, were made to recruit untrained volunteers to work under the direction of trained staff; surgical work had been abandoned or at least restricted in many regions and finally a rigorous admissions policy to hospitals applied to ensure the best use of accommodation and medical resources. Outpatient and assessment centres received mention suggesting their provision in certain circumstances, but most casualties still ended up with home nursing or in improvised rest areas. This all culminated in the overall conclusion, 'Shortages of essential material for the proper treatment of patients and inadequate diet are rapidly creating in hospitals an unhealthy atmosphere of depression and despair'.[24]

Critically, the narrative not only concentrated on the breakdown of the hospital system, but shifted the problem to the area of public health that hitherto had been a concern, but not necessarily billed as an apocalyptic disaster that could overtake the initial destruction. Contaminated water, infestations of fleas and lice, poor nutrition, as well as vomit and excrement from radiation-sufferers in overcrowded living conditions and a broken sewerage system raised the sceptre of a secondary disaster with the conditions ripe for plague conditions. The deterioration in the post-attack environment came with the admission that the local authority health services in England and Wales had been overwhelmed with the cascading hazard of dysentery, gastro-intestinal infections, septicaemia of wounds and finally a full blown tuberculosis outbreak or worse still smallpox, cholera or typhus epidemic. Significant in this 1965 picture of total horror was the complete lack of any medical practitioner plan on the one hand and the expectation on the other, announced by the Minister of Health in the pre-attack period, that councils were authorised to assume responsibility of the organisation of general medical services in accordance with previously prepared arrangements.

From that abyss of desolation CIVLOG finally cast the local authorities and their Medical Officers of Health as the rescuers of the nation from the plague and pestilence forecast, as well as setting up the rudimentary structure of a new National Health Service plan. They were to provide advice through mobile teams or broadcasts on improvised systems of sanitation, hygiene disciplines, refuse disposal and finally establish a rudimentary medical care system which the narrative envisaged in these terms:

> The general health picture over the whole country shows a shift of emphasis towards home care with the local authorities re-organising the local medical and nursing services accordingly. The peacetime pattern whereby a patient chose his own doctor has virtually disappeared, and general practitioners have been allocated streets, areas or districts in which they are responsible for the medical care of all inhabitants: they are assisted by the nursing staff of the local authority, home nurses, midwives, health visitors and unskilled volunteers.[25]

Emphasising the burgeoning medical supremacy of the MOH, the Ministry of Health extended and underpinned this governance role through regional exercises undertaken as desk top studies by councillors and their chief officers. One of the most radical and important came in STUDY GRASS SEED that took place in the southwest civil defence region to consider the implications of a hydrogen bomb falling close to Bristol. On the medical side, particular attention focussed on the radiation problem and the need to deal with thousands of irradiated individuals who had little hope of survival and posed a threat to public health. This especially illustrated the extent to which the so-called 'home nursing' scheme was applied as a key measure in the casualty plan. Moreover, those local authority medical officials involved in the GRASS SEED conundrum thoroughly demonstrated their position by heralding the social model as an answer to the public health catastrophe in all its permutations.[26]

Like erstwhile alchemists, Medical Officers of Health applied their skills to impose some kind of public health control over the disaster. The MOH Swindon looked to mass containment on the logic that a family that had been together would also succumb together to radiation sickness. Camps were to be outside the town, ideally located close to a communal burial ground, thereby avoiding large numbers of bodies being transported through any unaffected areas. Attempting to overlay a vestige of dignity over the arrangements, they also came with the idea that local priests should run centres of the kind described. Another slant to the war game was given by the MOH Somerset who felt that refugees crossing into the county should be dispersed to avoid the spread of disease and billeted with householders, all the sick being concentrated into one room of the house. Teams of volunteers skilled in home nursing would then visit and provide advice, but it was pronounced that no doctors could be spared. However, during that exercise the conclusion of the Medical Officer of Health for Bristol, who advocated keeping radiation victims in the city and home nursing applied, vividly provides the most startling epitaph of what the Government had achieved as he responded to the organisational dilemma presented: 'The concept of the local authority taking control of the situation in the event of an emergency such as nuclear war is welcome because it seems potentially workable'.[27] This bold, simple statement reflecting on nuclear war as an achievable challenge rather than a preordained tragedy shows the inherent optimism which continued to exist out there.

Furthermore, studies such as these illustrate the way local authorities revelled in their new role. STUDY PHOENIX FIVE held at the Staff College was no exception. Also designed to assess the reactions of the new control system, councillors of the South East Region and their senior officers, that included the Medical Officer of Health, engaged with the after effects on their population of a nuclear strike assumed to take place in 1971. The main target area involved an arc that stretched from Guildford to Folkestone with seven nuclear weapons used, the fallout running southwards to the south coast between Dover and Portsmouth. A vital ingredient of the study included the need for the local authority control organisation to demonstrate its resilience, 'to handle the tasks arising from the 'emergency regulations'. Highlighting the point, the notes remarked that in the early stages of the operation 'it would become increasingly difficult to draw a clear distinction between the functions of 'central' government and those of local government'. Amongst the many issues thrown at them, the controllers were empowered to assume responsibility of a general practitioner service. Accordingly, the exercise notes hypothesised that some general practitioners reported to the Regional Hospital Boards for duty and approximately 1,880 doctors were available on the list for general medical services though of these 250 had perished in the attack. Overshadowing everything, the ferocity of the new laws emerged as an open secret with the message that emergency courts would administer 'summary justice' and little left to the imagination as to what lay ahead.[28]

So the GRASS SEED study in 1966 and PHOENIX FIVE in 1967 reveal what the secret state achieved by that time. A new form of 'the nuclear health service' made its appearance in quite an extraordinary way given the history of failures. Whitehall, quite unofficially, had actually adopted the last mobilisation agreement for general practitioners as a kind of virtual working model on the one hand, but with the vital backing of the Defence Regulations on the other. The way that the MOH sector jumped with relish to take up the baton of leadership under such terms was not surprising. As far as general practitioners were concerned, the arrangements represented the outlandish symbol of the centralised state medical system they had fought hard to resist during the formative years of the NHS. It now materialised in its most blatant form and the losers of their medical status in peace, the Medical Officers of Health, regained that in the health service prepared for war. Their inheritance involved the total state control of medicine and its application to the needs of the state. Local authorities received unlimited powers of direction and the position of Medical Officers of Health made the essential hub of control over general practice along with responsibility for public health, domiciliary services, the ambulance service and the dead; one might say the final health centre for a stricken community.

Placebo Effects

Using 'the nuclear health service' for propaganda purposes certainly produced a paradox as between the reality of its icons such as the hospitals and Medical Officers of Health and the fictional pictures of hope that resulted from the organisational mix. The hope generated in the nuclear context did not mean just physical survival, but more and more became about the survival of the human spirit to survive, an addictive ideal in the search for comfort zones during the early years of the hydrogen bomb age. As a psychological comfort weapon it produced a placebo effect which could be both politically strong and welcome; but at times its very strength turned into potential political embarrassment requiring restorative action towards reality.

In 1965 that psychological statement of nuclear hope came under threat with the production of a film called the *The War Game*, but it also produced certain reactions very much pertinent to its importance.[29] Written, directed, and produced by Peter Watkins for the BBC's The Wednesday Play series, a horrific scene, forcefully projected through a docudrama format, was especially important in the context of mass compassion. This emerged from the collapse of the medical services after a nuclear war leaving the seriously injured and those suffering radioactive sickness left to die. The story line then involved the police being ordered to start mercy killing by shooting the masses caught in such severe agony.[30] With that scene, the prospect compellingly appeared that the mythologies of humanness and ethicality hitherto promoted would be destroyed if the mass killing regime was transmitted on television into genteel sitting rooms around the country.

New visions of the unthinkable had been put together with the help of an advisory panel to the film consisting of three members of civil defence, two strategists, a doctor, a bio-physicist and a physician. Nonetheless, the extensive working papers for the production at the BBC archive at Caversham, under the working title of *After the Bomb*, divulge that the idea of mercy killing was actually introduced completely speculatively. Peter Watkins, the producer himself confirmed that it was 'almost impossible to get any hard and fast evidence' for such behaviour, in a sense illustrating the era of trust that still existed. He admitted that he was influenced by the practice of euthanasia through some doctor friends who had confessed to it as a behavioural model and applied this to circumstances that would be magnified many times over.[31] Causing a media furore, the film was banned from television screens and its showing restricted to cinema audiences under an 'X' certificate.

Chapman Pincher in the *Daily Express* conjured up a CND plot and wrote, 'The film, which depicts the effects of a nuclear attack on Britain, is so super-horrific it could not possibly be shown on television.'[32] Attacks on Watkins could not grasp the inference of an ultimate betrayal of society and the idea of both police and those shot by them as victims in the same game. They debunked his thesis as nothing more than open-ended violence which served no other purpose than to leave society in a state of utmost misery and providing fuel for the 'better red than dead' protagonists. Support for such a view came in the *Financial Times* which accused Watkins of inserting the executions only for horror value, concluding the film played to what was termed 'the pacifist solution'.[33] Watkins had, of course, reassembled the relationship between the public, the police and the law that presented social violence in an uncompromising manner and which was neither gratuitous nor wrong, but for him involved experimenting in a dangerously provocative area. It produced the idea new moralities would surface to meet the needs of post-attack society, a radical departure from the kind of nuclear reality depicted in civil defence practices. In an important way it did show the success the Government had achieved in blocking out both the horrific images of nuclear war and also its own draconian measures to deal with the aftermath.

As chairman of the Central Religious Advisory Committee, the Bishop of Bristol 'admitted' in the *Bristol Diocesan Gazette* to being one of those whom the BBC had invited to see the film and had agreed with the decision taken to keep it off the television screens. He said he had found particular fault with it and suggested that there was a lack of depth to its message which represented a betrayal of human nature thereby turning it from art to propaganda.[34] The point says much about *The War Game* incident and the propaganda position of 'the nuclear health service' insofar as it did represent a national beacon of defiance. Taken in the context of the Cold War, those who criticised it could be denounced as defeatist and sympathisers of the communist cause. That sense of defiance through the humanitarian struggle which 'the national health service' portrayed also had far reaching consequences in other ways. Concerned not to be left out of the hope equation, the main church denominations in the country subscribed to the idea of imposing their spiritual layer of humanity by becoming involved in civil defence so they could undertake their pastoral duties as they had during the Second World War. As well as wanting to provide consolation to their congregations before an attack, they were also anxious to be involved at critical pinch points afterwards such as at FAMUAs where the great battles of medical survival were destined to take place. A journey, therefore, started towards finalising the most comprehensive, ecumenical agreement ever produced that eventually manifested itself through a manual titled *Clergy in War.* Designed to provide a spiritual backbone to the nation during its darkest hours, the scheme came complete with armbands for distribution to denote the wearer as a 'Minister of Religion'.[35]

This extraordinary achievement resulted from the Main Churches Committee (a group founded to present a common front in dealings with the Government) showing complete support for the project. A special working committee had been established with representatives of the main denominations sitting on it, including the Church of England, the Church of Scotland, the Roman Catholic Church, the Baptist Union of Great Britain and Ireland, the Presbyterian Church of England, the Congregational Union of England and Wales, plus representatives from the Jewish faith and the Methodist Church. As the pact between the churches and the Government was reached about the clergy's role in civil defence, its terms were sealed by a promise that although powers might be taken in a precautionary period to close places of entertainment or restrict public assembly, such powers would not apply to church premises. Regional Seats of Government, and their deep bunkers, also received a symbolic blessing of approval by the proposed appointment of a clergyman to act as both chaplain and religious adviser and to broadcast to the region in its hour of greatest need.[36]

Conversely, during the exercise newspaper interest in the proceedings of the working group did surface. The *Sunday Citizen* called for 'this absurd committee' to disband at once, or 'examine something worthwhile such as the morality of nuclear warfare!'[37] A *Daily Herald* reporter brought the most sarcastic note of disbelief under the headline 'Four-minute allies', a reference to the dreaded four minute warning the population would have before the missiles struck:

> What a splendid idea! Priests, perhaps may like to try their hands at writing a simple piece of liturgy about three minutes long, suitable for commemorating the end of Western civilisation. You may see that I am not really able to take this Armageddon-planning very seriously. Next thing, I suppose, we shall have special courses for barmen – 101 Drinks You Can Serve in Four Minutes. Come to think of it the only useful thing the clergy can do when IT happens is to try to get the decision reversed.[38]

Ridicule of this kind did not sit well with the new Labour Government. When they took over power from the Conservatives enthusiasm for the final dissemination of some 71,000 copies of the manual across the country to clergy and civil defence authorities began to dim. Home Secretary Sir Frank Soskice eventually expressed severe misgivings about the scheme. There had always been concerns at the publication falling into the wrong hands, but Soskice recognised wider political sensitivities:

> I do not wish to cause offence, but I feel there is something unpleasantly incongruous between religious institutions and the havoc of war, particularly nuclear war. Probably I am wrong, but I feel the public might be offended by the idea of a training handbook for clergymen on what to do in a war situation. Is it not better to say as little about it as possible and avoid any press statement or reference?[39]

Finally, the decision emerged through much political manoeuvring that the best way to avoid any kind of friction was to scrap the manual and the scheme altogether. The end, therefore, in many respects echoed the experience surrounding the general practitioners and government being comfortable about dealing with civil defence at institutional level, but not at 'the grassroots level' with its attendant problem of entering unknown territory. The Bishop of Lichfield, a leading supporter of civil defence, tried to fan the flames of enthusiasm in the House of Lords and argued about what the superhuman cleric could do for government:

> As we know, sometimes the Church can be written off as not being particularly relevant to the modern situation. But when you come to consider the matter, you find that in almost any locality the person who will be known by the greatest number of people is probably the parson, because he lives among his people in the community in which he works and is there all the time. I believe that this man, if used properly, could be of the greatest assistance in these terrible circumstances.[40]

Fine rhetoric was, however, not enough. The production of this play in the theatre of deception had ended and whilst the bishop provided its last soliloquy, the script of the whole affair in the form of the report was finally consigned for destruction. Although the years of work never ended in a public document, the continual debate created a sense of institutional passivity on civil defence by the churches (though not by individuals) that proved a valuable political commodity in itself.

The trouble was that the ingredient of logic folded into the facade could not just create a placebo effect, but also risk its destruction. In other words, the possibility existed of the facade as a propagandist structure actually becoming believable by those involved in its construction. Childbirth arrangements, which had largely remained unchanged since the atomic plan, exhibited distinct signs of succumbing to that danger. These had become the subject of a heated debate in Scotland around the new conditions of hydrogen bomb warfare which increased the likelihood of not enough beds being available in the right places for the post attack population, let alone maternity facilities. With the attendant risk that it would also be difficult and probably dangerous to encourage childbirth in overcrowded homes and billets, a school of thought emerged that the previous hospital-based policy for maternity services should be reversed. Highly provocative, the U-turn envisaged making local authorities responsible for establishing special local maternity hostels to deal with uncomplicated confinements.[41] Local authority domiciliary midwives, it was suggested, might then manage the hostels with visits made, arranged through a pool of general practitioners. The debate also boiled over into other areas such as the possible use of the FMAU as a maternity facility in addition to its formal role for casualty sorting.[41] London, however, remained categorical opposed to any changes whatsoever on the grounds that childbirth was a perfectly natural process which did not require any further support. Adopting this as their philosophy, the Ministry of Health opposed any diversion of medical facilities from the main task of helping casualties. In their eyes the place of midwives, district nurses or health visitors was to provide leadership in first aid parties dealing with the injured and nothing else.[42]

Again, Major General Richardson stepped into the breach and made an impassioned plea about the skewed ethics that in his judgement needed addressing. He suggested that even in nuclear war the process of childbirth should not be subordinated to the needs of casualties and made his point in characteristic manner:

> Medical services exist not merely to treat casualties but to support public morale. Doctors may regard childbirth as a normal physiological process, but to some 80 per cent of the public it is cause for alarm. (Admittedly soldier's wives of the Peninsula could leave the line of march to have their babies, and rejoin the regiment in bivouac that same day) But before any male suggests that our women, in the primitive conditions following nuclear attack, could or should develop a similar toughness, let him ask himself if, in these days when a public outcry may follow the caning of a schoolboy, any of us, like Wellington's soldiers according to Sir Arthur Bryant, could take three or four hundred lashings without a groan, chewing on a musket ball or a bit of leather to keep themselves from crying out while the blood ran down their backs.[43]

Richardson believed that the preservation of the lives and the health of women of childbearing age and their infants deserved a very high priority in the medical pecking order. He considered that even in any evacuation policy, whether it was for the priority classes or hospitals, the midwifery element should not be dismissed, but accentuated as a vital element of the long term survival regime. This meant the transfer of pregnant women to expanded maternity hospitals in reception areas and as much equipment as possible being removed for this task from the target areas. In the case of evacuation of would be mothers it was equally essential, in his opinion, that midwives should accompany the priority classes to deal with any emergency confinements along the way and eventually link up with the child welfare services in the reception areas. If there was a brutal ethic at all, the General maintained it existed in the fact that midwives should not be used for medical purposes where many people would end up crippled through injury, but rather to deal with the nation's future citizens.[44]

The reversal thesis, therefore, meant that Hospital Area Officers could keep their existing maternity hospitals, but only for complicated cases.

For most other situations domiciliary confinement appeared as the answer in what the General called 'Lambing Pens'. Separated from the gross conditions in domestic dwellings and arranged in hostels, such measures would come under the direction of the Medical Officer of Health.[45] Of course, faced with a proposal that had all the ingredients to risk the stability of 'the nuclear health service', if not the NHS itself, a senior civil servant at the Ministry of Health indicated his dismay, 'We can't suddenly turn a memo putting responsibility for maternity on to LA's after years of saying it is a hospital authority task'.[46] Fortunately for Whitehall the issue never erupted into a full blown war of words as it surely might have done if civil defence had survived longer. Very much reflecting that potential conflict area, at the end of 1967 Sir Douglas Baird of the Medical Sociology Unit, Aberdeen University, advised strongly that by that time local authorities such as Aberdeen had little to do with childbirth arrangements and the system should be kept firmly in the hands of hospitals.[47]

The management of maternity services may have eluded the Medical Officer of Health, but the nature of the decision making processes to maintain the status quo in the interests of harmony kept his nuclear inheritance intact. Flattery of domain power in all these ways provided those involved with a sense they could perhaps turn that towards a positive form of nuclear salvation. For those that were not flattered, they were swept along by peer pressure or simply through their contractual duty to comply. The truth of the matter was 'the nuclear health service' only existed as part of the facade and although it might have seemed real enough at times, its institutional attachment merely hung there by a thread of political opportunism. This tenuous position became all too apparent when, without any prior warning, Prime Minister Harold Wilson informed Parliament on 16 January, 1968 the civil defence budget had to be cut from around eight million pounds to just one million pounds. Drastic in every sense, the reduction left only enough to keep local authority control centres on a 'care and maintenance' basis, which operationally meant mothballing them and leaving very little money for anything else. Adding insult to injury, conspicuous failure by the Prime Minister at the time to thank civil defence volunteers for their past service ended the organisation in a most undignified way. Once reassuringly known as 'The Fourth Arm of Defence' it found itself bundled up unceremoniously into the Post Devaluation Measures that involved a swathe of cuts and showed little respect for historical attachments. Backed only by political promises civil defence, without contractual liabilities, made it a soft target, unlike the Concorde project which survived to eventually fly.[48] 'The nuclear health service' as it had been constructed effectively came to an end after enduring for nearly twenty years.

At its demise civil defence, which still had the overtones of the Second World War organisation, had not fallen to a crisis of confidence, but rather to a general crisis of economic confidence. If that had not happened, it might well have continued until the end of the Cold War, if not beyond. (As the Civil Defence Corps has survived in the Isle of Man to deal with civil disasters) Nearly 2000 civil defence volunteers and 150 members of the Auxiliary Fire Service, representing local authorities throughout England and Wales, protested by marching in London on the 25 February 1968 against the plans to disband the two services. They paraded in Trafalgar Square, held a short service at the Cenotaph and then handed in a petition at 10 Downing Street.[49] The gesture in many respects portrayed the final result that government had achieved insofar as the occasion marked the celebration of a system which outwardly displayed the fight for democracy, but hid the abject form of totalitarianism if deterrence failed.

Ironically, the sense of loss echoed one more time when civil defence was brushed away, but then caused Burke Trend, the Cabinet Secretary, to write on 3 July 1968 to the Prime Minister expressing the disquiet of the Home Defence Committee over the country's future ability to respond to the threat of a nuclear attack:

> The results suggest that our home defence arrangements are now seriously deficient and that, as things stand, it would be difficult, if not impossible, to activate an effective home defence organisation within the period which we may expect, or even within a much longer period.[50]

That last discernible squeak of protest illustrates just what a psychological prop the system represented to those who still held a responsibility for home defence in government. Fleetingly, the facade achieved the status of a reality, even when it no longer existed, a fitting testament to its uncanny power of providing comfort.

Medical Notes

If the bedrock on which mass compassion was constructed had to be identified it seems reasonable to point to that emotional amalgam which the wartime generation still felt where the past was a natural pathway to seeing the future. Between 1948 and 1968 'the nuclear health service' appeared to grow out of that kind of mixture of thoughts and reactions unique to an era fast disappearing. Labour Prime Minister Clement Attlee, himself a veteran of the Gallipoli campaign of the First World War, provided an early glimpse of that emotive attachment to a previous age when addressing his military leaders in 1949 during EXERCISE BRITANNIA. As the country's top brass pondered the future around a model of Bristol before and after an atomic attack, generals, field marshals, admirals and air marshals were urged by Britain's first 'nuclear leader' to be ready to support the civil population. Attlee emphasised his message that most in the room would have understood by telling them, 'The lesson of the First World War and the Second World War is that you have got to be prepared in every possible way'.[51] Though used in the context of a war cry of vigilance, the emotional value of preparedness linked to the past had a much wider application. When employed to create the illusion of a cohesive medical civil defence system that same sentiment allowed the past to flood into the planning process enabling organisations, individuals and politicians to use it in ways that most suited their needs.

In the construction of the medical side of 'the facade' experiences were, as the history showed, frequently pulled out as comforting notations of conquering the unknown terrors of the future. A remarkable example of that kind of optimism is in the way Major General Richardson also added his experience of the Second World War when he prepared the Scottish bible of casualty sorting by suggesting 'the holding unit' within the Forward Medical Aid Unit did not automatically constitute the pathway to a painful and lingering death. Instead, he argued limited movement rather than long ambulance journeys was often preferable and cited the Battle of Alamein where the casualties amongst tank crew left out all night fared better than infantry soldiers collected and treated early.[52]

Difficult as such a belief system might seem from today's perspective, Hans J. Morgenthau, an influential US commentator on nuclear politics, observed in a contemporary paper written in 1964, that whilst the nuclear era had started with a vengeance, people still actually lived through thoughts and institutions of an age that had passed. He extended his philosophy into the area of nuclear survival, describing the approach as being in the nature of a specific psychological defence mechanism that took the fallacious view nuclear war was possible to regard as a staged progression from conventional war. Conventional thinking, according to Morgenthau created answers in logical ways, but failed to accept the scale of the impact on society and its possible annihilation. Crucially, it is this kind of search for 'logical' pathways which allowed adaptions of past practice to be incorporated into the facade, even when the degree of destruction increased.[53] Over time the main problem related to the need to balance a limited budget with transmitting the message of compassion in the most efficient way. The exercise reached its zenith during the last stages of civil defence that still used a version of Second World War protocols to create the masterpiece of deceptive emotional architecture in the most audacious package of all. On the one hand the secret state recognised the impossibility of pulling together much in the way of medical support and finally relied on draconian Defence Regulations to muster any vestiges of physical, mental or organisational effort still available. Yet on the other, the sheer awfulness of that nuclear reality remained hidden by the benign framework of civic structures, which included the Medical Officer of Health. This represented the redefinition of the nuclear holocaust from the indefinable into a highly-focussed ethical space of localism that could not have been more in step with the experience of the Second World War.

For all that, although conventionalism could do much in one direction to redefine the impossible into the possible, in another way it held massive dangers. Whilst allowing the reassurances of the past to enter the equation it also risked conventionalist fears to infiltrate the belief system with damaging, if not fatal consequences. The fears continuously harboured by the British Medical Association over state intervention of some kind and its fight to protect general practitioners against that possibility is a notable area of potential disaster. A matter of some irony lay in the fact that whilst the latent potential for friction always remained, the tensions underneath were often harnessed productively and allowed 'the nuclear health service' to develop through a delicate balance of inclusion and exclusion. Organisationally, the National Health Service, characterised by its three components that included the hospital services, health authorities and general practitioners, provided exactly the right framework for those relationships to be managed. The hospital service did not need any formal induction into the facade through new legislation since Regional Hospital Boards had a legal obligation under the *National Health Service Act 1946* to administer their regions as agents for the Ministry of Health. Reshaping the hospital plans to meet the changing patterns of attack were, therefore, put into the hands of Senior Administrative Medical Officers and cascaded down through a compliant system that would regard it as another part of routine administration.

The *Civil Defence Act 1948* also played a key role in sustaining that critical process of preventing friction. Doctors, surgeons and nurses were not allowed to join the civil defence services, but able to offer their medical expertise in giving civil defence lectures or training the mobile units. Therefore, the hospital service could be projected in public using the vicarious role of the National Hospital Service Reserve and the volunteer Ambulance Service instead. These organisations thus acted out the casualty procedures that promised nuclear care to their communities and presupposed access to a supportive medical system. Accordingly, the resources of the National Health Service were integrated through the interplay of illusion and reality and the effect profitably harnessed as part of the Government's visible support of taking civil defence seriously. A paradox resulted between a highly centralised medical bureaucracy and the discretionary decision making allowed to sympathetic medical and nursing staff, in a small but critical area of civil defence. This process successfully maintained equilibrium in the medical profession and prevented any hostility ever attaining institutional status.

Keeping the British Medical Association a bystander played a critical role in that separation process as between voluntary and enforced participation. By allowing the organisation to keep its bespoke control structure of committee networks produced a valuable political dividend of continued passivity. Deeply-held suspicions of doctors becoming a powerful anti-civil defence lobby made deployment an issue so sensitive that made it unworkable. Against the backdrop of disputes with general practitioners and fears that the civil defence issue could become a bargaining tool they were effectively consigned into a no man's land and yet left the BMA seemingly ambivalent to the idea of their membership becoming part of 'the nuclear health service'. By default, the principle of surrogacy also applied. Only sympathetic doctors became involved in lecturing or exercises, but could signal the wider profession being equally committed to 'the nuclear health service'.

Medical Officers of Health, on the other hand, actively sought to become involved as a profession. Unlike general practitioners, most had attended courses at the Sunningdale Staff College and Taymouth Castle and were ready to take up their positions and become medical overlords. They were the ideal candidates for this propagandist entrapment who had lost much prestige and power during the establishment of the National Health Service and were willing to reverse that position in the parallel service designed for nuclear war. The tension was perfect to sustain a publicly acceptable model of post-nuclear attack conditions. Behind the benign model of universal care, the coercive side was possible to establish as an insurance policy for the survival of state. With that production, all its trappings of raw power were hidden and terms like home nursing, first aid, priority classes, which had been defended as moral protocols, would dissolve in the acid conditions of mass destruction. In particular, the medical aspect secretly reversed from the delivery of mass compassion through the casualty chain or hospital services to fighting plague and pestilence. The most potent of cures for the ills of the facade had been found in the 'alternative medicine' prescribed by the secret state that would give a new and sinister meaning to the 'National' Health Service.

Whilst an awesome vehicle for disseminating propaganda, 'the nuclear health service' was not without its medical detractors. The Medical Association for the Prevention of War, which had already shown its hand over the hydrogen bomb, continued to be a key antagonist. Having said that, the association's approach mainly involved attempting to influence other practitioners through the wider narrative of opposing war more generally.[54] Conference papers sometimes appeared, somewhat incongruously, in the *Lancet* stamped with revolutionary dedication by titles such as 'Prevention of War'[55] and the 'The Pathogenisis of War'.[56] This activity did, nevertheless, contribute to an increasingly articulate and more informed climate of dissent, eventually giving rise to probably the most coherent of all critiques. Published by the *New Statesman* in 1960 under the self-explanatory title of 'The Civil Defence Fraud', Morris Berenbaum, the pathologist who earlier challenged the optimism of the casualty sorting procedures, set out the inconsistencies between civil defence and medical practice with incontrovertible clarity. He especially found it unbelievable that even the simple relationship between the likelihood of several million casualties and only 50,000 doctors to deal with them did not in itself destroy the mythology. His final pitch came with the following reasoning for the situation:

> It is also claimed that Civil Defence is necessary as part of the deterrent, that an aggressor will hesitate if he knows the population is prepared. In other words, Civil Defence 'makes the deterrent more credible'. But credible to whom? To the possessor of a stockpile sufficient to destroy us fifty times over? Obviously not. To our military authorities who are presumably aware of these facts? That may be doubted. The answer must be that the main purpose of Civil Defence is to soothe the fears of the electorate and to win support for the deterrent policy – a policy for which we have to pay now with our money and in the future maybe with our lives.[57]

Berenbaum's deep sense of frustration reflects just how the politics of fear still resonated with the embers of collective wartime memory and needed to be indulged; if for no other reason than to show the nuclear button was in the hands of a moral and caring state. Well-argued as many medical papers may have been on the impossibilities of coping with a nuclear war, they never managed to assail the civil defence ethos to the same extent the *Protect and Survive* campaign eventually suffered during the 1980s. Very much a different political climate, some anti-government postures of that later era serve as a useful reminder of what could occur when deference to the nuclear system no longer existed. Those delivered through the professional institutions were most damaging. Adopting Bristol as their model city, the nurses in a paper *Report of an RCN Working Party Nuclear War Civil Defence Planning, The Implications for Nursing* (1983) disputed the thesis of medical attention being possible following a nuclear strike and suggested that the only defence was nuclear disarmament.[58] In a similar mood of belligerence the British Medical Association, published the, *Board of Science and Education Inquiry into the Medical Effects of Nuclear War* (1983) which took up the same point that in nuclear war half of Britain's doctors would be dead or missing and lethal fallout likely to preclude any assistance from those surviving.[59]

The fact that this kind of direct institutional irreverence never occurred on a similar basis during the early years of the Cold War adds the essential uniqueness of the way 'the nuclear health service' had been formed within an environment that still tipped the scales towards conformity, rather than confrontation. A propaganda device of iconic proportions developed, a matter that did not escape the attention of Bertrand Russell (1969). The eminent philosopher and anti-bomb campaigner observes in his autobiography how an array of misinformation had been used to support civil defence. Important to the history of the era, he confirms this as being encompassed in a pervasive power able to mislead, but being so insidious and pervasive to the degree it was impossible to counteract:

> It is difficult to make the facts known to ordinary men and women, because governments do not wish them known and powerful forces are opposed to dissemination of knowledge which might cause dissatisfaction with government policies. Although it is possible to ascertain the probabilities by patient and careful study, statements entirely destitute of scientific validity are put out authoritatively with a view to misleading those who have not time for careful study.[60]

Russell's concerns reflect the creation of a reality by what he calls the product of 'artificial ignorance', adding the further observation: 'and from public men this ignorance trickles down to become the voice of the people'.[61] The last reference to 'the voice of the people' perhaps reflects the most important political attribute of civil defence in general and 'the nuclear health service' in particular. Even in latent apathy it could suddenly crystallise into a symbolic civil right and a rallying point of defiance against the Soviet threat.

Mass compassion was an integral part of that complex mix of emotional propaganda described by Russell. In a sense it represented the final conventionalist tilt at the nuclear windmill and as a historical phenomenon stands out as a unique and distinctive element of British Cold War history. Having been implanted as an ideology its roots could indeed be exceptionally deep and resilient. An image illustrating the point is contained in a commentary written in the *Nursing Mirror* as late as 1966. Produced by a retired Sister, who had joined the National Hospital Service Reserve at Wembley Hospital, Middlesex, she appealed for retired nurses to join the Reserve and support the NHS in its role as the provider of mass compassion at the frontline of nuclear devastation. In her article, she described aspects of the casualty chain and how it was to be rolled out across the country and provide the appropriate treatment before the wounded were dispatched to hospital. Her chosen scenario centred on two aspects, namely the NHS and its doctors and nurses were ready to deal with a nuclear emergency and the seriously injured had nothing to fear insofar the service would operate in war as it did in peace. Describing the Forward Medical Aid Unit being the key sorting point in the system, she confirmed its purpose having three functions: 'To give emergency treatment to the most seriously injured before removal to hospital; to give supportive treatment to those as yet unable to stand the journey to hospital; and to give treatment to the slightly injured'.[63]

As demonstrated in the historical journey, even the idealised medical service really did not exist at all. Few doctors or nurses were nuclear ready in the sense that they had never participated in civil defence and certainly 'the seriously injured' faced abandonment rather than scarce resources wasted on them. In fact, the message delivered through a respected nursing journal and by a volunteer supporting the NHS, but not part of it, really provides the perfect allegory as to exactly how the Government used voluntarism and patriotic duty as external supports for deterrence policy. All told, a very British deception had been built through a binary process at many levels of behavioural strategy which involved the contrived possible hiding the impossible reality. It epitomised a Britain of the past that clung on to the old ethics and for a while this eclipsed the new world of mass destruction. Its position as a social phenomenon should not be consigned to the realms of a banal footnote of Cold War history, but recognised for what it became which was a psychological weapon in every way as real as the Vulcan bombers ready 24/7 to take their lethal cargoes deep into the Soviet heartland.

The legacy of the Cold War remains in certain sectors of the NHS, such as the improvements in the blood transfusion organisation. Above all, it continues to be a political weapon that weaves its psychological power through the medium of universal compassion. A relentless battle rages to deliver this in line with its founding charter, and arguments abound as to whether the NHS is being broken up or improved. Successive governments and opposition parties embrace it to secure the moral high ground by fighting over which side can be trusted as its political custodian. Today, advances in medical practice and life expectancy have moved our own expectations to different levels that include more complex and expensive healthcare procedures. But a new vocabulary that includes privatisation, cover-ups, patient dignity, targets, whistleblowing, bullying, response times and special measures has seemingly provided an ever-increasing pathway of stepping stones away from the core value of universal care originally laid down. For all those machinations, however, the humanitarian credentials of the National Health Service do rise above that cacophony through television fly on the wall documentaries allowing us to witness the work of midwives or surgeons that projects the picture of compassion outside the amorphous bureaucracy of the system. Wounded soldiers from Iraq and Afghanistan have had their bodies put together in extraordinary ways and events such as the British Paralympics provided the ultimate pinnacle of that achievement. During the Cold War, it was the fear of government about the fear of the people over deterrence that directed sentiments into ways that were unique to that era. Taking a leaf out of that history, perhaps we should be aware of our vulnerability to the emotional politics of healthcare and their value as a distractive device that shapes our thinking both in peace and for war.

REFERENCES

Introduction

1. TNA, CAB 21/4920, Nature and the Threat to the United Kingdom-HDR (60)3(Revise), Annex to JIC/1760/62.
2. John Hersey, *Hiroshima* (New York) 19460, p.73.
3. TNA, CAB 134/81. CD(M)(50) 2nd Meeting, 'Training Manual on Atomic Welfare', 15 March 1950.
4. BATH RECORD OFFICE, Unregistered Folder, Civil Defence Chief Officers, 1966.
5. TNA, CAB 21/4920, Nature and the Threat to the United Kingdom-HDR (60)3(Revise), Annex to JIC/1760/62.
6. Home Office, *Nuclear Weapons*, HMSO, 1959.
7. TNA, CAB 21/4920, Nature and the Threat to the United Kingdom-HDR (60)3(Revise), Annex to JIC/1760/62.
8. J. A. Scott, D.J.B. Cooper and S. Seuffert, *The National Health Service Acts, 1946 and 1949*, (London, 1950), pp. xxv-lxi.
9. Ibid.
10. CUMBRIA RECORD OFFICE (KENDAL), RHB(CD) 1952/2, 'Civil Arrangements at hospital premises', February 1952.
11. CND, *Telling Britain, From Now to the Election*, 1963.

Chapter 1: Atomic Reactions

1. Ministry of Health, *Report Part I, 1. The National Health Service, 2 Welfare, Food and Drugs, Civil Defence, for the period 1 April, 1950 to 31 December 1951, p.108.*
2. TNA, MH 131/55. WP(MA)(50) Conclusions 1, February 1950.
3. *The Times*, 3 December 1951.
4. TNA, CAB MH 131/54. Minutes of meeting of 5 November 1948: also the papers before regarding the membership of the Sub-committee.
5. TNA, MH 131/54. Douglas to Rock Carling 29 October 1948.
6. TNA, CAB 128/13. CM(48) 44th Conclusions, 28 June 1948.
7. TNA, MH 131/54. Ministry of Health, 'Sudden attack without warning', undated.
8. *The Lancet*, 11 February 1950.
9. Ibid., 5 August 1950.
10. *The Lancet*, 9 December 1950.
11. CUMBRIA RECORD OFFICE (KENDAL), RHB(CD) 1950/1, Civil Defence Hospital and First Aid Service, 23 May 1950.

12. NRS, HH 51/332. 'Emergency Medical Services'.
13. TNA, MH 131/54. Ministry of Health, WP(MA)(48)1, 29 October 1948, 'Terms of Reference and Composition.'
14. Lieut. Colonel C. L. Dunn, *The Emergency Medical Services, Volume I, England and Wales* (London, 1952), p. 44.
15. Ibid., p. 43.
16. TNA, MH 131/54. Undated paper headed 'Task' and numbered 20.
17. Ibid., WP(MA)(4)3, Estimated Scale of Casualties and Provision of Hospital Beds, 3 February 1949.
18. Ibid., WP(MA)(49)3, 'Estimated Scale of Casualties and Provision of Hospital Beds'.
19. C. L. Dunn, *The Emergency Medical Services, Volume 1, England and Wales* (London, 1952), p. 203.
20. Ibid., p. 94.
21. TNA, MH 131/54. WP(MA)(49)3-Addendum, Estimated Scale of Casualties and Provision of Hospital Beds, 19 February 1949.
22. Ibid., WP (MA)(49)3, 'Estimated Scale of Casualties and Provision of Hospital Beds'.
23. Percy Craddock, *Know Your Enemy, How the Joint Intelligence Committee Saw the World* (London, 2002), p. 54.
24. TNA, CAB 134/137. CD(O)(49)15, 'Scale and Nature of Initial Air Attack on the United Kingdom-1957', Note by the Joint Secretaries, 12 May 1949.
25. Royal College of Physicians of Edinburgh, Obituary of Dr John Smith, 13 July 1913 – 10 August 2010.
    John Smith was born in Glasgow and educated at the High School of Glasgow and Sedburgh School. At Christ's College, Cambridge he read for the Natural Sciences Tripos in pre-clinical medicine, graduating BA in 1935 and MA in 1943. After clinical studies at Glasgow he graduated MB BChir (Cambridge) and MB ChB (Glasgow) in 1938. When war broke out he was in the Royal Artillery (TA) and was called up as a gunner officer, transferring six months later to the RAMC. He was briefly a Company Commander with a Field Ambulance before being appointed to a staff post. Rapid promotion followed. As Assistant Director of Medical Services (ADMS), 2nd Army, he wrote the medical orders for the D-Day Landings. As ADMS of 21 Army Group he planned, with his staff, the move of 34,000 hospital beds, plus infrastructure, from France to Belgium. In April 1945, at age 31, he was youngest full Colonel in the RAMC and as Deputy Director of Medical Services (Operations and Planning) he was responsible for disbanding the Wehrmacht Medical Services in the British Zone.

26. TNA, MH 131/54. WP(MA)(49)14, 'Hospital Staffing under Conditions of Atomic, Biological and Chemical Warfare', Enclosure, 26 May 1949.
27. TNA, MH 131/55. 'Equipment of Mobile Surgical Units', Note by Dr J.G. Johnstone, 2 February 1950.
28. TNA, MH 131/54. WP(MA)(49)18, Hospital Staffing under Conditions of Atomic, Biological and Chemical Warfare, 30 June 1949, Enclosure.
29. TNA, MH 131/55. WP(MA)(49) Conclusions 8, August 1949, 'Hospital Staffing – Further action on WP(MA)(49)18.
30. Ibid.
31. TNA, MH 131/55. (WP)(MA)20, Paper by Sir Claude Frankau. 'On the length of stay of casualties in acute hospitals'. 21 September 1949.
32. TNA, MH 131/54. WP (MA)48 Conclusions 5, Notes of Conclusions, 2 December 1948.
33. TNA, MH 131/55. Note to S.F. Wilkinson, 1 April 1950.
34. TNA, MH 131/56. Muston to Brown 2 February 1952, Attached Note 'Evacuation of Hospitals.'
35. TNA, MH 131/54. WP(MA)(49)9, Control of Medical Manpower in War, 19 March 1949, Attached Skeleton Plan March 1949.
36. CUMBRIA RECORD OFFICE (KENDAL), RHB(CD) 1950/1, 23 May 1950.
37. Ibid.
38. TNA, CAB 134/791. CD(O)(53)20, 'Ambulance Trains', Note by the Chairman of the Civil Defence Joint Planning Staff, 29 August 1953.
39. TNA, CAB 134/84. CD(O)(50)16, 'Atomic Weapons – Scale of attack on the United Kingdom in the period up to the end of 1951', Note by the Chairman of the Civil Defence Joint Planning Staff, 23 May 1950.
40. TNA, MH 131/90. DM 10/50, The Wartime Hospital and First Aid Service-'Central Zones of Target Areas', June 1950.
41. CUMBRIA RECORD OFFICE (KENDAL), RHB(CD) 1950/1, Civil Defence Hospital and First Aid Service, 23 May 1950.
42. Ibid.
43. CUMBRIA RECORD OFFICE (KENDAL), RHB(CD) 1950/1, Civil Defence Hospital and First Aid Service, 23 May 1950.
44. Ibid.
45. TNA, MH 131/64. Note 29 August 1952.
46. Ibid., 'Evacuation of Hospitals', Attached to letter 2 February 1952, Muston to Brown. The removal equation is quoted in RHB(CD)1952/5 deposited at the Cumbria Record Office (Kendal).

47. NRS, HH 51/332. Wilson to Main, 'Expansion of Hospital and First Aid Services', (copy undated).
48. NRS, HH 51/15. 'Arrangements for Tuberculosis Beds in an Emergency', (Undated).
49. CUMBRIA RECORD OFFICE (KENDAL), RHB(CD) 1950/3, Civil Defence Hospital and First Aid Service, 23 May 1950.
50. CUMBRIA RECORD OFFICE (KENDAL), Appendix (revised) to RHB (CD) 1950/3.
51. TNA, CAB 134/789. Report on Civil Defence Planning 1952, 'Inter-hospital Transport', p. 15.
52. TNA, MH 131/55, WP(MA)(50)11, 'Revised Memorandum, by Dr J. Smith of the Department of Health for Scotland', 26 June 1950.
53. TNA, MH 131/55. 'Importation of Doctors from Overseas', Note by the Ministry of Health', Undated.
54. Ibid,. Hospital Staffing under Conditions of ABC Warfare, 'Note of a Meeting on 12 September' (1950).
55. TNA, HO 357/4. CDJPS(51)7, Basic Assumptions for Planning Civil Defence and Due Functioning Measures in Selected Industries, 6 March 1951.
56. Ibid., Civil Defence Joint Planning Staff, Report on Civil Defence Planning to the Official Committee on Civil Defence.
57. CUMBRIA RECORD OFFICE (KENDAL), RHB(CD) 1952/11, 'Mobile Teams', 19 November 1952.
58. TNA, HO 357/5. CDJPS main papers and minutes 1952. Contains much background of the planners struggling to come to terms with the atom bomb threat.
59. TNA, MH 131/93. 'Radiotherapy Services', Note of a meeting at the Ministry of Health, 12 October 1951. Also this file contains background of the arrangements made.
60. Ibid.
61. LONDON METROPOLITAN ARCHIVES, H2/WH/A57/6, RHB(CD) 1953/4. 'Radiotherapy, radio diagnosis and pathology in hospitals in wartime', 18 May 1953.
62. TNA, MH131/67. Divisional Memorandum, 'The Hospital and Casualty Services in Wartime'. February 1956.
63. Lieut. Colonel C. L. Dunn, *The Emergency Medical Services, Volume I, England and Wales* (London, 1952), p. 247.
64. NRS, HH 51/332. Civil Defence Training School, Taymouth Castle, Casualty Services Study 28 to 31 October 1957, 'Mobile First Aid Units'.
65. Ibid.
66. Ibid.

67. NRS, HH 51/343, Note for Commander Galbraith's Meeting with Mr T. Steele M.P. and Mr C. Bence M.P..
68. TNA, MH 131/54. WP(MA)(48)3, 'Ambulance Service', 9 November 1948.
69. TNA, MH 131/43. Ministry of Health, 'Ambulance Service,' December 1948.
70. Ibid., Ambulance Service, CDJPS (49) 4, Comments on Departmental Observations, 17 March 1949.
71. TNA, MH 131/43.CD(O)(49)14, 'Ambulance Service, Scotland'. Memorandum, 22 April 1949.
72. TNA, MH 131/54. WP(MA)(48) Conclusions 6, 11 December 1948.
73. Ibid.
74. Ibid., WP(MA)(49) Conclusions 4, 18 March 1949.
75. TNA, MH 131/54. WP(MA)(48)3, Ambulance Service, 9 November 1948.
76. Home Office, *Manual of Basic Training, Volume 1, Ambulance Section*, HMSO, 1950, p. 3.
77. TNA, MH 131/57. WP(MA)(51)14, Note on the operation of the casualty services, 'Control', 26 July 1951.
78. Ibid.
79. NRS, HH 51/332. Division 8, Divisional Memorandum No. 1, 'The Hospital and Casualty Services in War-time', February 1956.
80. TNA, MH 119/9. Ministry of Health Circular 13/55, Civil Defence (Casualty Collection) Regulations 1954, 29 September 1955.
81. TNA, MH 131/54. WP(MA)(49)19, Final Report by Sub Committee, 13 July 1949.
82. CUMBRIA RECORD OFFICE (KENDAL), RHB(CD) 1950/4, 'Emergency Maternity Units', 16 November 1950.
83. CUMBRIA RECORD OFFICE (KENDAL), RHB(CD) 1952/6, 'Hospital Group Officers', 4 July 1952.
84. LONDON METROPOLITAN ARCHIVES, H2/WH/57/6, Report on Park Prewett Hospital, near Basingstoke, Hants., 1 September 1953.
85. Ibid., Moule to Eade, 'Civil Defence', 27 February 1953.
86. Ibid., Scheme for a Casualty Transit Centre in Wartime, 1 September 1953.

Chapter 2: Cold Comfort War

1. TNA, MH 131/43. Ministry of Supply to Ministry of Health, 8 July 1949.
2. TNA, HO 322/14. Chuter Ede to Prime Minister, 4 July 1950.
3. Lieut. Colonel C. L. Dunn, *The Emergency Medical Services, Volume I, England and Wales* (London, 1952), pp. 334-355.

4. TNA, MH 131/54. 'Expansion of the Blood Transfusion Service,' Draft Memorandum for the Civil Defence Joint Planning Staff, March 1949.
5. Ibid., WP (MA)(49) Conclusions 2, Wartime expansion of the Blood Transfusion Service – Paper WP(MA)(49)2, 9 February 1949.
6. TNA, HO 357/2. 'Expansion of the Blood Transfusion Service', Memorandum by the Civil Defence Joint Planning Staff, (undated)
7. Ibid.
8. TNA, MH 131/54. WP(MA)(48) Conclusions 3, 7 November 1948.
9. CUMBRIA RECORD OFFICE (KENDAL), RHB (CD) 1950/2, National Blood Transfusion Service, 'Expansion', 16 October 1950.
10. Ibid.
11. Ibid., RHB(CD)1952/10, National Blood Transfusion Service, 'Expansion', October 1952.
12. TNA, MH 131/64. Notes on the availability of accommodation for hospital services in wartime, July 1952.
13. Michael Dockrill, *British Defence Since 1945* (London, 1988), p. 43.
14. TNA, CAB 134/139. DTC (51) 1st Meeting, 1 January 1951, 'Hypothesis for Defence Preparations'.
15. TNA, CAB 134/81. CD(M)(50) 5th Meeting, 'Civil Defence Expenditure over the next four years', 21 July 1950.
16. Ibid.
17. TNA, CAB 134/84. CD (O) (50)24, 'Civil Defence Expenditure over the next four years', Report to the Ministerial Committee, 18 July 1950.
18. TNA, MH 131/64. Note to Sir John Wrigley, 'Expenditure on Civil Defence', 19 July 1950.
19. TNA, CAB 134/64. Note to Sir John Wrigley, 19 July 1950.
20. TNA, MH 131/2. CD(H)91/2/1, Purchase of Equipment for Emergency Ward Units and Nurses' Accommodation Units, 3 December 1951.
21. Ibid., D.3/1/19, 'Civil Defence Hospital Service'.
22. TNA, 131/2, RHB(CD) 1950/5, 'Civil Defence Hospital and First Aid Services Provision of Emergency Hospital Ward Units, 16 December 1950.
23. TNA, CAB 134/81. CD(M)(51) 1st Meeting, Civil Defence Expenditure Over the Next Four Years, 18 January 1951.
24. Ibid., CD(M)(51) 2, 'Civil Defence Preparations', Annex1, Memorandum by the Home Secretary, 29 January 1951.
25. Ibid.
26. TNA, MH 131/2. RHB(CD) 1950/5, 'Civil Defence Hospital and First Aid Services Provision of Emergency Hospital Ward Units, 16 December 1950.

27. TNA, CAB 134/81. CD(M)(51) 1st Meeting, Civil Defence Expenditure Over the Next Four Years,' 18 January 1951.
28. TNA, MH 131/24. CD 93/1/, 'Note on Supply of Equipment', August 1951.
29. TNA, MH 131/2. 'Civil Defence Building Proposals', 1951.'
30. Ibid., Note to Brown, Civil Defence Emergency Accommodation, Programme Stage I, February, 1951.
31. Ibid., Ministry of Works note, Headquarters Building Committee, 15 February 1952.
32. TNA, CAB 129/45. *Economic Survey for 1951*, March 1951. 'Confidential Proof'.
33. TNA, CAB 129/52. C(52)166, 'Economic Policy', Memorandum by the Chancellor of the Exchequer, 17 May 1952.
34. TNA, CAB 134/809. DP(M)(53) 1st Meeting, 'The Future Course of Defence Expenditure', 18 June 1953.
35. TNA, MH 131/64. Draft note to Official Committee, March 1953, 'Capital Expenditure for Civil Defence Hospital, First Aid and Blood Transfusion Service'.
36. Ibid., 'Note for Meeting of the Official Committee on Civil Defence on Wednesday 6 May'.
37. Ministry of Health, *Report Part I, 1. The National Health Service, 2, Welfare, Food and Drugs, Civil Defence, for the period 1 April, 1950 to 31 December 1951, p.109.*
38. NRS, HH 51/343. See correspondence between 17 August 1951 and 15 February 1952.
39. Ibid.
40. TNA, CAB 134/789. Civil Defence Planning 1952, 'Hospital and First Aid Services'.
41. TNA, MH 131/64. Note on the availability of accommodation for the Hospital Services in war-time, July 1952.
42. TNA, CAB 134/813. DTC(53)4, 'Use of Schools in War by Other Departments', 21 May 1953.
43. Ibid.
44. Ibid., DTC(53) 3rd Meeting, Cabinet Defence (Transition) Committee, Minutes, November 1953.
45. TNA, CAB 139/50. C (52)100, 'Employment in the Textile and Clothing Industries', Memorandum by the Home Secretary and the Minister of Defence, 2 April 1952.
46. TNA, MH 131/64. Prime Minister to Home Secretary, 20 March 1952.
47. Ibid., Strath to Armer, 26 March 1952.
48. TNA, CAB 134/57. Report on Civil Defence Planning 1952, 'Health Departments'.

49. Ibid.
50. Ibid., WP(MA)(53) Conclusions 1, 'Paragraph 2(b)'.
51. Ibid., 'Raw Opium', May 1951.
52. TNA, HO CDJPS(54)6, Report on Civil Defence Planning 1953, 224 – 227.
53. TNA, MH 131/57. Note to Dr Clark, 'Supply of Oxygen,'7 May 1954.
54. Ibid., Ross to Ellerington, 23 June 1954.
55. TNA, MH 131/57. WP(MA)(53) Conclusions 6, 'Reserves of First Aid Equipment (Item 4(b)).
56. TNA, CAB 129/54. C(52)253, 'The Defence Programme', Memorandum by the Minister of Defence, 22 July 1952.
57. TNA, DEFE 7/719. Minute Sheet, ref TS 309/08/49, 19 March 1952.
58. TNA, PREM 11/606. D(52) 5th Meeting, 'Civil Defence and War Plans of Civil Departments', 14 May 1952.
59. Ibid.
60. House of Commons, *First Report from the Select Committee on Estimates, Session 1953-54, Civil Defence*, pp. 48, 1331 and 1333.
61. TNA, PREM 11/606. *First Report of the Select Committee on Estimates Session 1953 - 54, Civil Defence.*
62. Ibid.
63. TNA, PREM 11/606. Norman Brook to Prime Minister, 23 December 1953.
64. Ibid.
65. TNA, CAB 134/789. CD(M)(54)1st Meeting, 'The First Report from the Select Committee on Estimates on Civil Defence', 19 January 1954.
66. TNA, HO 312/3. Civil Defence Circular 3/54, 'First Report from the Select Committee on Estimates Session 1953/54', 29 January 1954.
67. TNA, CAB 134/938, HDC(53)1, Home Defence Committee, 'Terms of Reference and Composition'.
68. Ibid.
69. Ibid.
70. Ibid., HDC(53)8, 24 July 1953, Annex 10, 'Hospital Services in England and Wales', Memorandum by the Ministry of Health.
71. Ibid., HDC(53)7, The Initial Phase of a War, 'Morale', 24 July 1953.

Chapter 3: Surgical Spirits

1. TNA, MH 131/54, WP(MA)(49)9. 'The Skeleton Plan' agreed internally along with the strategy for its approval.
2. C. L. Dunn, *The Emergency Medical Services, Volume 1, England and Wales* (London, 1952), p. 391.

3. The Ministry of Health, *On the State of the Public Health during the six years of war, Report of the Chief Medical Officer of the Ministry of Health 1939-1945* (London, 1946), p. 191.
4. Ibid.
5. C. L. Dunn, *The Emergency Medical Services, Volume 1, England and Wales* (London, 1952), p. 391.
6. Ibid., p. 390.
7. The Ministry of Health, *On the State of the Public Health during the six years of war, Report of the Chief Medical Officer of the Ministry of Health 1939-1945* (London, 1946), p. 192.
8. Ibid.
9. Ibid. p. 193.
10. Ibid.
11. Ibid., p. 193.
12. Ibid., p. 195.
13. Ibid., p. 194.
14. C. L. Dunn, *The Emergency Medical Services, Volume 1, England and Wales* (London, 1952), p. 397.
15. The Ministry of Health, *On the State of the Public Health during the six years of war, Report of the Chief Medical Officer of the Ministry of Health 1939-1945* (London, 1946), p. 193.
16. Ibid., p. 194.
17. C. L. Dunn, *The Emergency Medical Services, Volume 1, England and Wales* (London, 1952), p. 399.
18. Ibid., p. 71.
19. Richard M. Titmuss, *Problems of Social Policy*, (London, 1950), p. 493.
20. J. A. Scott, D.J.B. Cooper and S. Seuffert, *The National Health Service Acts, 1946 and 1949*, (London, 1950), pp. xxv-lxi.
21. TNA, 131/54. WP(MA)(48)13, 'Use of Medical Manpower', Memorandum by Sir Alexander Hood, 27 November 1948.
22. TNA, MH 131/54. WP(MA)48 Conclusions 51, Note of Conclusions reached at the Fifth Meeting held on November 25th, 1948, 4(h) – 'Staffing of Hospitals'.
23. TNA, MH 131/45. Note of a Meeting at the Ministry of Health, 11 September 1950.
24. TNA, MH 131/54. WP(MA)(48)13, 'Use of Medical Manpower', Memorandum by Sir Alexander Hood, 27 November 1948.
25. TNA, 131/54. WP(MA)49)1, 8 January 1949, 'Use of Medical Manpower', paper by Mr. Clark-Turner.
26. TNA, MH 131/54. Control of Medical Manpower in War, Skeleton Plan, May 1949.
27. Ibid.

28. Ibid. The suggestion of 'other ranks' appears in WP(MA)(48) Conclusions 3.
29. TNA, AIR 20/8686. Points from meeting of Ministry of Defence Working Party on Medical Establishments of the Services, 21 November 1947.
30. TNA, AIR 20/8687. MSC/P(48)12, Annex, Draft, Medical Services Co-Ordinating Committee, 'Directive to Local Commands'.
31. TNA, MH 79/632. MSC/P(50)8, Medical Services Coordinating Committee, 'Shortage of Specialists in the RAMC,' Note by the Director General Army Medical Services, 23 May 1950.
32. Ibid.
33. TNA, MH 131/44. Medical Services Co-Ordinating Committee, 'The Organisation of Medical Services in War', Draft Report by the Standing Sub-committee, 2 July 1949.
34. Ibid., 'The Organisation of Medical Services in War', Report by the Standing Sub-Committee, 6 August 1949.
35. Ibid., MSC/M(49)5, Medical Services Co-Ordinating Committee, Minutes of Meeting 11 August 1949.
36. TNA, MH 131/54. Suggested Amendments to WP(MA)(49)9,'Approval of the Plan', Attached to letter Graham to Wilkinson, 2 April 1949.
37. TNA, MH 131/44. MSC/M(49)5, Ministry of Health internal memo, 31 August 1949.
38. Ibid., Ministry of Health internal memo, 9 September 1949.
39. Ibid., Letter marked 'secret' to William Daley, Chairman, Society of Medical Officers of Health, 13 September 1949.
40. On the issue of medical politics see Marina Rintala, *Creating the National Health Service, Aneurin Bevan and the Medical Lords* (London: 2003).
41. TNA, MH 131/44. File note, 7 October 1949.
42. Ibid., 'Control of Medical Manpower in War', Minutes of Meeting 10 October 1949.
43. Ibid., Ministry of Health internal memo, 23 November 1949.
44. Ibid., Letter from British Medical Association to Russell Smith, 29 December 1949.
45. Ibid., Ministry of Health internal memo, 30 December 1949.
46. TNA, MH 131/45. Medical Women's Federation to The Ministry of Health, 2 March 1950.
47. Ibid., 'Comments of Representatives of the Medical Profession', position as at 15 February 1950.
48. TNA, MH 131/44. Wilkinson to Nash, 7 July 1949.
49. TNA, LAB 6/367. Note to Sir Harold Wiles, 7 October 1949.
50. TNA, MH 131/44. Nash to Russell-Smith, 9 December 1949.

51. Ibid.
52. TNA, MH 131/45. Nash to Russell-Smith, 20 January 1950.
53. Ibid., Ministry of Health internal memo, Wilkinson to Russell Smith, 16 March 1950.
54. Ibid.
55. TNA, MH 131/45. Norman Brook to Sir Godfrey Ince, 27 March 1950.
56. Ibid., Notes of Meeting 'Control of Medical Manpower in War', 5 April 1950.
57. Ibid.
58. TNA, MH 131/45. 'Skeleton Plan for Control of Medical Manpower in War, Comments and Suggestions of Ministry of Labour'.
59. TNA, MH 131/45. Memo by Wilkinson, 31 August 1950.
60. Ibid., Note of meeting 11 September 1950.
61. Ibid., 'Skeleton Plan for Control of Medical Manpower in War, Comments and Suggestions of Ministry of Labour'.
62. Ibid.
63. James Stirling Ross, *The National Health Service in Great Britain* (London, 1952) Chapter 26, The Course of Expenditure.
64. BMA ARCHIVES, Council Documents 1948-1950, Supplementary Council Agenda, 22 November 1950.
65. James Stirling Ross, *The National Health Service in Great Britain* (London, 1952) PostScript: November 1951 to June 1952.
66. TNA, MH 131/45. Milne to Zachary Cope, 21 September 1950.
67. Ibid., A Macrae to Russell-Smith, 25 September 1950.
68. TNA, MH 131/46. Note of Discussion with the Medical Profession on 20 October 1950.
69. Ibid., Ministry of Health internal note, Bliss to Milne, 25 November 1950.
70. Ibid.
71. Ibid.
72. Ibid.
73. TNA, MH 131/46. Control of Medical Manpower in War, Skeleton Plan Revised January 1951.
74. BMA ARCHIVES, Committee on Control of Medical Manpower in War Session 1951-52, Minutes of meeting, 1 March 1951.
75. TNA, MH 131/46. Macrae to Milne, 20 March 1951.
76. Ibid.
77. Ibid., Note for meeting on 28 March 1951.
78. BMA ARCHIVES, CMWC Documents. 1946-52, Report of the Services Committee for the year 1951.
79. TNA, LAB 6/383. Report reference M. 2806/21/48, 5 February 1951.

80. Ibid., Major-General Bainbridge to Nash, 7 February 1951.
81. Ibid., Macrae to Russell-Smith, 14 February 1951.
82. BMA ARCHIVES, Council Documents Session 1952-53. Report of the Services Committee for the year 1951, 'VI. Screening of General Practitioners on the Reserves of H.M Forces.'
83. BMA ARCHIVES, Minutes and Documents ARM London 1951. Annual Representative Meeting. 16 June 1951, Item 242.
84. Ibid.
85. TNA, MH 131/47. Notes of discussion at the Ministry of Health, 28 March 1951.
86. Supplement to the *BMJ*, 2 February 1952.

Chapter 4: Facade Fatigue

1. TNA, HO 322/44. 'South-Western Region, Regional Report for Quarter ended 31 December 1952'.
2. TNA, HO 357/7. CDPS, 'Report on Civil Defence Planning 1953'.
3. *Civil Defence*, January and February 1954.
4. TNA, DEFE 7/706. 'Memorandum by the Ministry of Health on the Organisation and Operational Control of the Civilian Casualty Services', January 1957.
5. Guy Oakes, *The Imaginary War* (New York, 1994), pp. 60-61.
6. *Daily Express,* 1 April 1954.
7. TNA, CAB 134/789. CD(M)(54) 5th Meeting, 20 May 1954, 'Draft Statement on Civil Defence Plans To Be Made By The Home Secretary In The House Of Commons'.
8. TNA, CAB 134/808, DP(54) 3rd Meeting, 'Defence Policy', 17 June 1954.
9. TNA, CAB 134/792. CD(O)(54) 3rd Meeting, 'First Review of Civil Defence Plans', 12 May 1954.
10. Doctors Support Coventry, *Peace News*, 19 July 1954.
11. TNA, CAB 134/940. 'The Defence Implications of Fall-Out from a Hydrogen Bomb, Report by a Group of Officials', 8 March 1955.
12. Ibid., Section V, 'General Implications'.
13. Ibid., Section XV, 'Summary of Conclusions and Recommendations'.
14. Ibid., Section X, 'Machinery of Control'.
15. TNA, CAB 134/940. HDC(55)3, 'Fall-Out', Report of a Working Group. 'Medical and Relief Services'.
16. TNA, CAB 134/940. HDC(55) 1st Meeting, Home Defence Committee, 'Report of the Strath Group on the Defence Implications of Fall-Out from a Hydrogen Bomb', 17 March 1955.

17. Ministry of Health, Report Part I,I. *The National Health Service, 2, Welfare, Food and Drugs, Civil Defence, for the year ended 31 December, 1956*, p.7.
18. TNA, MH 119/11. HM(CD)(57)1, 'Organisation of Hospital Services in War-Time', March 1957.
19. Although the National Archives catalogue file MH 131/57 is referenced as being on Medical Aspects planning from 1951 to 1957, in fact the bulk of the file ends in 1954 with a somewhat 'rogue letter' dated 1957 having been inserted In effect a complete section of planning history has been destroyed between 1955 and 1957.
20. TNA, MH 131/67. War Plans of the Health Departments, July 1955.
21. Ibid.
22. TNA, MH 119/11. HM(CD)(57)1, 'Organisation of Hospital Services in War-Time', March 1957.
23. Ibid.
24. TNA, DEFE 7/706. 'Memorandum by the Ministry of Health on the Organisation and Operational Control of the Civilian Casualty Services', January 1957.
25. NRS, HH 51/342, 'The Organisation of the Hospital Service in South-Eastern Region in Wartime', February 1968.
26. TNA, MH 119/11. HM(CD)(57)1, 'Organisation of Hospital Services in War-Time', March 1957.
27. Ibid.
28. NRS, HH 51/334. SHM(CD)59/1. 'Organisation of Hospital Services in Scotland,' 1959.
29. Ibid.
30. TNA, DEFE 7/706. MSC(MP)/M(56)1, 'Manpower', 24 December 1956.
31. TNA, DEFE 10/231. MSC(MP)/P(57)10, Co-ordination of Service and Civilian Medical Services in Great Britain, 10 April 1957.
32. TNA, DEFE 7/706. 'War Office', Extract from MSC(MP)M(56)1, 11 December 1956.
33. Ibid.
34. TNA, DEFE 20/231. MSC(MP)/M(58), 'Co-ordination of Service and Civilian Medical Services in Nuclear War', 21 April 1958.
35. TNA, CAB 134/1248. HDC(S)(55)18, Annex C 'Medical Supplies', 23 September 1955.
36. Ibid.
37. TNA, CAB 134/1248. HDC(S)(55)13,'Medical Supplies,' 7 September 1955.
38. Ibid.
39. Ibid.

40. TNA, PREM 11/1260. Ministry of Defence, Selwyn Lloyd to Prime Minister, 14 November 1955.
41. TNA, CAB 134/940. HDC(55)20, Home Defence Committee, 'Stockpiling for Home Defence', 30 September 1955.
42. TNA, CAB 134/1245. HD(M)(55)10, Home Defence (Ministerial) Committee, 'Shelter Policy, Memorandum by the Home Secretary', 25 October 1955.
43. TNA, CAB 129/63. C(53)355, 'Civil Supply 1954-55, Memorandum by the Chancellor of the Exchequer', 6 December 1953.
44. TNA, CAB 134/1245. HD(M)(55) 5th Meeting, Home Defence (Ministerial) Committee, 20 December 1955.
45. TNA, PREM 11/1260. (DP(54)9), 'Civil Defence Plans. Norman Brook to Prime Minister, 23 June 1954. See also CAB 134/1245. HD(M)(55) 2nd Meeting, Home Defence Committee, Defence Expenditure by Civil Departments and Shelter Policy', 27 October 1955.
46. *Daily Express*, 18 April 1956.
47. TNA, CAB 134/1207. CD(O)(56)10, 'Defence expenditure by Civil Departments', Memorandum by the Central War Plans Secretariat, 26 July 1956.
48. TNA, DEFE 7/706. MH/MSC(SS)/P(57)3, Report attached 'Existing Civil Defence Reserves for Hospitals'.
49. TNA, CAB 134/1207. CD(O)(56)5, 'Memorandum by the Health Departments', 10 September 1956.
50. Ibid.
51. Ibid.
52. Ministry of Health Report, 1956.
53. TNA, MH 131/65. Official Committee on Civil Defence, Agenda note, 21 October 1958.
54. Home Office, *Manual of Fire Appliances for Mobile Fire Columns* (HMSO, 1956).
55. NRS, HH 51/339. Ministry of Health, 'Training Vehicles-review of arrangements', 26 August 1959.
56. Ibid.
57. TNA, DEFE 7/231. 'Memorandum by the Ministry of Health on the Organisation and Operational Control of the Civilian Casualty Services'. January 1957.
58. TNA, MH 119/11. HM(CD)(57)1, 'Organisation of Hospital Services in War-Time', March 1957.
59. TNA, MH 131/126. Notes on the organisation of the Casualty Services, 'Expansion of the Hospital Service for war purposes'.

60. TNA, DEFE 7/231. 'Memorandum by the Ministry of Health on the Organisation and Operational Control of the Civilian Casualty Services'. January 1957.
61. TNA, CAB 134/1207. CD(O)(56) 1st Meeting, 'Accommodation', 16 March 1956.
62. TNA, DEFE 7/231. 'Annex to MSC (MP)/P(57)9, Interim Report'.
63. Ibid., Letter from the Ministry of Defence to the Ministry of Health, Ref.145/094/56. 21 January 1958.
64. TNA, MH 131/64. 'Tentage-Production Position', Undated Memo.
65. Ibid., Greenhalgh to Mitchell, 13 January 1954.
66. Ibid., Firth to Kirkman, 6 July 1955.
67. NRS, HH51/342. 'The Organisation of the Hospital Service in South-Eastern Region in Wartime', Revised 1968.
68. TNA, MH 131/65. 'Hutted Hospitals', Attached to Review of Home Defence Expenditure, 3 August 1956.
69. TNA, CAB 134/1476. CD(57) 1st Meeting, Ministerial Committee on Civil Defence, 'Home Defence Policy', 16 April 1957.
70. TNA, CAB 134/1436, C(O)D(58)7 'Home Defence Policy-Estimates 1959/60', 15 October 1958.
71. TNA, HO 322/157. Note by General Sir Sidney Kirkman to Sir Charles Cunningham and the Home Secretary, 7 August 1958.
72. Ibid., Memorandum to the Home Secretary, 15 October 1958.
73. Ibid., Hand written note by the Home Secretary on the above memo.
74. TNA, CAB 134/1476. CD(57), 1st Meeting, 'Home Defence Policy,' 16 April 1957.

Chapter 5: Admission Impossible

1. TNA, CAB 134/1436. C(O)D(58)7, 'Home Defence Policy-Estimates 1959/60', 15 October 1958.
2. TNA, DEFE 7/759. Draft Minute from the Home Secretary to the Prime Minister, date stamped 5 January 1960.
3. Ibid., Paper attached to memorandum by J.H. Nelson to Lawrence-Wilson, 4 February 1960.
4. Ibid., Norman Brook to Prime Minister, Home Defence Policy, 14 December 1960.
5. TNA, CAB 21/4441. Draft Report by the Home Defence Policy Review Committee 1960, 'Home Defence Policy'.
6. TNA, CAB 134/2040. 'Review of Emergency Medical Services', Paper by the Ministry of Health. Attached to note by the Secretaries, 7 June 1960.
7. TNA, CAB 134/1437. C(O)D(61) 2nd Meeting, 'Use of Educational Premises', 12 September 1961.

8. TNA, CAB 134/1477. CD(62), 'The Education Service in War', Note by the Chairman, 27 May 1962. Also see attached report by the Official Committee on Civil Defence.
9. Ibid.
10. Ibid.
11. Ibid., CD(M)(63)6. 'The Education Service in War', Memorandum by the Secretary of State for Scotland and the Minister of Education, 6 December 1963.
12. NRS, HH 51/252. Circular 3/64, 'The Education Service and Nuclear Attack', 20 March 1964.
13. TNA, MH 131/117. Regional Hospital Board Civil Defence Officers Meeting, 1 May 1963.
14. Ibid., Note of Meeting with Regional Hospital Board Representatives on Civil Defence Matters, 'Inter hospital transport', 20 January 1966.
15. *Report of the Ministry of Health 1963*, p. 56.
16. *Report of the Ministry of Health 1964*, p. 64.
17. TNA, CAB 21/5184. 'Functions and Organisation of the Civil Defence Corps and the Auxiliary Fire Service', Memorandum by the Home Office.'
18. Ibid.
19. TNA, CAB 134/2040. 'Review of Emergency Medical Services', Paper by the Ministry of Health. Attached to not by the Secretaries, 7 June 1960.
20. TNA, MH 131/107. Ministry of Health Letter of the Senior Administrative Medical Officer, South East Metropolitan Regional Hospital Board, 31 March 1960.
21. Ibid.
22. TNA, MH 131/107. Ministry of Health letter, 'Care and Custody of Civil Defence Stocks', 25 June 1965.
23. TNA, MH 131/117. Meeting with Regional Hospital Board Representatives, 20 January 1966. 'Notes on the Agenda.'
24. TNA, MH 131/122. Internal report by Hewitt to Harrison, 'Civil Defence', 24 December 1963.
25. Ibid., Note by Parliamentary Secretary, 'Civil Defence', 3 January 1964.
26. TNA, CAB 134/2042. HDR(64)10, Medical Services, 'Medical Supplies', 23 November 1964.
27. TNA, MH 131/110. Correspondence, 'Long-Acting Analgesics – South Western RHB'.
28. SOMERSET ARCHIVE, D/H/yeo 1/3/5. 'South - Western Regional Hospital Board, Defence and Mobilisation Plan 1967'.

29. TNA, MAF 313/34. The file contains extensive discussions as to how the hospital service was to be supported by food supplies provided by local food officers.
30. TNA, HO 322/186. STUDY BULL RING, 29 May to 21 June 1956.
31. Ibid.
32. Ibid.
33. TNA, CAB 134/1493. STUDY MEDICAL CARAVAN, 15 May 1957.
34. Ibid.
35. Ibid.
36. TNA, MH 131/59. 'Functions of Forward Medical Aid Units', Annexures A-D.
37. TNA, MH 131/64, CD(O)2, Official Committee on Civil Defence, 'Veterinary Surgeons'.
38. Ministry of Health Circular 9/60, 'The organisation and operational control of the Ambulance and Casualty Collection Services', 2 June 1960.
39. Ibid.
40. Ibid.
41. ROYAL SOCIETY OF MEDICINE ARCHIVE, Proceedings of the Royal Society of Medicine, Volume 50, 967, Sectional Pages 21-22, United Services Section, Discussion on the Management of Mass Casualty Situations in Time of War, 6 June 1957.
42. Ibid.
43. British Medical Journal, 9 August 1958 pp. 379-382.
44. Ibid., 1 November 1958. p. 1101.
45. Ibid., p. 1102.
46. BRISTOL RECORD OFFICE, Box 40795/16, Civil Defence, Civil Defence Weekend Course for Senior Hospital Administrators, 10 - 11 November 1956.
47. Ibid.
48. TNA, MH 131/59. EXERCISE RELIANCE, 13 July 1958.
49. Ibid.
50. Ibid.
51. TNA, MH 131/117. Draft Home Defence Preparations, 'Interim Planning', (undated).
52. TNA, DEFE 7/706. 'Co-ordination of Service and Civilian Medical Services in Nuclear War', Extract from MSC/M(57)2, 27 July 1957.
53. TNA, MH 119/12. HM(CD)(58), Ministry of Health Memorandum, 'Blood Transfusion Service in War', 30 May 1958.
54. TNA, MH 131/59. 'The Initial Management of Mass Casualties', Lecture given by the Senior Medical Officer, South Western Regional Hospital Board.

55. Ibid., HM(59) D, 'Forward Medical Aid'.
56. Ibid., Memorandum by the Working Party on the Organisation and Equipment of Forward Medical Aid Units, (Undated).
57. Ibid.
58. TNA, MH 119/14. HM(CD)(60), 'Forward Medical Aid', 15 September 1960.
59. TNA, BD 2/16. Civil Defence and First Aid Services, 'Operation Fall' Series of Forward Medical Aid Exercises, 1960-65.
60. TNA, MH 131/97, Note of a meeting with Representatives of Regional Hospital Boards at the Ministry of Health, 28 November 1962.
61. TNA, MH 119/17. HM(CD)(63)1, Extended First Aid and Additional Life Saving Techniques, 31 December 1963.
62. *The Independent,* Obituary 16 September 1996.
63. TNA, MH 131/105. 'Priorities and Casualty Sorting in Civil Defence', (2nd Draft).
64. NRS, HH 51/163. Wayne to Smith, 23 March 1964.
65. Ibid., Handwritten note by Richardson to Smith, 26 March 1964.
66. TNA, MH 131/97, L.H.Murray to Illingworth, 'Guidance to Doctors on Management of Mass Casualties'. 23 October 1964.
67. Ibid.
68. NRS, HH 51/163. Ministry of Health to South Western Regional Hospital Board, 19 May 1964.
69. NRS, HH 51/163. Internal note, the Department of Health Edinburgh, 13 October 1964.
70. Ibid., Smith to Hume, 18 November 1964.
71. TNA, BD 2/23. Welsh Hospital Board, 5 January 1967, HM(CD)(63)1, 'Mass Casualty Care'.
72. NRS, HH 51/163. *The Management of Mass Casualties,* Scottish Home and Health Department, April 1967, p. 27.
73. TNA, MH 131/105. Priorities and Casualty Sorting in Civil Defence, Hand written note attached to draft addressed to Colonel Barton by Newman Illingworth.
74. NRS, HH 51/163. *The Management of Mass Casualties,* Scottish Home and Health Department, April 1967, p. 14.
75. Ibid., Notes on the Management of Mass Casualties, p. 2.
76. Ibid., p. 4.
77. Ministry of Health, *Guidance Notes for Doctors Teaching Mass Casualty Care (Previously Extended First Aid).* p. 7.
78. Ibid., p. 24.
79. TNA, DEFE 10/231. MSC/P((57)13, 8 November 1957, Medical Services Coordinating Committee, 'Lessons of the SHAPE medical conference', Comments by the Ministry of Defence.

80. NRS, HH 51/163. *The Management of Mass Casualties,* Scottish Home and Health Department, April 1967, p. 32.
81. Ibid., p. 33.
82. CUMBRIA RECORD OFFICE (KENDAL), Report on STUDY SURVIVAL and paper presented by Mr D.A. Sandford FRCS.
83. Ibid.
84. NRS, HH 51/163. *The Management of Mass Casualties,* Scottish Home and Health Department, April 1967, p. 13.

Chapter 6: Body Language

1. TNA, HO 357/10. CDJPS(M)(50)(18), 'Issue of personal gamma ray dosimeters to the public', Note by Sir John Hodsoll, 24 November 1950.
2. TNA, MH 131/65. Contains much information on the introduction of home nursing as does file TNA,MH 131/116. Also TNA, CAB 134/1437. CD(59)6, Home Defence Budget 1960/61, 3 December 1959.
3. Home Office, Manual of Civil Defence: Vol.1, *Nuclear Weapons* (London, 1956),p. 13. Also Medical Research Council, *The Hazards to Man of Nuclear and Allied Radiations* (London, 1956), pp. 13-23.
4. NRS, HH51/173. Fraser to Hodges, 25 June 1956.
5. Ibid., 'Training Syllabus'.
6. Ibid., 20 December 1961, Draft Civil Defence (Training in Nursing) (Scotland) Regulations, 1961.
7. Ibid., St Andrew's Ambulance Association to Department of Health for Scotland, 9 January 1962.
8. Ibid., 'Syllabus', Appendix to DHS Circular No. /62.
9. *Reynolds News*, 13 September 1959.
10. RVS ARCHIVE, Box 85. AA3c CO, Packet 2, Publicity One-in-Five, 'Yellow Door Poster', 1 August 1961.
11. Nursing Times, 26 September 1958,p.1139.
12. NRS, HH 51/337. RHB(CD)(66) 2, Wartime Responsibilities of Local Health Authorities, Note by Scottish Home and Health Department.
13. TNA, CAB 134/1477. CD (62)1st Meeting, 'Advice to the Public-Booklet', 18 July 1962.
14. Ibid.
15. Ibid.
16. TNA, MH 131/117. Regional Hospital Board, 'Civil Defence Officers Meeting', 1 May 1963.
17. Ibid., Note of a meeting with representatives of Regional Hospital Boards, 'Civil Defence Matters,' 13 December 1963.

18. *The Times*, 26 November 1963.
19. Ibid.
20. TNA, CAB 134/2027. HDC (64)6, 'Official Announcements in a Precautionary Stage', Note by the Chairman of the Public Information in War Sub Committee. 11 September 1965.
21. Ministry of Defence, *Statement on Defence, 1956*, p. 25.
22. TNA, CAB, 134/1437. C(O)D(60)3, 'Evacuation,' Note by the Home Office, 24 March 1960.
23. TNA, CAB 134/1437. C(O)D(59)17, 'Hospital Evacuation,' Note by the Health Departments, 30 December 1959.
24. TNA, CAB 134/2040. HDR(60)33, 9 August 1960, 'Evacuation', Note by the Secretary.
25. TNA, CAB 129/108. C(62)62, 'Home Defence: Dispersal Policy', Memorandum by the Secretary of State for Home Department, the Secretary of State for Scotland and Minister of Housing and Local Government and the Minister for Welsh Affairs, 9 February 1962.
26. TNA, CAB 134/2045. HDR (65)4, 'Dispersal,' Note by the Secretaries, 5 July 1965.
27. NRS, HH 51/334. Ministry of Health to Regional Hospital Secretaries (England), 25 July 1962.
28. Ibid.
29. NRS, HH 51/332. Note of a meeting with representatives of Regional Hospital Boards, 8 May 1956.
30. NRS, HH 51/334. Illingworth to Mackay, May 1963.
31. NRS, HH 131/176. Scottish Home and Health Department to Secretary Regional Hospital Board, 23 October 1964.
32. TNA, CAB 134/2042. HDR(64)10, 'Medical Services', 23 November 1964.
33. TNA, CAB 134/2883. HD(M)(66)2, 'Hospital Evacuation Policy', Note by the Secretary of State for Scotland and the Minister of Health, 28 September 1966.
34. Ibid.
35. TNA, HO 312/3, Home Office Civil Defence Circular 31/56, 'Radioactive Fall-out Provisional Scheme of Public Control'.
36. Lorna Arnold, *Britain and the H-Bomb* (Basingstoke,2001), pp. 235-236.
37. TNA, CAB 130/129, 3rd Meeting, Cabinet Disarmament Committee 18 June 1957, Minute 19 June 1957.
38. TNA, CAB 21/4920. CD(58)2, 'Form and Duration of a Major War', 19 March 1958.
39. TNA, HO 226/71. Scientific Advisers Branch, 'Casualties from a Heavy Nuclear Attack'.

40. NRS, HH 51/338. Civil Defence Study of the Casualty Services, Taymouth, October 1957.
41. NRS, HH51/336. Western Regional Hospital Board, 'Protection of Hospital Buildings', 15 December 1960.
42. Note of a meeting with representatives of Regional Hospital Boards, 31 May 1962, 'Arrangements for clearing Hospitals in Z-Zones'.
43. TNA, MH 131/117. Notes for Civil Defence Officers meeting, 1 May 1963.
44. Ibid., Note of a meeting with representatives of Regional Hospital Boards, 1 May 1963, 'Clearance of Hospitals in Z Zones'.
45. Ibid., Meeting with Regional Hospital Board representatives, 'Radiac Instruments', 20 January 1966.
46. TNA, HO 322/339. STUDY MINERVA 65, Held at Civil Defence Staff College 23 – 25 March 1965.
47. TNA, HO 322/340. STUDY MINERVA 65, Held at Civil Defence Staff College 23 – 25 March 1965.
48. Ibid.
49. NRS, HH51/277. SI, 1949 No. 2139 (S.147) *Civil Defence (Burial) (Scotland) Regulations 1949.*
50. Ibid., Ministry of Health Circular 98/50, 20 September 1950.
51. Ibid. Summers to MacRobbie, 27 October1950.
52. Ibid. 'Disposal of the Dead', Draft Report, (Undated).
53. TNA, HLG 120/1400. Report of the Working Party on Disposal of Civilian War Dead in War, 24 September 1952.
54. Ibid.
55. Ibid.
56. Ibid.
57. Ibid.
58. Ibid.
59. TNA, HLG 120/922. Compton to Mitchell, 17 December 1965.
60. Ibid., Ministry of Housing and Local Government, 'Disposal of the Dead', To all Local Authorities.
61. TNA, HLG 120/1400. Hoard to Howard, 1 February 1961.
62. Ibid., Note to Hoffman, 13 April 1961.
63. Ibid.
64. Ibid.

Chapter 7: Nursing Numbers

1. TNA, MH 131/43. WP(MA)(48)Conclusion 2, 16 November 1948.
2. TNA, MH 131/55. WP(MA)(49)22, 'Supply of Nurses for the Casualty Services', Note by G.T. Milne Nursing Division, 3 November 1949.

3. J. S. Ross, *The National Health Service: An Historical and Descriptive Study* (London, 1952), p. 285.
4. Ibid., p. 290.
5. TNA, MH 55/2648. Report of the Sub-Committee on the National Reserve of Nurses, Paper 2.
6. Ibid., Civil Nursing Reserve Advisory Council Sub-Committee, Minutes of first meeting, 24 June 1946.
7. Ibid., Department of Health for Scotland to the Scottish Branch of the Red Cross Society, 23 June 1947.
8. TNA, MH 131/75. Bliss to Leopold, 26 January 1950.
9. TNA, MH 131/78. Riddle to Mitchell, 20 August 1949.
10. TNA, MH 131/137. Newspaper cutting, *Daily Worker* in Ministry of Health file.
11. TNA, MH 131/81. 'National Hospital Service Reserve', Outline of Approved Scheme.
12. Ibid., 'National Hospital Service Reserve', Outline of Approved Scheme.
13. TNA, MH 55/982. Ministry of Health, 21 December 1950.
14. Ibid., 'Civil Defence Recruitment', Notes of Meeting 1 September 1950. Also MH 55/983. Civil Defence Recruitment, Campaign Guide, October 1950.
15. TNA, MH BD 2/1. Welsh Regional Executive Committee, 'Letter to Visitors', 8 October 1951.
16. WARWICKSHIRE COUNTY RECORD OFFICE, CR2564/83, South Warwickshire Hospital Group (no. 14) Birmingham Regional Hospital Board, Minutes of NHSR Local Publicity Committee, 14 June 1950.
17. Ibid., 17 July 1950.
18. Ibid., 13 December 1950.
19. TNA, MH 131/80. National Health Service Reserve Leaflet, 'Improved Conditions'.
20. TNA, MH 55/989. Campaign Bulletin, Wales and Monmouthshire, November 1951.
21. TNA, 131/143. Note by Heald to Mrs White, 20 August 1952, 'Parliamentary Secretary's visit to Cumberland, 25 August'.
22. TNA, BD 2/25. Recruitment for N.H.S.R., Campaign Guide, National and Local Publicity 1952-53, p. 1.
23. TNA, MH 118/8. HM(55)4, National Hospital Service Reserve, 'Sick Pay Scheme', 14 January 1955.
24. TNA, BD 2/25. Recruitment for NHSR, Campaign Guide, National and Local Publicity 1952-53.
25. Ibid.
26. TNA, MH 131/143. Internal note to Jamieson, 22 March 1954.

27. Ibid., 'Let Women Combat Apathy', 2/2/53-No. 3.
28. Ibid., 'Nursing Badges as 'Peace Symbols', 26/1/53-No. 9.
29. TNA, BD 2/25. Campaign BULLETIN No. 4/52, Exercise Savile.
30. Ibid., Campaign Bulletin No. 5/52, 'Bombs fall on Wrexham'.
31. TNA, MH 55/987. Hospital Management Committee, Hackney Group (No. 6), Extract from Report of Group Secretary to Local Committee, 19 June 1952.
32. TNA, MH 131/134. Sub Committee on Publicity, Minutes of Fourth Meeting, 6 May 1953.
33. TNA, MH 55/981. Outline of publicity campaign attached to Ministry of Health letter, 30 April 1953.
34. LONDON METROPOLITAN ARCHIVES, HA/NW/E1/1-24, Copy Letter from Rose Walker, 28 February 1956.
35. TNA, BD 2/26. National Hospital Service Reserve, Welsh Committee, WEC(57) 1st Meeting, 'Hospital Training and Refresher Courses'.
36. TNA, MH 55/983. Nursing Auxiliaries – Hospital Training, List of the Duties which should be practised and performed.
37. TNA, MH/55. Recommendations of the Advisory Committee, 13 February 1950.
38. TNA, MH 131/88. Internal note to Wilkinson and Hawton, 'Auxiliary Nursing Reserve: Uniforms'. 23 July 1949.
39. Ibid., Note to Mr Rossington, 28 October 1954, Reference 93290/54/2.
40. Ibid., 'Uniforms for Auxiliary Members of the NHSR', Ministry of Health Memorandum for Discussion.
41. TNA, MH 55/986. *News of NHSR*, No. 2.
42. Also, *More Ways Than One of Fighting a War* by Eric Claxton (Aldershot, 1944), gives a history of the formation of the Casualty Union.
43. *Bristol Evening World*, 10 October 1960.
44. TNA, BD 2/26. National Hospital Service Reserve Welsh Committee, WEC(56) 2nd Meeting, 'Publicity'.
45. LONDON METROPOLITAN ARCHIVES, H2/WH/A57/39. South West Metropolitan Regional Hospital Board, 'Mobile First Aid Unit Competition 1957'.
46. TNA, MH 131/77. Birmingham Regional Hospital Board, 22 July 1955, 'Mobile First Aid Unit Competitions'.
47. OXFORDSHIRE HEALTH ARCHIVES, Banbury and District Hospitals Management Committee, NHSR Local Co-ordinating Committee, 19 November 1962.
48. TNA, MH 131/131. General Background to the re-organisation outlined in memorandum HM(CD)(57)2.

49. TNA, MH 131/77. Note of Meeting with Co-ordinating Officers, 24 May 1957.
50. Ibid.
51. TNA, MH 131/70. Hodges to Clark, Cockayne and Heald, 'Future of the National Health Service Reserve', 19 June 1956.
52. Ibid.
53. Ibid., National Hospital Service Reserve, 'Future Policy'.
54. Ibid., Hancock to Hodges, 2 July 1956.
55. Ibid., Minutes prepared by Hodges and signed by Clark, Dimond, Cockayne and Heald.
56. Ibid., p. 4.
57. TNA, MH 10/180. HM(CD)2, National Health Service Reserve, 31 December 1957.
58. Ibid.
59. Ibid.
60. Ibid.
61. NRS, HH 51/177. National Hospital Service Reserve, 'Administration and Records', 26 April 1963.
62. TNA, MH 131/132. Notes of Meeting to discuss the NHSR and Civil Defence, 26 February 1960.
63. Ibid.
64. Ibid., Agenda for meeting on 26 February.
65. TNA, HH 51/177. Macdonald to Strachan, 26 June 1963.
66. TNA, MH 131/151. Mackay to Aldridge, 13 February 1963.
67. TNA, BN 10/203 to 204 and BN 10/36. Folders of campaign material and posters.
68. TNA, MH 131/142. Reprint from the *Nursing Times*, 9 June 1961.
69. Ibid.
70. TNA, INF 6/91. 'Operation Shuttlecock', Final Commentary, 21 May 1959.
71. TNA, BD 2/3. Welsh Hospital Board, 'Press Publicity', 15 March 1963.
72. Ibid.
73. Ibid., Welsh Hospital Board to National Federation of Woman's Institutes, 29 November 1962.
74. Ministry of Health, *Report Part I, 1. The National Health Service, 2, Welfare, Food and Drugs, Civil Defence, for the year ended 31 December 1959, p.207.*
75. TNA, MH 131/113. South East Metropolitan Regional Hospital Board, 2 November 1960, Forward Medical Aid Units, Return for the year ended 30 September 1960.
76. TNA, MH 131/132. Minister's Cup Competition 1961, Rules and also Amendments to rules for Minister's Cup Competition 1961.

77. TNA, MH 131/152, Birmingham Regional Hospital Board, 'Report on FMAU Competition 1964, 7 January 1965.
78. Ibid.
79. TNA, DEFE 13/848. Briefing note Ministry of Health, 3 November 1965.
80. NRS, HH 51/177. Minutes of Meeting 10 January 1967.
81. Ibid.
82. Ibid.
83. Ibid.
84. Ibid., Note of a meeting with the Voluntary Aid Societies, 19 October 1967.
85. Ibid.

Chapter 8: Alternative Medicine

1. Even the preparation of a special manual for doctors ended in disaster because of delays and the eventual appearance of the hydrogen bomb. See TNA, MH 131/57. WP(MA)(54) Conclusion 3, Minutes of Meeting 20 May 1954, 'Manual for Doctors'.
2. BMA ARCHIVES, Council Documents 1959-60, Central Medical Recruitment Committee, Report of the Services Subcommittee for 1960-61.
3. LONDON METROPOLITAN ARCHIVES, H2/WH/A57/31. Ministry of Health, 'Use of Dental Surgeons in the Wartime Hospital and First Aid Services, 12 October 1955.
4. BMA ARCHIVES, Committee on Control of Medical Manworking in War Sessions 1951-55, Minutes of Meeting, 25 May 1955, 'Evidence for Willink Committee'.
5. Ibid.
6. Ibid.
7. TNA, ADM 1/25650. Central Medical Recruitment Committee, 'Classification of Register of Profession-England and Wales and Scotland on 31 December 1953'.
8. NRS, HH 51/331. This file contains the history of a complex set of debates and draft ideas about the control of medical manpower in war. The main principles have been extracted.
9. Ibid., Turnbull to Dodds,'Remuneration of General Medical Practitioners in Wartime'. 20 August 1956.
10. Ibid., Russell-Smith to Armer, 20 October 1955.
11. Ibid., Control of Medical Manpower, Allocation and Mobilisation of Medical Manpower for Wartime needs of the Health Departments, p. 4.
12. Ibid., Lister to Rowland, 15 June 1959.

13. TNA, MH, 131/125. Handwritten file note to Dr Murray dated 24 November.
14. NRS, HH 51/418. Hume to Hewitt, 'Allocation of Medical Manpower', 13 September 1961.
15. TNA, MH, 131/125. Handwritten file note to Dr Murray dated 24 November.
16. NRS, HH 51/331. Draft agreement attached to letter initials NCR to Dodds, 25 August 1955.
17. Ibid., Medical Manpower requirements for civil defence, CD/8/48/1, 5 November 1956.
18. BMA ARCHIVES, Annual Representative Meetings, Minutes and Documents, Brighton, 9 July 1956.
19. TNA, MH 131/124. Oxford Regional Hospital Board to Ministry of Health, 7 December 1956.
20. TNA, HO 322/186. Civil Defence Staff College, Home Office and Ministry of Health Study, EXERCISE BULL RING, Comments by General Sir Sydney Kirkham, 18 July 1956.
21. TNA, MH 131/124. Matthews to Murray, 29 May 1959.
22. Ibid., Letter (1st March, 1960) from the Ministry of Health.
23. Ibid.
24. TNA, MH 131/125. This file contains a whole range of correspondence between the BMA and the Ministry of Health regarding the issue of further inclusion of general practitioners into the hospital plan.
25. Ibid., Woodlock to Hedgecock, 8 February 1961.
26. Ibid., Goodale to Hewitt, 17 May 1962.
27. NRS, HH 55/331. This file contains the incredibly complex history of the development of the distribution concepts of the medical profession between 1951 and 1961.
28. NRS HH51/318. Note of Departmental Meeting on Medical Manpower in War, 7 November 1961.
29. NRS, HH 51/328. Paper A No. 194, 'Allocation of Medical Manpower'.
30. Ibid., National Medical Manpower Committee, Minute No. 37, 6 February 1963.
31. NRS, HH 51/318. Teleprinter note Macdonald to Robertson and Scottish Central Medical Recruitment, Memorandum by the Scottish Home and Health Department, SCMRC 1965.
32. Ibid., Letter to Haughney, 11 January with enclosed draft papers.
33. Ibid.
34. Ibid., Teleprinter note 'para 15 revised as follows', 28 January 1963.
35. Ibid., Illingworth to Mackay, 1 March 1963.

36. Ibid., Hewitt to Macdonald, 13 September 1963 and note of meeting of the National Medical Manpower Committee, 10 April 1963.
37. TNA, CAB 134/1479. CD(M)(64) 2nd Meeting, 'Selection of General Medical Practitioners for Transfer to the Hospital Service', 27 February 1964.
38. NRS, HH 51/318. House of Commons, Non-oral answer, 23 March 1964.
39. Ibid., p. 48.
40. BMA ARCHIVES, Council Documents. 1955-56. Control of Medical Manpower, p. 46.
41. Ibid.
42. Ibid.
43. TNA, CAB 134/1479. CD(M)(64)2nd Meeting, 27 February 1964, 'Selection of General Medical Practitioners for Transfer to the Hospital Service'.
44. NRS, HH 52/327. Central Medical Recruitment Committee, 'Selection of Doctors for Transfer to Wartime Hospital Services, Suggested Quotas for Executive Council Areas'.
45. Ibid., Illingworth to Grey-Turner, 12 January 1965.
46. Ibid., Central Medical Recruitment Committee Minutes, 'Proposed Scheme for the Selecting Doctors for Wartime Transfer to the Hospital Service', 2 April 1965.
47. Ibid., Note of meeting on the allocation and utilisation of medical manpower in war, 9 December 1964.
48. Ibid., Richardson to Raeburn, 21 February 1966.
49. Ibid.
50. TNA, MH 131/125. Illingworth to Edwards, 7 April 1965.
51. Ibid.
52. BMA ARCHIVES, Council. 1965-66. Vol. 1, Area Health Boards and A Proposed Pilot Plan Applicable to Wales.
53. Ibid.
54. Ibid., Council. 1964-65, Vol.2, British Medical Guild.
55. Ibid.
56. Ibid., Central Consultants and Specialists Committee, 'An appraisal of the Hospital Service'.
57. NRS, HH 51/327. Written file note by Richardson at the beginning of file dated 12 February (1965).
58. Ibid., Richardson to Falconer, 31 March 1966.
59. TNA, HLG 120/922. Emergency Civil Defence Measures 1961. The file provides an insight into the emergency measures that were to be put into effect.
60. TNA, MH 131/117, Note of meeting with representatives of Regional Hospital Boards, 13 December 1963.

61. TNA, CAB 134/1478. Report on Civil Aspects of EXERCISE FALLEX 62, Appendix B, (Undated).
62. TNA, HO 322/231. Home Office, Civil Defence Corps, 'Deployment for Operations in England and Wales', May 1963.
63. *The Economist*, 29 December 1962.
64. TNA, HO 312/4. Civil Defence Circular 21/1964, 'Mobilisation and Deployment for Operations'.
65. TNA, MH 131/117. Illingworth to Hewitt, 26 January 1965.
66. TNA, CAB 21/4886. DTC(L)59, Defence (Transition) Committee, War Legislation Sub Committee, R.A.Butler to Prime Minister, 'Emergency Legislation', 7 February 1959.
67. Ibid., 'Emergency Legislation, Memorandum by the Chairman of the Defence (Transition) Committee, 8 January 1959.
68. TNA, CAB 134/1478. CD(65)9, Cabinet Ministerial Committee on Civil Defence, Emergency Legislation.
69. Ibid.
70. Ibid.
71. Ibid
72. TNA, HO 322/275. Draft Handbook.
73. Ibid.
74. TNA, HO 322/333. Draft May 1965, Defence (Administration of Justice) (England) Regulations.
75. TNA, HO 322/331. Defence (Administration of Justice) (England) Regulations, Draft Instructions for Revised Regulations.
76. TNA, HO 322/335. (WPC)(64)6, War Planning Committee, 'Law and Order, Note by the Secretary'. 14 July 1964.
77. TNA, HO 353/33. Drafting commentary by Brennan, 13 July 1964.
78. TNA, HO 322/333. Lord Stoneham to Minister of State and Secretary of State, Defence (Administration of Justice) (Regulations) 10 May 1965.
79. TNA, HO 322/331. Defence Regulations-Series 14(1). Draft.
80. Ibid. Draft (Undated) to Sir Charles Cunningham.
81. TNA, HO 322/333. Defence (Administration of Justice) (England) Regulations, 11 May 1965.
82. TNA, HO 322/275 Draft Handbook.

Chapter 9: Which Doctors

1. TNA, HO 352/40. Draft, The Home Defence Review 1965, p. 3.
2. TNA, CAB 134/2045. HDR(65)27, 'Future Home Defence Policy', Note by Chairman, 17 March 1965, p. 8.

3. TNA, 'DEFE 13/848. Papers attached to letter by Allen to the Secretary of State for Defence, 11 January 1966. 'The Civil Defence Corps: Public Confidence'.
4. TNA, CAB 134/2045. Home Secretary to the Paymaster General, 22 December 1965.
5. TNA, DEFE 13/848, Home Defence Review Committee, Commentary on the paper by the Paymaster General, 14 December 1965.
6. TNA, DEFE 13/848. Home Defence Review Committee, Note of a meeting to discuss the Civil Defence Corps, 29 November 1965.
7. TNA, PREM 13/1386. 'Statement of Civil Defence', 14 December 1966.
8. TNA, HO 322/311. 'Ministry of Housing and Local Government'.
9. TNA, HO 322/309. STUDY JANUS 63 Draft Report, Held at the Staff College 19 to 21 November 1963.
10. TNA, HO 322/311. Central Government STUDY JANUS 63, 'Housing and Health'.
11. Ibid., 'Essential for Survival II'.
12. TNA, HO 322/309. STUDY JANUS 63, Draft Report.
13. TNA, CAB 134/1438. C(O)D(64)5, Official Committee on Civil Defence.
14. WILTSHIRE AND SWINDON RECORD OFFICE, F2/1400/19. A Synopsis of Civil Defence Circular 1/67, 'The Control System, The Civil Defence Corps'.
15. TNA, HO 322/706. Home Office Report, Annex E. 'The Control Structure'.
16. TNA, HO 312/7. CDC 1/1967, Local Authority Controls, Appendix A, Annex II.
17. TNA, MH 131/117. Meeting with Regional Hospital Board representatives, 20 January 1966.
18. NRS, HH 51/337. 'The Wartime Responsibilities of Local Health Authorities', 1966.
19. Ibid., Note by the Scottish Home and Health Department, 28 February 1966.
20. Ibid., 'The Wartime Responsibilities of Local Health Authorities', 1966.
21. TNA files MH 131/129, MH 131/130 and MH 131/131 contain comprehensive evidence of the way Medical Officers of Health were provided with courses at the Civil Defence Staff College.
22. NRS, HH 51/270. Civil Defence Study for Medical Officers of Health, 21 to 25 October 1963.
23. TNA, CAB/1478. CD(65)3, CIVLOG-UNITED KINGDOM NARRATIVE, 3 May 1965.

24. Ibid.
25. Ibid.
26. BATH RECORD OFFICE, Box STUDY GRASS SEED, 'City and County of Bristol Report, Civil Defence Study, 1966'.
27. Ibid.
28. TNA, HO 322/351. Civil Defence Staff College, STUDY PHOENIX FIVE, 10-13 July 1967.
29. *The War Game*, 1965, Directed by Peter Watkins.
30. Ibid.
31. BBC Written Archive, T 56/263/2. 14 January 1965, List of Experts.
32. *Daily Express*, 5 March 1966.
33. Financial Times, 18 May 1966.
34. Bristol Diocesan Gazette. Vol. XLIV 530, March 1966.
35. TNA, HO 322/564. CW(63)1, 'Home Office Committee on Clergy in War'.
36. Ibid.
37. TNA, HO 322/564. Newspaper cutting file.
38. Ibid.
39. TNA, HO 322/720. Handwritten note by Home Secretary, Committee on Clergy in War, 6 January 1965.
40. TNA, HO 322/571. Extract from Hansard.
41. TNA, MH 131/121. Hospital Civil Defence Meeting, 8July 1964.
42. Ibid.
43. NRS, HH 51/337. Note by Frank Richardson, 'Maternity Services in War', 27 January 1965.
44. NRS, HH 51/346. Handwritten note at front of folder by General Richardson, 29 April 1966.
45. Ibid.
46. NRS, HH51/37. Handwritten note 24 February (1966) on file memo by Richardson, 21 February 1966.
47. NRS, HH 51/346. Sir Douglas Baird to John Smith, 16 August 1967.
48. TNA, CAB 128/43. CC(68)3rd Conclusions, 'Home Defence', 9January 1968.
49. *The Times*, 26 February 1968.
50. TNA, DEFE 13/848. 'Home Defence and the Security of the United Kingdom Base', Burke Trend to the Prime Minister, 3 July 1968.
51. TNA, WO 216/819, War Office EXERCISE BRITANNIA, Report May 1949, p. 241.
52. NRS, HH 51/163. *The Management of Mass Casualties*, Scottish Home and Health Department, April 1967.p.14.

53. Hans Morgenthau, 'The Fallacy of Thinking Conventionally About Nuclear Weapons', in Carlton and Schaerf (eds.), *Arms Control and Technological Innovation* (New York, 1976), pp. 255-7.
54. UNIVERSITY OF BRADFORD, Archive Of the Medical Association for the Prevention of War. Statement made at meeting of 130 doctors in London March 1951. *Physicians' Forum Bulletin* December *1951,* pp.11-13.
55. *The Lancet,* 17 May 1952, p.1015.
56. Ibid., 29 July 1961, pp. 259-261.
57. *New Statesman*, 3 September 1960, pp.292-293.
58. Royal College of Nursing, *Report of an RCN Working Party, Nuclear War Civil Defence Planning, The Implications for Nursing.*
59. British Medical Association, *Board of Science and Education Inquiry into the Medical Effects of Nuclear War.*
60. Bertrand Russell, *The Autobiography of Bertrand Russell, Volume III, 1944-1967* (London, 1969), p. 108.
61. Ibid., p. 141.
62. TNA, DEFE 7/759. 'The influence of C.D. measures in the United Kingdom on the effectiveness of the deterrent'. (Undated, but is a background paper prepared for the Home Defence Review 1960).
63. *Nursing Mirror*, 4 March 1966, pp. x to xii.

Appendices

Appendix 1: TNA, HO 357/4.
Appendix 2: TNA, MH 131/54.
Appendix 3: TNA, MH 131/116.
Appendix 4: TNA, CAB 134/1477.
Appendix 5: BMA, Council Minutes. Vol. 1 1964-65.

APPENDIX 1: Atomic Aiming Points, March 1951

Bomb	Location	Selected Aiming Point
1	London	Royal Albert Dock Basin.
2	London	River entrance, Royal Victoria Dock.
3	London	Shadwell New Basin.
4	London	Parliament Square.
5	London	Fulham Power Station.
6	London	Dalston Junction.
7	London	Junction of Camberwell Road and Camberwell New Road.
8	London	Junction of Mitcham Road, Hardcroft Road and Factory Lane, Croydon.
9	London	Western Avenue road bridge over railway between West Acton and North Acton stations.
10	Liverpool	Alexandra Dock.
11	Liverpool	In centre of river opposite entrance to Birkenhead Docks.
12	Hull	City centre.
13	Manchester	Manchester Docks.
14	Bristol	City centre.
15	Glasgow	In river between Queen's and Princess Docks.
16	Middlesbrough	Western end of Middlesbrough Docks.
17	Cardiff	Rail junction ¼ mile north of Bute West Dock.
18	Southampton	City centre.
19	South Shields	In river between Tynemouth and South Shields Docks.
20	Birmingham	City centre.

APPENDIX 2: Diagrammatic representation of Skeleton Plan A for mobilising the Medical Profession

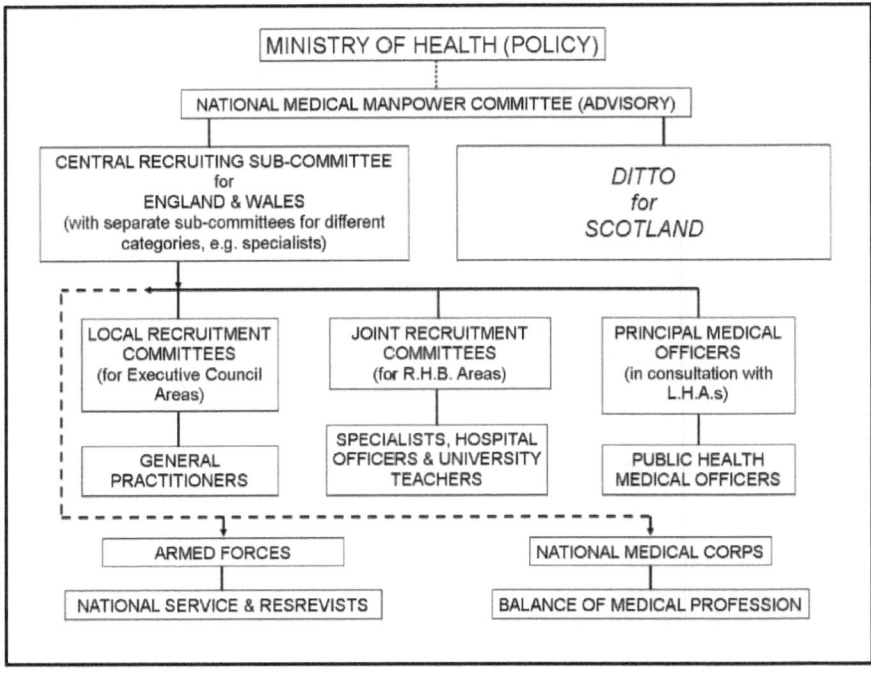

APPENDIX 3: Idealised casualty flow within a Forward Medical Aid Unit

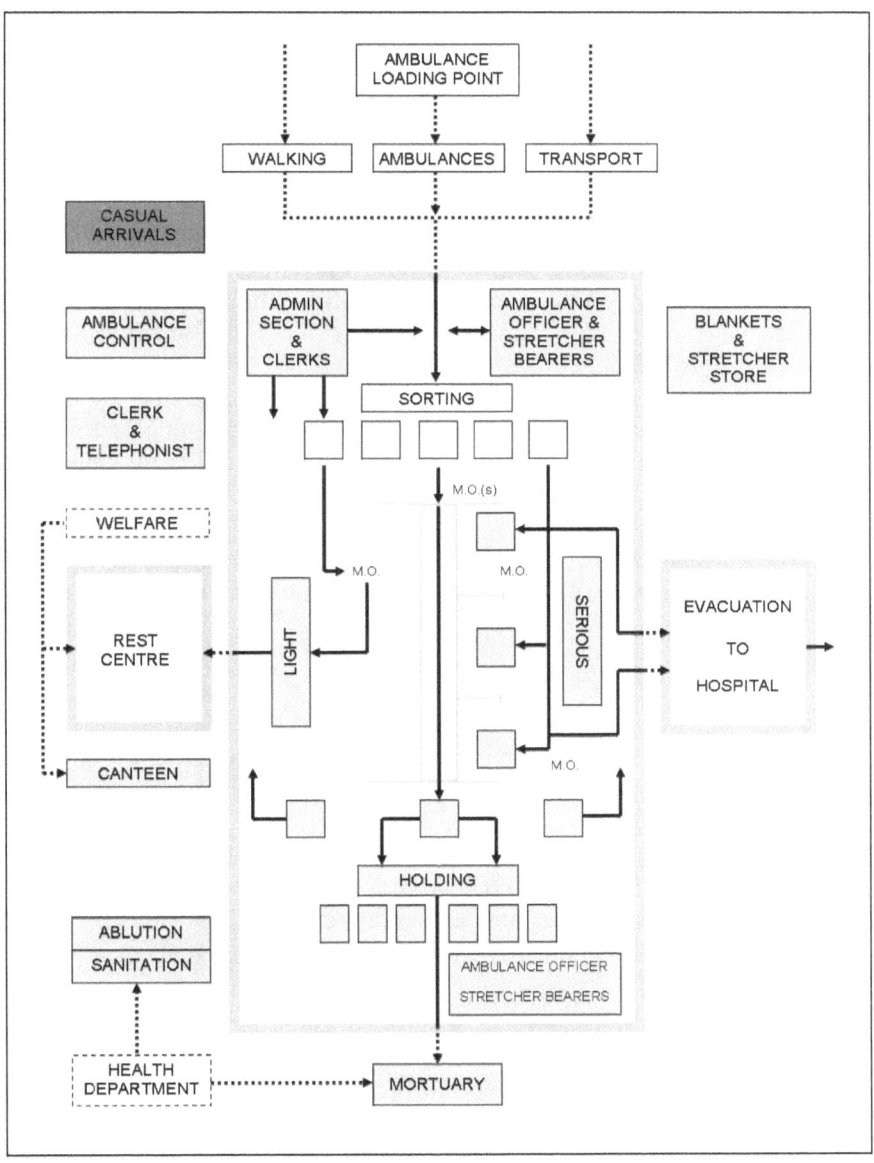

APPENDIX 4: First Aid and Home Nursing Advice to the Public

APPENDIX B

DRAFT SECTION ON FIRST AID AND HOME NURSING

THE SICK AND INJURED

After a nuclear attack many casualties may have to be looked after at home, possibly for some days, without the help of a doctor or nurse. Blocked roads or fall-out may prevent skilled help from reaching you sooner.

This section gives simple instructions on how to care for the sick and injured and is intended for those who have had no training in first aid or home nursing. The advice it contains is to help you deal with emergencies and injuries until you can obtain skilled attention.

Follow the instructions carefully. The simple treatments may well save live(s) or minimise the effects of injuries and the risk of disease.

FIRST AID

Shock
    This may be caused by emotional upset or injury and may be serious. The patient looks pale and frightened, feels cold, is clammy to the touch and may be shivering.
    Lay him down, make him as comfortable as possible, and reassure him.
    Attend to any injuries (see below).
    Give him sips of drinks such as tea, but do not give drinks of any kind if there are abdominal injuries (see wounds of the abdomen).

Burns
    Within a wide area round a nuclear explosion everyone out-of-doors or near unprotected windows may suffer some degree of burning of the exposed skin. Generally, the effects will be fairly superficial as in sunburn. For such burns no special treatment will be required. If blisters occur they should not be broken.
    For large and more serious burns do not try to clean the areas affected; just cover them with dressings, clean sheets or towels.

DO NOT prick or cut out the blisters unless they are tense and very painful; if they are, sterilise the point of a needle by holding it in flame, let it cool and then prick the blister.

DO NOT apply oil or any kind of ointment to the burned areas of the body. If the eyelids are burnt smear a little face or shaving cream on their edges.

In the case of large burns covering the whole of the area or any areas which together total as much as ten times the size of the patient's palm, it is important that the fluid which the body loses from the injured areas should be replaced. Give the patient a special drink made by adding one level teaspoonful of bicarbonate of soda to two pints of water. This drink can be sweetened or flavoured by sugar or cordial.

Encourage the patient to take this in small drinks, but in the first 8 hours the total amount should not exceed one half pint for infants, 5 pints for an adult female and 6 pints for and adult male. Similar quantities should not be exceeded in the following 16 hours, and during the second day not more than half these quantities should be allowed. If by the third day the doctor has been unable to reach you continue to give the patient the special drink sufficient in amounts to satisfy his thirst.

Injuries

Bleeding

First, control the bleeding. Uncover the wound, if necessary by cutting the clothing up the seams. If any large object such as a piece of glass or fragment of brick or wood is lying in the wound remove it but do not try to remove objects which are embedded or look for small fragments in the wound. Press a dressing firmly upon the wound. Preferably this should be sterile but if you have not such a dressing use a clean handkerchief, cloth or towel. This should control the bleeding; then fix it position by a bandage.

Wounds of the Abdomen

Cover the wound with a sterile dressing or a clean folded cloth, towel or handkerchief fixed in place with a bandage or adhesive plaster. DO NOT give anything to drink; if the patient becomes very thirsty let him wash out his mouth. If medical attention cannot be obtained, small quantities of water can be swallowed from the second day.

Wounds of the Chest

If the lungs are penetrated, breathing will be difficult, and you may hear sucking of air or see blood-stained froth coming from the wound opening. Cover the wound with a large clean dressing fixed firmly by a bandage or adhesive plaster and prop the patient up with pillows, cushions, etc.

Fractures

If there is a wound, or a bone is protruding through the skin, apply a sterile dressing or a clean cloth.

If the broken bone does not pierce the skin, it can usually be detected by deformity or by the unnatural position of the affected limb. There may be no outward sign beyond some local swelling but the patient will complain of pain on movement of the limb. Handle the injured limb very carefully to avoid the broken end of the bone coming through the skin. Place the limb in its natural position. Do this very gently, and on no account use any force or further damage may be caused. Relieve the pain and prevent further injury by supporting the broken limb including the joints above and below the fracture. The lower limb may be supported on both sides by rolled blankets or firm pillows.

If the patient cannot move, his spine may be fractured. Do not move him unless it is absolutely necessary. If he must be moved, move him in the posture in which he is found.

Radiation Sickness

Those who have been exposed to a moderate amount of radiation may, after three hours or more, feel sick and even vomit. Usually this feeling passes off. Reassure and rest the patient and give him plenty of sweet drinks.

If the dose of radiation has been severe, he may after a further three to eight days, complain of sickness and suffer from vomiting and diarrhoea. In that case medical aid should be sought.

NURSING CARE

The Basic needs of the Sick and Wounded

These are
  (1) Sleep, rest and reassurance.
  (2) Nourishment.
  (3) Attention to personal hygiene.
  (4) Attention to sanitary needs.

Rest: Particularly sleep, are very important. You should appear calm, confident and sympathetic. Keep the patient quiet and in a comfortable position. Hot drinks will help him to rest and sleep.

Nourishment: Whatever the patient fancies will as a rule do him no harm in moderation, but he may have to be coaxed to take nourishment. See that he gets 3 pints of fluid in each period of 24 hours, given little at a time and as often as possible. It may be given with milk powder or beaten up egg, thin gruel as thin as soup.

Personal Hygiene: Personal cleanliness is of great importance. Sponge the patient occasionally from head to foot with warm water. Dry well, massage the areas subjected to pressure with methylated or surgical spirit, and then powder or apply Vaseline or skin cream to prevent bed-sores.

Care of the Mouth: A very ill or unconscious patient will soon develop a dry bad-smelling and painful mouth unless special care is taken. Rub the lips gently with Vaseline or skin cream. At intervals clean the inside of the mouth with a small piece of cotton wool or clean cloth wrapped round a thin piece of wood, such as an orange stick. Dip this in weak soda bicarbonate solution and use it to clean the tongue and around the teeth.

Use of the Bedpan: A person confined to bed will need help in using the bedpan. Brown paper can be used as a mackintosh, and newspaper may be useful in cases where there is loss of control of the bladder or bowel. Clean the patient carefully after the use of the bedpan, if possible with soap and water.

Observation and Reporting: For very sick people keep notes of the following, for the use of the doctor or nurse when they arrive:-
   (1) The amount food and drink taken.
   (2) The amount of sleep and rest.
   (3) If the patient has pain, and if so, where.
   (4) If bowel and bladder action is normal or if anything unusual is noticed.
   (5) If there is any bleeding or vomiting.

FIRST AID KIT

APPENDIX 5: Memorandum for the Allocation and Utilisation of Medical Manpower for the Civilian Health Services in War

APPENDIX
IN CONFIDENCE

Allocation and utilisation of medical manpower
for the civilian health services in war

Introduction

This memorandum deals with the anticipated war-time needs of the civilian health services. Planning has reached a stage at which it is desirable to agree with the medical profession on a number of matters affecting doctors in particular the methods of meeting the staffing needs of the hospital service (which would be considerably expanded to deal with the casualty situation) and the organisation of general practitioner services in war.

(1) The War-time Hospital Service
Recommendations of the National Medical Manpower Committee

In the light of information supplied by the Health Departments, the National Medical Manpower Committee has made the following recommendations for staffing the war-time hospital service -

(a) Part-time hospital medical staff should work full-time.

(b) On the assumption that the teaching of medical students would be suspended in war, the medical teaching staffs of universities should work in the hospital service.

(c) The bulk of the additional doctors required for the hospital service should come from doctors engaged in general practice in the National Health Service.

Deployment of doctors in the war-time hospital service

Existing hospital medical staff and doctors transferred to the hospital service from other fields would have to be deployed within the expanded service to the best advantage. It would be for Regional Hospital Boards, through the Senior Administrative Medical Officer, to assign war-time duties and locations.

Arrangements for the selection of general practitioners for transfer to the hospital service in war

The National Medical Manpower Committee have recommended that selection should be undertaken through the machinery of the Central Medical Recruitment Committee, that it should be undertaken in peace-time, and that doctors selected for transfer should be notified and given instructions on where to report if called upon.

The arrangements proposed are as follows. Based on the National Medical Manpower Committee's recommendation as to the number of general practitioners to be transferred, the Ministry of Health would work out and agree with the C.M.R.C. quotas to be provided by the Local Medical Recruitment Committee. In fixing quotas they would have regard to a number of considerations: the number of additional acute beds to be provided in the hospital region, the number of general practitioners in the area, and whether the area was a dispersal, neutral or reception area for the purposes of the civil dispersal scheme. The quotas would be fixed so that as many as possible of the general practitioners required would be supplied by dispersal areas, leaving a comparatively small number in those areas to provide a home cover service.

The Central Medical Recruitment Committee would notify the Local Committee concerned and ask them to select individual doctors to meet the quota. It is hope that the Local Committee would have the co-operation of individual doctors and that those volunteering for work in hospitals or with Forward Medical Aid Units would be accepted for transfer. Local Committees would have regard to appropriate personal factors, e.g. age, and, in the case of married women doctors, family; and to the desirability of maintaining a reasonable geographical distribution of general practitioners within their area.

Those accepted or selected for transfer would be told, and their names passed to the appropriate Regional Hospital Board. The Regional Hospital Board would issue to those selected 'instructions' on where to report in the event of an emergency. Arrangements would be made for the regular review and revision of the lists.

It is considered that the process of selection should be put in hand as soon as the necessary arrangements have been made.

It will be apparent that the implementation of these proposals depends on the voluntary co-operation of the profession, although it can be assumed that any powers of direction of manpower that the Government of the day might decide to take in the event of an emergency would apply to doctors as to other members of the community.

(2) <u>Organisation of general practitioner services in war</u>

The transfer of large numbers of general practitioners to the hospital service in the period before an attack, and the implementation of the civil dispersal scheme if this were ordered by the Government, would disorganise the present general practitioner service based on doctors' lists. As a result of an attack there would be mass casualties and further movements of population, including many homeless. Because the hospital service would be more than fully stretched in caring for the more seriously injured, very many sick and injured would have to be cared for at home, in billets or in whatever improvised arrangements it were found possible to make. General practitioners would have to give what medical care and treatment was possible on an emergency basis, and they would need help in obtaining medical supplies and all available assistance from people with some training in home nursing. Communications would be disrupted, and the efforts of the community for survival would have to be directed and co-ordinated by the regional and local system of civil defence controls that are planned.

In such a situation the peace-time system of administering general practitioner services could not operate. Nor would it be adequate for the task. The services would have to be organised by a body in possession of information about damage, casualties and fall-out, and with access to Civil Defence communications. The Medical Officer of Health as medical adviser to the control at county or county borough level would have access to this information. Councils of counties and county boroughs would also have responsibilities for home nursing services.

It is accordingly proposed that local health authorities should have the responsibility for organising general practitioner services to cover the period following attack and that general practitioners should be in contract with and remunerated by them. The normal terms of service of general practitioners would be suspended during the period of the emergency, and instead they would accept an obligation to provide whatever medical services to patients were practicable in the circumstances, and to do so in whichever area or for whatever groups of people the local health authority might determine through the Medical Officer of Health in consultation so far as practicable with the Chairman or other representative of the Local Medical Committee. These arrangements would be without prejudice to whatever arrangements it was found possible to make in the longer term.

Movement of doctors in the post-attack period

After an attack it might be found necessary to reinforce the medical services in one area by sending doctors from other areas. Such movements would be arranged on instruction from Region or Sub-Region where there would be senior medical officers of the Ministry of Health acting as advisers to the Commissioner. Instructions would be given to the Senior Administrative Medical Officer, in the case of doctors in the hospital service, and to the Medical Officer in the case of local authority medical staffs and general practitioners.

The timing of a decision to release from the hospital service general practitioners that had been transferred to it would depend on circumstances and relative needs. The release would be arranged through the Senior Administrative Medical Officer or his representative and the Medical Officer or his representative and the Medical Officer of Health.

Local Authority Medical Staff

The National Medical Manpower Committee recommended that in war local authority medical staffs should remain at about their peace-time level but then if the Civil Dispersal scheme were put into operation, it would be necessary to reinforce staff in reception areas by transferring a proportion from dispersal areas. Further consideration is being given to this recommendation.

Remuneration

If these plans ever have to be put into operation it would clearly be impossible to continue the peace-time basis of remuneration for general practitioners and it seems inequitable to distinguish between those transferred to the hospital service and those remaining in general practice. The Government cannot at this stage say on what basis it would be practicable to remunerate doctors and others undertaking emergency civilian duties in the aftermath of an attack. These are matters which would have to be decided in the light of the conditions prevailing. Until these decisions are taken it is proposed that general practitioners whether transferred to the hospital service or remaining in general practice would be remunerated on a salaried basis, at a rate equivalent to the standard average net income of the day of general practitioners.

General practitioners transferred to the hospital service would be remunerated by the hospital authority; those remaining as general practitioners by the local health authority.

University medical teaching staffs transferred to the hospital service would continue to be remunerated at their university rates by the Regional Hospital Board to which they were transferred.

Existing hospital medical staffs would be remunerated at their whole-time as part-time contracts would be converted to whole-time, and would carry out whatever hospital duties were assigned to them.

BIBLIOGRAPHY

Primary Sources

THE NATIONAL ARCHIVES (TNA)

Admiralty, and Ministry of Defence, Navy Department

ADM 1. Medical Services Co-ordinating Committee

Air Ministry

AIR 2. Policy and Administration Papers
AIR 20. Air Historical Branch Papers

Department of Health and Social Security

BN 10. Publicity Material
BN 29. Children

Cabinet Papers

CAB 12. Home [Ports] Defence Committee Minutes
CAB 21. Machinery of Government papers
CAB 124. Secretariat Files
CAB 125. Radio Board and Committees
CAB 126. Atomic Energy Files.
CAB 128. Cabinet Minutes
CAB 129. Cabinet Memoranda
CAB 130. Ad-Hoc Committees Papers
CAB 133. Conferences and Visits
CAB 134. Cabinet Committee Papers
CAB 139. Central Statistical Office
CAB 164. Theme Series
CAB 165. Secretariat Papers
CAB 175. War Books

Colonial Office

CO 986. Defence and Security of the Colonies

Ministry of Defence

DEFE 7. Registered Files: General Series
DEFE 8. Chiefs of Staff Committees and Sub-Committees
DEFE 10. Major Committees: Minutes and Papers.
DEFE 11. Chiefs of Staff Committee
DEFE 13. Private Papers
DEFE 15. Research & Development Technical Reports
DEFE 20. British Joint Services Mission

Foreign Office

FO 371. General Correspondence: Political
FO 953. Foreign Publicity

Ministry of Housing and Local Government

HLG 120. General Policy and Procedure

Home Office

HO 45. Domestic Matters
HO 97. Secretary's Office Books and Papers
HO 197. Chief Engineer's Department Files
HO 205. Public Shelter in Wartime
HO 225. Scientific Adviser's Branch: Reports
HO 226. Scientific Adviser's Branch: Reports
HO 227. Scientific Adviser's Branch Reports
HO 228. Scientific Adviser's Branch: Reports
HO 255. Radio Department: Registered Files
HO 303. Publicity and Public Relations
HO 310. Traffic Files
HO 312. Civil Defence Circulars
HO 322. Civil Defence Files
HO 338. Scientific Adviser's Branch
HO 353. Police, War Emergency Matters
HO 356. Administration of Local Government
HO 357. Civil Defence Joint Planning Staff

Central Office of Information

INF 12. Publicity

Ministry of Labour

LAB 6. Military Recruitment
LAB 12. Establishments

Ministry of Agriculture, Fisheries and Food

MAF 313. Rationing Arrangements
MAF 325. Storage and Transport
MAF 357. Emergency Feeding

Metropolitan Police

MEPO 2. General Police Work
MEPO 4. Police Regulations and Administration

Ministry of Health

MH 79. Pay and Pensions
MH 117. Regional Medical Officers
MH 119. Health Circulars
MH 123. Specialist Hospital Services
MH 131. Civil Defence
MH 163. SAMO Meetings

Prime Minister's Office

PREM 8. Attlee Labour Administration
PREM 11. Conservative Administration
PREM 13. Harold Wilson Administration

Treasury

T 221. Regional Files
T 227. Social Services Division
T 229. Central Economic Planning Section
T 233. Home Finance Division
T 326. Finance, Home and General papers

War Office

WO 195. Scientific Advisory Council Papers
WO 216. Correspondence with Prime Minister

Welsh Hospital Board

BD 2. Civil Defence and NHSR

BATH RECORD OFFICE

Bath Civil Defence Training Paper for Chief Officers 1966
Civil Defence Staff College Notes for Senior Water Engineers 1957
Civil Defence Staff College Notes for Senior Officers 1963

BBC WRITTEN ARCHIVE CAVERSHAM

R 78/2620/1   *The War Game* Part 1
T16/679/1   Television Policy, *The War Game*, File 1a-1963-65
T16/679/2   Television Policy, *The War Game*, File 1g-1966-68
T16/748   Television Policy, *War Game* Dossier & Appendix 1067
T 56/263/1   *The War Game*, Internal Correspondence
T 56/263/2   *The War Game*, Internal Correspondence
T 56/263/1   *The War Game*, Internal Correspondence
T 56/264/1   *The War Game*, Talks Not Broadcast

BEDFORDHIRE AND LUTON ARCHIVES

HO/NB32 NHSR Special Sub-Committee

BRITISH MEDICAL ASSOCIATION ARCHIVE (BMA)

Committee on Control of Medical Manpower in War Session 1951-52
Committee on Control of Medical Manpower in War Sessions 1951-55
CMWC Documents 1946-52
Council Documents 1948-49
Council Documents 1949-50
Council Documents, Session 1950-51
Council Documents, Session 1952-53
Council Documents 1951-52
Council Documents 1955-56
Council Documents 1959-60
Council 1965-66, Vol. 1
Council 1964-65, Vol. 1
Council 1964-65, Vol. 2
Medical Manpower Evidence (Steering) Committee 1954-55
Metropolitan Regional Medical Recruitment Committee, Session 1952-53
Minutes & Documents A.R.M. London 1951

Minutes & Documents A.R.M. 1952
Minutes & documents A.R.M. Glasgow 1954

CUMBRIA RECORD OFFICE (KENDAL)

WDSo. Civil Defence Welfare Papers
WC/H/A1816. Civil Defence Papers

LONDON METROPOLITAN ARCHIVES, CITY OF LONDON

H2. Westminster Hospital
HA. North West Metropolitan RHB

ARCHIVE OF THE MEDICAL ASSOCIATION FOR THE PREVENTION OF WAR (UNIVERSITY OF BRADFORD)

H3 Pamphlets 3. MAPW Annual General Meeting 1955
H3 Pamphlets 4. MAPW Bulletin Supplement 1955
H3 Pamphlets 6. The Pathogenesis of War 1961
H3 Pamphlets 8. The Doctor and Situations of Tension 1966

ROYAL COLLEGE OF NURSING ARCHIVE

RCN/15/1/3/32. RCN Working Party on Nuclear War 1980s
RCN/5/1/W/5. One in Five Scheme aimed at nurses

ROYAL SOCIETY OF MEDICINE ARCHIVE

Proceedings of the Royal Society of Medicine, United Services Section
Annual Representative Meetings 1950-1968

ROYAL VOLUNTARY SERVICE ARCHIVE (RVS)

Box 3. Packet 1   Home Office General Correspondence
Box 9. Packet 2   Civil Defence Uniform
Box 9. Packet 6   Civil Defence Staff College
Box 9. Packet 7   Welfare Section Training Policy
Box 10. Packet 5 Civil Defence Studies at HQ and in Regions
Box 10. Packet 10 Civil Defence Policy 1949-57
Box 11. Packet 7 Courses with Home Office and other Ministries
Box 22. Packet 7 Federal Civil Defense Administration
Box 35. Packet 7 One-in-Five, Nuclear Disarmament

Box 85. Packet 2   Publicity One in Five
Box 85. Packet 7   Welfare Section of the Civil Defence Corps

NATIONAL RECORDS OF SCOTLAND (NRS)

HH 51. Civil Defence

OXFORDSHIRE HEALTH ARCHIVES

OHA HMC 4 C1/1. Records of Banbury and District Management Committee: National Hospital Service Reserve.

SOMERSET ARCHIVE

C/CD/3/152-54. Civil Defence Pamphlets
D/H/yeo/1/3/4.   Staff College Notes for Hospital CD Officers 1965
D/H/yeo/1/3/4.   South Western RHB, Mobilisation Plans

WARWICKSHIRE COUNTY RECORD OFFICE

CR2564. Nursing Services and Catering Committee Minutes

WILTSHIRE AND SWINDON RECORD OFFICE

F2/1400/10. Civil Defence Control Systems and War Duty Establishment

Periodicals

Local Newspapers

Peace News
Birmingham Gazette
Coventry Evening Telegraph

National Newspapers

Daily Express
Daily Herald
Daily Mail
Daily Sketch
Daily Telegraph
Daily Worker
Financial Times

The Scotsman
The Sunday Telegraph
The Times
Manchester Guardian
News Chronicle
Reynolds News

Other Periodicals

Civil Defence
The British Medical Journal
The Economist
Fission Fragments
Forward
The Lancet
The Municipal Journal
The New Statesman
Nursing Mirror
Nursing Times
Peace News

Official Publications

Home Office, *Civil Defence Manual for Basic Training, Volume II Atomic Warfare* (London: HMS0, 1950).
Home Office, *First Aid Manual* (London: HMSO, 1951).
Home Office, *Radioactive Fall-out: Provisional Scheme of Public Control* (London: HMSO, 1956).
Home Office, *Manual of civil defence: Vol.1. Pamphlet no1, Nuclear Weapons* (London: HMSO, 1956).
Home Office, *Manual of civil defence Vol. I pamphlet No 2 Radioactive Fall-out provisional scheme of public control* (London: HMSO, 1956).
Home Office, *Nuclear Weapons* (London: HMSO, 1959).
Home Office, *Civil Defence Training Memorandum No. 8, Civil Defence Corps (England and Wales) Deployment for Operations* (London: HMSO, 1965).
Home Office, Ambulance and First Aid Section Training Bulletin no.1 (London: HMSO, 1960).
Home Office, *Police War Duties Manual* (London: HMSO, 1965).
Home Office, *The Hydrogen Bomb* (London: HMSO, 1957).
Home Office, *Advising the Householder on Protection against Nuclear Attack* (London: HMSO, 1963).

Ministry of Health, *Statement Relating to the Hospital Organisation, First Aid Posts and Ambulances* (London: HMSO, 1939).
Ministry of Health, *Report for the year ended March 1944* (London: HMSO, 1944).
Ministry of Health, *Report for the year ended March 1945* (London: HMSO, 1945).
Ministry of Health, *On the State of the Public Health During the Six years of war, Report of the Chief Medical Officer of the Ministry of Health 1939-45* (London: HMSO, 1946).
Ministry of Health, *Life Blood, The Official Account of the Transfusion Services* (London: HMSO, 1945).
Ministry of Health, *Report Part I, 1. The National Health Service, 2, Housing Local Government, Civil Defence, Welfare, Water, for the year ended 31 March 1950* (London: HMSO) September 1951.
Ministry of Health, *Report Part I, 1. The National Health Service, 2, Welfare, Food and Drugs, Civil Defence, covering the period 1 April 1950 to 31 December 1951* (London: HMSO, September 1951).
Ministry of Health, *Report Part I, 1. The National Health Service, 2, Welfare, Food and Drugs, Civil Defence, covering the period 1 April 1950 to 31 December 1951* (London: HMSO, September 1952).
Ministry of Health, *Report Part I, 1. The National Health Service, 2, Welfare, Food and Drugs, Civil Defence, for the year ended 31 December, 1952* (London: HMSO, 1953).
Ministry of Health, *Report Part I, 1. The National Health Service, 2, Welfare, Food and Drugs, Civil Defence, for the year ended 31 December, 1953* (London: HMSO, 1954).
Ministry of Health, *Report Part I, 1. The National Health Service, 2, Welfare, Food and Drugs, Civil Defence, for the year ended 31 December, 1954* (London: HMSO, 1955).
Ministry of Health, *Report Part I, 1. The National Health Service, 2, Welfare, Food and Drugs, Civil Defence, for the year ended 31 December, 1955* (London: HMSO) 1956.
Ministry of Health, *Report Part I, 1. The National Health Service, 2, Welfare, Food and Drugs, Civil Defence, for the year ended 31 December, 1956* (London: London: HMSO, 1957).
Ministry of Health, *Report Part I, 1. The National Health Service, 2, Welfare, Food and Drugs, Civil Defence, for the year ended 31 December, 1957* (London: HMSO, 1958).
Ministry of Health, *Report Part I, 1. The National Health Service, 2, Welfare, Food and Drugs, Civil Defence, for the year ended 31 December, 1958* (London: HMSO, 1959).

Ministry of Health, *Report Part I, 1. The National Health Service, 2, Welfare, Food and Drugs, Civil Defence, for the year ended 31 December, 1959* (London: HMSO, 1960).
Ministry of Health, *Report Part I, 1. The National Health Service, 2, Welfare, Food and Drugs, Civil Defence, for the year ended 31 December, 1960* (London: HMSO, 1961).
Ministry of Health, *Report, Part I, The Health and Welfare Services, for the year ended 31 December, 1961* (London: HMSO, 1962).
Ministry of Health, *Report, The Health and Welfare Services, for the year ended 31 December, 1962* (London: HMSO, 1963).
Ministry of Health, Report, *The Health and Welfare Services, for the year ended 31 December 1963* (London: HMSO, 1964).
Ministry of Health, *Report, for the year 1964* (London: HMSO, 1965).
Ministry of Health, *Report, for the Year 1965* (London: HMSO, 1966).
Ministry of Health, *Report, for the Year 1966* (London: HMSO, 1967).
Ministry of Health, *Report, for the Year 1967* (London: HMSO, 1968).
Ministry of Health, *Guidance Notes for Doctors Teaching Mass Casualty Care (Previously Extended First Aid)*.
Ministry of Health, *Emergency Home Care* (London: HMSO, 1964).

Contemporary Books and Pamphlets

Association of Scientific Workers, *Atomic Attack, Can Britain be Defended* (London: Association of Scientific Workers, 1950). [pamphlet]
Atomic Scientists' Association, *Atom Train*, (London: Atomic Scientists' Association, 1947). [pamphlet]
Admiralty, *Notes on Atomic Energy for Medical Officers* (London: HMSO, 1957).
American Psychiatric Association Committee on Civil Defense, *Disaster Fatigue* (Washington: American Psychiatric Association, 1956).
U.S, Department of Defense and U.S. Atomic Energy Commission, *The Effect of Atomic Weapons* (Washington, 1950).
Baker, J. O., *Civil Defence and You* (London: Jordan and Sons, 1951).
Baynes, John, *Morale: A Study of Men and Courage* (London: Leo Cooper, 1967).
Bertrand, Russell, *The Autobiography of Bertrand Russell 1944-1967* (London: George Allen and Unwin, 1969).
Blackett P.M.S., *Studies of War, Nuclear and Conventional War* (Edinburgh and London: Oliver & Boyd, 1962).
Blackett P.M.S., *Fear, War and the Bomb, Military and Political Consequences of Atomic Energy* (New York: McGraw-Hill, 1949).
Bradley, David, *No Place to Hide* (Boston: Atlantic Monthly Press, 1948).

British Red Cross Society, *Mental Health Manual* (London: British Red Cross Society, 1958).

Brockway, Fenner, *Outside the Right* (London: George Allen & Unwin, 1963).

Brown, J. A. C. Brown, *Techniques of Persuasion From Propaganda to Brainwashing* (Middlesex: Penguin Books, 1963).

Burhop, S, *Ban Those Bombs* (London: The British Peace Committee, 1954). [pamphlet]

Butler, David, *The British General Election of 1955* (London: Macmillan, 1955).

Central Office of Information, *Britain: An Official Handbook* (London: HMSO, 1967).

CND, *Telling Britain From Now Until The Election* (London: CND, circa 1962). [pamphlet]

CND, *Civil Defence and Nuclear War* (London: CND, circa 1962). [pamphlet]

Clements, Roger, *Local Notables and the City Council* (London: Macmillan, 1969).

Beaton, Leonard and John Maddox. *The Spread of Nuclear Weapons* (London: Chatto and Windus, 1962).

Clitheroe, G.W., *Coventry under Fire* (Gloucester: The British Publishing Company, 1941).

De Kadt, Emanual, J, *British Defence Policy & Nuclear War* (London: Frank Cass, 1964).

Claxton, Eric C., and W.J. Maelor Evans, *Realistic Battle Training for Civil Defence* (Aldershot: Gale and Polden, 1944).

Department of Scientific and Industrial Research and Fire Offices' Committee, *Fire and the Atomic Bomb* (London: HMSO, 1954).

Downie, R. S., *Government Action and Morality, Some Principles and Concepts of Liberal Democracy* (London: Macmillan, 1964).

Dunn, C.L., *The Emergency Medical Services, Volume I, England and Wales* (London: HMSO, 1952).

Dunn, C.L., *The Emergency Medical Services, Volume II, Scotland, Northern Ireland and the Principal Air Raids on Industrial Centres in Great Britain* (London: HMSO, 1952).

Hodgkinson, George, *Sent to Coventry* (London: Robert Maxwell, 1970).Home Office, *Air Raid Shelter Policy* (London: HMSO, 1938).

Home Office, *Notes on German Civil Defence* (Inspector General's Department, 1946).

Ickle, Fred Charles, *The Social Impact of Bomb Destruction* (Oklahoma: University of Oklahoma, 1958).

Irving, David, *The Destruction of Dresden* (London: William Kimber, 1963).

Elliot, Mabel, A. and Merrill, Francis, E., *Social Disorganisation* (New York and London: Harper and Row, 1961).
Fallout from Nuclear Weapons Tests, *Hearings before the Special Subcommittee on Radiation of the Joint Committee on Atomic Energy Congress of the United States Eighty-Sixth Congress, May 5, 6, 7 and 8, 1959.*
Federal Civil Defense Administration, *Health Services and Special Weapons Defense* (Washington: 1950, Reprinted 1952).
Federal Civil Defense Administration, *Emergency Medical Treatment* (Washington: 1950, Reprinted 1952).
Frank, Jerome, *Sanity and Survival* (New York: Random House, 1967).
Gatland, Kenneth W., *Development of the Guided Missile* (London: Iliffe and Sons, 1954).Graham, Virgnia, *The Story of the WVS* (London: HMSO, 1958).
Grosser G. H. et. al., *The Threat of Impending Disaster* (Cambridge, Massachusetts: The M.I.P. Press, 1964).
Goure, Leon, *Civil Defense in the Soviet Union* (Berkeley: University of California Press, 1962).
Halperin, Morton H., *Limited War in the Nuclear Age* (New York: John Wiley and Sons, 1963).
Hanunian, Norman, *Dimensions of Survival: Post-Attack Survival Disparities and National Viability* (Santa Monica: Rand Corporation, 1966).
Hersey, John, *Hiroshima* (New York: Alfred A. Knopf, 1946).
H.M. Treasury: *Statements Relating to the Atomic Bomb* (London: HMSO, 1945).
Home Office, *Manual of Fire Appliances for Mobile Fire Columns* (London: HMSO 1956).
Janis, Irving, *War and Emotional Stress* (New York: McGraw-Hill Book Company, 1951).
Home Office, *Police War Duties Manual* (London: HMSO, 1965).
Joint Committee on Atomic Energy, *Civil Defense Against Atomic Attack: Preliminary Data* (Washington: United States Government Printing Office, 1950).
Jungk, Robert, *Brighter Than a Thousand Suns* (New York: Harcourt, Brace and Company, 1958).
Kahn, Herman, *On Thermonuclear War* (Princeton: Princeton University Press, 1960).
--- *Thinking about the Unthinkable* (London: Weidenfeld and Nicolson, 1962).
King-Hall, Stephen, *Defence in the Nuclear Age* (London: Victor Gollancz, 1958).

Kissinger, Henry A., *Nuclear Weapons and Foreign Policy* (New York: Harper Brothers for Council on Foreign Relations, 1957).
Labour Party Joint Committee, *Report of the Labour Party Joint Committee on Civil Defence* (Labour Party, 1955).
Lapp, R.E., *Must We Hide* (Cambridge, Mass.: Addison- Wesley, 1949).
Lapp, Ralph, E, and Jack Schubert, Radiation, *What it is and how it affects you* (New York: Viking Press, 1957).
Lawson, D. I., *Fire and the Atomic Bomb* (London: HMSO, 1954).
Lifton, Robert Jay, *Death in Life* (London: Weidenfeld and Nicolson, 1968).
Lowry, Ira. S., *The Post Attack Population of the United States* (Santa Monica: Rand Corporation, 1966).
MacInnes, M. C, *Bristol at War* (London: Museum Press Limited, 1962).
Martin, Thomas L., and Donald C. Latham, *Strategy for Survival* (Tucson: The University of Arizona Press, 1963).
Medical Research Council, *The Hazards to Man of Nuclear and Allied Radiations* (London: HMSO, 1956).
Melman, Seymour, (ed.) *No Place to Hide, Fact and fiction about fallout shelters*, (New York: Grove Press,1962).
Milne R. S. and H. C. Mackenzie, Marginal Seat, 1955, *A Study of Voting Behaviour in the Constituency of Bristol North East at the General Election of 1955* (London: The Hansard Society for Parliamentary Government, 1958).
Ministry of Health, *Emergency Home Care* (London: Ministry of Health, 1964).
Montgomery, John, *The Fifties* (London: George Allen & Unwin Ltd, 1965).
Muhkin A. P. (ed.), *Medical and Civil Defense in Total War* (The Israel Program for Scientific Translations: 1961).
Newman, R., James, *The Rule of Folly* (New York: Simon and Schuster, 1962).
Parkin, John, *Middle Class Radicalism, The Social Bases of the British Campaign for Nuclear Disarmament* (Manchester: University of Manchester, 1968).
NATO, *Emergency War Surgery* (Washington: United States Department of Defence, 1958).
Pogrund, R. S., *Nutrition in the Post-Attack Environment* (Santa Monica: Rand Corporation, 1966).
Powell C., *The Hydrogen Bomb and the Future of Mankind* (London: F.H Radford, 1955).
Report of the British Mission to Japan, *The Effects of the Atomic Bombs at Hiroshima and Nagasaki* (London: HMSO, 1946).

Pirie, A., (ed.) *Fall out, Radiation Hazards from Nuclear Explosions* (London: Macgibbon and Kee, 1958).
Ross, James Sterling, *The National Health Service in Great Britain, An Historical and Descriptive Study* (London: Oxford University Press, 1952).
Russel Bertrand, *The Autobiography of Bertrand Russell 1944-1967*, (London: George Allen and Unwin, 1969).
Rust, H., John, and D. J. Mewissen, *Exposure of Man to Radiation in Nuclear Warfare* (New York: Elsevier Publishing Company, 1963).
Scott, J. A., Cooper D.J.B., Seuffert S., and Sturgess and H. A. C. Sturgess, *The National Health Service Acts, 1946 and 1949* (London: Eyre & Spottiswoode, 1950).
Sears, Thad P., *The Physician in Atomic Defense* (Chicago: The Year Book Publishers, 1953).
Shipley, S. Paul, *Bristol Siren Nights* (Bristol: Rankin Bros., 1943).
Shute, Nevil, *On the Beach* (London: Heinemann, 1957).
Slessor, John, *The Great Deterrent* (London: Cassell, 1957).
Smelser, Neil, J., *Theory of Collective Behavior* (London: Routledge & Kegan Paul: 1962).
Sokolovsky, V. D., *Military Strategy* (London: 1969).
Stella Reading, *Voluntary Service* (WVS, undated).
Stonier, Tom, *Nuclear Disaster* (Middlesex: Penguin Books, 1964).
Takashi, Nagai, *We of Nagasaki: The Story of Survivors in an Atomic Wasteland* (New York: Duell, Sloan and Pearce, 1951).
Tax Research Institute, *Improving Your Chances for Survival Under Thermonuclear Attack* (New York: 1961).
Thomson, Daniel; 'Civil Defense in the United Kingdom' *New York State Journal of Medicine,* June 1963, 1841-1844.
Titmuss, Richard M., *Problems of Social Policy* (London: HMSO, 1950).
Essays on 'The Welfare State' (London: Unwin University Books: 1964).
War Office, *A Field Surgery Pocket Book* (London: HMSO: 1962).
WVS, *It's The Job That Counts 1939-1953, A Selection from the speeches and writings of the Dowager Marchioness of Reading* (Private Publication, 1954).
WVS, *Notes for Guidance on the Distribution and Care of WVS Clothing* (London: WVS, 1959).
WVS, *Report on 25 Years' Work* (London: 1963).
Zuckerman, Solly, *Scientists and War, the Impact of Science on Military and Civil Affairs* (New York: Harper Row, 1967).

Regulations made under the Civil Defence Act 1948 relating to Local Authority Functions

S.I. 1949 No. 1432 C.D. (General) Regulations 1949.
S.I. 1949 No. 2145 C.D. (Burial) Regulations 1949.
S.I. 1951 No. 1223 C.D. (Emergency Feeding) Regulations 1951.
S.I. 1952 No. 2138 C.D. (Billeting) Regulations 1952.
S.I. 1953 No. 1777 C.D. (Grant) Regulations 1953.
S.I. 1954 No. 252 C.D. (Police) Regulations 1954.
S.I. 1956 No. 469 C.D. (Shelter) (Maintenance) Regulations 1956.
S.I. 1960 No. 502 C.D. (Disease) Regulations 1960.
S.I. 1963 No. 926 C.D. (Training in Nursing) Regulations 1963
S.I. 1965 No. 362 C.D. (Emergency Feeding) Regulations 1965.
S.I. 1965 No. 1104 C.D. (Casualty Services) Regulations 1965.

Secondary Sources (Works)

Addison, Paul, *Now the War is Over, A Social History of Britain 1945-51* (London: BBC, 1985).
Andrews, Elaine K., *Civil Defense in the Nuclear Age* (New York: Franklin Watts, 1985).
Arnold, Lorna, *Britain and the H-Bomb* (Basingstoke: Palgrave, 2001).
Atomic Scientists Association, *Atom Train: Guide to the Travelling Exhibition on Atomic Energy,* (London: Atomic Scientists' Association, 1947).
Aubrey, Crispin, *Nukespeak: The Media and the Bomb* (London; Comedia Publishing Group, 1982).
Barker, Rodney, *Hiroshima Maidens, A Story of Courage and Survival* (New York:V.King, 1985).
Barnett, Correlli, *The Verdict of Peace, Britain Between her Yesterday and the Future* (London: Macmillan, 2001).
Barnwell, S., (ed.), *Cold War, Building for Nuclear Confrontation 1946-1989* (Swindon; English Heritage, 2003).
Barthes, Roland, *Mythologies* (London: Vintage, 2000).
Beauman, Katharine Bently, *Green Sleeves* (London: Seeley Service, 1977).
Becket, Brian, *Weapons of Tomorrow* (London: Orbis Publishing, 1982).
Bensen, David W. and Arnold H. Sparrow (eds.), *Survival of Food Crops and Livestock in the Event of Nuclear War* (U.S. Atomic Energy Commission: Springfield, 1971).
Bidwell, Shelford (ed.), *World War 3* (Feltham: The Hamlyn Publishing Group, 1978).

Boyer, Paul, *By the Bomb's Early Light: American thought and Culture at the Dawn of the Atomic Age* (New York: Pantheon, 1985).
British Medical Association's Board of Science and Education, *The Medical Effects of Nuclear War* (Chichester: John Wiley and Sons, 1983).
Brown, Anthony Cave (ed), *Operation: World War III* (London: Arms and Armour Press, 1979).
Burtch, Andrew, *Give Me Shelter, The Failure of Canada's Cold War Civil Defence* (Vancouver and Toronto: UBC Press, 2012).
Calder, Angus, *The People's War* (London: Jonathan Cape 1969).
Carlton, David and Carlo Schaerf (eds.), *Arms Control and Technical Innovation* (New York: Wiley, 1976).
Campbell, Duncan, *War Plan UK: The Truth about Civil Defence in Britain* (London: Burnett Books, 1982).
Catterall, Peter, (ed.), *The Macmillan Diaries, The Cabinet Years 1950-1957* (London: Macmillan, 2003).
Catterall, Peter, (ed.), *The Macmillan Diaries, Prime Minister and After 1957-1966* (London: Macmillan, 2011).
Cheshire, Leonard, *The Light of Many Suns: The Meaning of the Bomb* (London: Methuen, 1985).
Churcher, John and Elena Lieven 'Images of Nuclear War and the Public in British Civil Defense Planning Documents' *Journal of Social Issues*, Volume 39, No.1 1983, 117-132.
Claxton, Eric C., *More Ways of Fighting a War* (Lewes: The Book Guild, 1990).
Connell, R W., *Gender* (Malden MA: Polity in association with Blackwell Press, (2002).
Craddock, Percy, *Know Your Enemy: How the Joint Intelligence Committee Saw the World* (London: John Murray, 2002).
Crofts, William, *Coercion or Persuasion: Propaganda in Britain after 1945* (London: Routledge, 1989).
Cumings, Bruce, *War and Television* (London: Verso, 1992).
Davis, Tracy C., Stages of Emergency, Cold War Nuclear Civil Defense (Durham and London: Duke University Press, 2007).
Davies, A J., *To Build a New Jerusalem, The British Labour Movement from the 1880s to 1990s* (London: Michael Joseph, 1992).
DeGroot, Gerard, *The Bomb, A Life* (London: Jonathan Cape, 2004).
Diacon, Diane, *Residential Housing and Nuclear Attack* (Beckenham: Croom Helm, 1984).
Dockrill, Michael, British Defence since 1945 (London: John Murray, 2002).
Donaoughue, Bernard and G. W. Jones, *Herbert Morrison: Portrait of a Politician* (London: Weidenfeld and Nicolson, 1973).

Doob, Leonard, *Propaganda, Its Psychology and Technique* (New York: Henry Holt, 1943).

Doss, Erika (ed), *Looking at Life Magazine* (Washington: Smithsonian Institution Press, 2001).

Dowling, John, and Evans M. Harrell (eds.), *Civil Defense: A Choice of Disasters* (New York: American Institute of Physics, 1987).

Duff, Peggy, *Left, Left, Left* (London: Allison and Busby, 1971).

Eagleton, Terry, *Ideology, An Introduction* (London: Verso, 1991).

Eckstein, Harry, Pressure Group Politics, The Case of the British Medical Association (Stanford, California: Stanford University Press, 1960).

Edwards, Oliver, *The USA and the Cold War* (London: Hodder and Stoughton, 2002).

Elshtain, Jean Bethke, *Women and War* (New York: Basic Books, Inc, 1987).

Ferris, Paul, *Sir Huge; The Life of Huw Wheldon* (London: Michael Joseph, 1990).

Figes, Eva, *Patriarchal Attitudes, Women in Society* (London: Faber and Faber, 1970).

Finnis, John, Boyle M. Jr., Joseph, Grisez, Germain, *Nuclear Deterrence, Morality and Realism* (Oxford: Clarendon Press, 1987).

Fishbein, Martin, and Icek Ajzen, *Belief, Attitude, Intention and Behaviour* (Philippines: Addison-Wesley, 1975).

Foot, Michael, *Aneurin Bevan 1945-1960* (London: Davis-Poynter, 1973).

Frazier R. W., *The Law Brigades and Air Raid Precautions* (London: The Solicitor's Stationery Society 1938).

Freedman, Lawrence, *The Cold War* (London: Cassell, 2001)

Grant, Matthew, *After the Bomb, Civil Defence and Nuclear War in Britain, 1945-68* (Basingstoke: Palgrave Macmillan, 2010).

Goudsblom Johan, *Fire and Civilization,* (London: Penguin, 1992).

Gourvish, Terry, and Alan O'Day, Britain since 1945 (London: Macmillan 1991).

Grossman, Andrew D., *Neither Dead Nor Read, Civilian Defense and American Political Development During the Early Cold War* (New York, Routledge, 2001).

Hackett, John, *The Third World War August 1985: A Future History* (London: Sidgwick and Jackson, 1978).

Haldane, J.B.S., *A.R.P.* (London: Victor Gollancz: 1938).

Harris, Kenneth, *Attlee* (London: Weidenfeld and Nicolson, 1982).

Harris, Peter (ed.) *Post War Bristol 1945-1965, Twenty Years that changed the city* (The Bristol Branch of the Historical Association)

Harrison, Tom, *Living Through the Blitz* (Reading: 1990).

Hartley, John, (ed.) Understanding News (London:Methuen,1982).

Hastings, Max, *The Korean War* (London: Michael Joseph, 1987).

Hennessey, Peter, *The Secret State* (London: Penguin, 2002).
Heuser, Beatrice, *Nuclear Weapons in Their Historical, Strategic and Ethical Context* (London: Longman, 2000).
Hill, Charles and Woodcock, John, *The National Health Service* (London: Christopher Johnson, 1949).
Hinton, James, *Women, Social Leadership, and the Second World War, Continuities of Class* (Oxford: Oxford University Press, 2002).
Hocking, William Ernest, *Morale and Its Enemies* (New Haven: Yale University Press, 1918).
Honeyman, Victoria, *Richard Crossman, A Reforming Radical of the Labour Party* (London: I.B. Tauris & Co Ltd 2007).
Honigsbaum, Frank, *Health, Happiness, and Security, The Creation of the National Health Service* (London: Routledge, 1989).
Jacobsen, C. G., *The Nuclear Era* (Cambridge, Mass: Oelgeschlager, Gunn and Hain, 1982).
James, Lawrence, *Warrior Race* (London: Little, Brown, 2001).
Johnson, Peter, *Frames of Deceit, The Study of the Loss and Recovery of Public and Private Trust* (U.S.A.: Cambridge University Press, 1993).
Keegan, John, *A History of Warfare* (London: Hutchinson, 1993).
Kerr J. Thomas, *Civil Defence in the U.S.: Bandaid for a Holocaust?* (Boulder Colo.: Westview Press, 1985).
Kirk, Robert, *Relativism and Reality* (London: Routledge, 1999).
Kosakai, Yoshiteru, *Hiroshima Peace Reader* (Hiroshima: Hiroshima Peace Culture Foundation, 1980).
Knightley, Phillip, *T First Casualty, from the Crimea to Vietnam: The* War *Correspondent as Hero, Propagandist, and Myth Maker*(New York: Harcourt Brace Jovanovich, 1975).
Kull, Steven, *Minds at War: Nuclear Reality and the Inner Conflicts of Defense Policymakers* (New York: Basic Books, 1988).
Langdon-Davies, John, *Air Raid* (London: Routledge, 1938).
Larres, Klaus, *Churchill's Cold War* (London: Yale University Press, 2002).
Lasswel, Harold Dwight, *Essays on the Garrison State* (Transaction Publishers: 1997).
Lasswel, Harold Dwight and Dorothy Blumenstock, *World Revolutionary Propaganda: a Chicago Study,1970 Reprint of 1939 Edition* (U.S.A.: First Greenwood Reprinting).
Laurie, Peter, *Beneath the City Streets* (London: Penguin, 1972).
Leaning, Jennifer, and Langley Keyes (eds.), *The Counterfeit Ark* (Cambridge, Mass: Bellinger, 1984).
Lee, Christopher, *The Final Decade* (London: Book Club Associates, 1981).
Levin, Bernard, *The Pendulum Years* (London: Jonathan Cape, 1970).

Liddington, J, *The Long Road to Greenham, Feminism & Anti-Militarism in Britain since 1820* (London: Virago Press, 1989).
Lindqvist, Sven, *A History of Bombing* (London: Granta Publications, 2001).
Lowi, Theodore J., *The End of Liberalism, The Second Republic of the United States*, Second Edition (New York: W.W. Norton & Company, 1979).
Lukes, Steven, *Power, A Radical View, Second Edition* (Basingstoke: Palgrave Macmillan, 2005).
Lustgarten, Laurence, and Ian Leigh, *In from the Cold, National Security and Parliamentary Democracy* (Oxford: Clarendon Press, 1994).
Marwick, Arthur, *The Sixties* (Oxford: Oxford University Press, 1998).
McEnaney, Laura, *Civil Defense Begins at Home Militarization Meets Everyday Life in theFifties* (Princeton: Princeton University Press, 2000).
Mclaine, Ian, *Ministry of Morale, Home Front Morale and the Ministry of Information in World War II* (London: George Allen and Unwin, 1979).
McNamara, Robert, *Blundering into Disaster Surviving the First Century of the Nuclear Age* (London: Bloomsbury, 1987).
Medical Campaign against Nuclear Weapons and Medical Association for the Prevention of War, *The Medical Consequences of Nuclear Weapons* (Cambridge: 1981).
Middlemas, Keith, *Power, Competition & the State, Volume 1 Britain in Search of Balance 1940-61* (London: Macmillan Press Ltd, 1986).
Moorehead, Caroline, *Troublesome People: Enemies of War 1916-1986* (London:Hamish Hamilton, 1981).
Morton, Adam, *A Guide through the Theory of Knowledge* (Oxford: Blackwell, 2003).
Musgrove, Gordon, *Operation Gomorrah* (London: Jane's Publishing Company, 1981).
Newhouse, John, *The Nuclear Age* (London: Penguin, 1989).
Oakes, Guy, *The Imaginary War* (New York: OUP, 1994).
O'Brien, Terrence H., *Civil Defence* (London: HMSO, 1955).
Oppenshaw, S. and Steadman, P., *Predicting the Consequences of a Nuclear Attack on Britain:Models, Results and Public Policy and Implications* (Environment and Planning C, Government and Policy, 1983).
Page, Robert M., and Richard Silburn, (eds.) *British Social Welfare in the Twentieth Century* (London: Macmillan, 1999).
Paris, Michael, *Warrior Nation* (London: Reaktion Books, 2000).
Pater, John E, *The Making of the National Health Service* (London: King Edward's Hospital Fund for London, 1981).
Penny, John, *Bristol at War* (Derby: The Breedon Books Publishing Company Limited, 2002).

Perry, Ronald W., *The Social Psychology of Civil Defense* (Lexington: Lexington Books, 1982).
Pigott, A. J. K., *The Second World War 1939-1945 Army: Manpower Problems* (The War Office, 1949).
Postgate, Oliver, *Thinking it through: the Plain Man's Guide to the Bomb* London: The Menard Press, 1982).
Postgate, Raymond, (ed.), *Air Raid Protection: The Facts* (London: Fact, 1938).
Radical Statistics Nuclear Disarmament Group, *The Nuclear Numbers Game* (London: Radical Statistics, 1982).
Rawls, John, *A Theory of Justice, Revised Edition* (Oxford: Oxford University Press, 1999).
Reiner, Robert, 'Dixon's Decline, Why Policing Has become So Controversial.' *Contemporary British History*, Volume 3, No.1 1989, 2-6.
Richardson, F. M., *Fighting Spirit, Psychological Factors in War* (London: Leo Cooper, 1978).
Richardson, Kenneth, *Twentieth-Century Coventry* (London: Macmillan Press Ltd, 1972)
Rintala, Marvin, *Creating the National Health Service, Aneurin Bevan and the Medical Lords* (London: Routledge, 2003).
Robin, Fear, *The History of a Political Idea* (Oxford: Oxford University Press, 2004).
Roberts, Ernie, *Strike Back* (Orpington: Ernie Roberts, 1994).
Roberts, Fred, *60 years of Nuclear History, Britain's Hidden Agenda* (Charlbury: Jon Capenter, 1999).
Rogers, Paul, and Malcom Dando and Peter van den Dungen, *As Lambs to the Slaughter: The Facts about Nuclear War* (London: Arrow books 1981).
Royal College of Nursing, *Nuclear War, Civil Defence Planning: The Implications for Nursing* (Royal College of Nursing Working Party, 1983).
Royal Air Force Historical Society at The University of Newcastle, Defending the Northern Skies 1915-1995, (UK: Royal Air Force Historical Society, 1996).
Russell-Smith, Enid, *Political Realities, Modern Bureaucracy: The Home Civil Service* (London: 1974).
Scheibach, Michael, *Atomic Narratives and American Youth, Coming of Age with Atom, 1945-1955* (Jefferson: McFarland and Company, 2003).
Selbourne, David, *The Principle of Duty* (London: Sinclair-Stevenson, 1994).
Sibley, Bruce Colin, *Surviving Doomsday* (London: Shaw and Sons, 1977).
Snook, I. A., (ed.), *Concepts of Indoctrination and Education* (London: Routledge and Kegan Paul, 1972).

Spender, Stephen, *Citizens in War and After* (London: George G. Harrap, 1945).

John Steinbach, 'Nuclear Threats and Civil Defence in Australia, 1951-1957,' *War and Society*, Volume 20, No. 2, October 2002, 1-106.

Taylor, John, *War Photography: Realism in the British Press* (London: Routledge, 1991).

The Boeing Aerospace Company, *Industrial Survival and Recovery after Nuclear Attack* (Washington: 1976).

The Report of the Greater London Area War Risk Study Commission, *London Under Attack* (Oxford: Basil Blackwell, 1986).

The Royal United Services Institute for Defence Studies, *Nuclear Attack: Civil Defence* (Oxford: Brassey's Publishers 1982).

Thompson, Dorothy, (ed.), *Over Our Dead Bodies: Women against the Bomb* (London: Virago Press, 1983).

Thompson, James, *Psychological Aspects of Nuclear War* (Chichester: The British Psychological Society, 1985).

Thomson, Oliver, *Easily Led* (Stroud: Sutton Publishing, 1999).

Truman, David, *The Governmental Process, Political Interests and Public Opinion, Second Edition* (New York: Alfred A. Knopf, 1971).

United States Army Nuclear Agency, *The Army Nuclear Survivability Program* (Texas:1974).

United States Army Nuclear Agency, *The Elctromagnetic Pulse (EMP)* (Texas: 1974).

United States Army Nuclear Agency, *Rainout* (Texas:1976).

Wheldall, Kevin, *Social Behaviour* (London: Methuen, 1975).

White, Mark J., *Missiles in Cuba* (Chicago: Ivan R. Dee, 1997).

Wicks, Ben, *No Time to Wave Goodbye* (New York: St. Martin's Press, 1988).

Wigner, Eugene P., (ed.) *Who Speaks for Civil Defense* (New York: Charles Scibner's Sons, (1968).

Williams, Bernard, *Truth and Truthfulness, An Essay in Genealogy* (Oxford: Princeton University Press, 2002).

Wood, Derek, *Attack Warning Red, The Royal Observer Corps and the Defence of Britain 1925 to 1992* (Portsmouth: Carmichael and Sweet, Revised Edition 1992).

Wood, Gordon S. *The Purpose of the Past, Reflections on the Uses of History* (New York: The Penguin Press, 2008).

Zuckerman, E., *The Day after World War III* (New York: Viking, 1984).

Zuckerman, Solly, *Scientists and War, The Impact of Science on Military and Civil Affairs,* (New York: Harper Row,1967)

----*Nuclear Illusion and Reality* (London: Collins, 1982).

Academic and Unpublished Papers

Clarke, R. B. M., (1978) *Britain and Thermonuclear War: the Chances for Survival,* Ph.D. thesis, University of Lancaster.
Cross, D. R., (1987) *Labour and the Bomb*: 1951 - 64, Ph.D. thesis, University of Lancaster.
Fox S. P., (2000) *Control Chain 1948-1968*, Private Paper.
Lonie, R., (1987) *Civil Defence: Social Control and Information*, Ph.D. thesis, University of Dundee.
Scott, G.E., (2006) *Caught in the Act: Bristol Civil Defence and the Political Abuse of Statutory Duty to Support Deterrence Policy 1948 -1968*, Ph.D. thesis, University of the West of England, Bristol.

CD, DVD and Video Resources

Archbishop Sees Civil Defence, Pathe News 1964, Cannister 64/5.
Bristol Civil Defence Our Good Neighbour, Bristol Cinematic Society.
Care of the Homeless, The Home Office and Scottish Home and Health Department, RHR Production, 1965.
CD Headquarters, Pathe News 1955, Cannister 55/96.
Civil Defence Bulletins 1-7, The Home Office and Scottish Home Department, RHR Production.
Fyfe Reviews Civil Defence, Pathe News 1953, Canister 53/59.
Sheffield Civil Defence, Recruitment Film 1958.
The Hole In The Ground, The Home Office and Scottish Home Department, RHR Production, 1962.
The Waking Point, Crown Film Unit 1951.
The War Game, 1965, BFI Video Publishing
The Warden and his Duties, The Home Office and Scottish Home Department, RHR Production, 1961.

INDEX

Abandonment and neglect of casualties, prospect of 19, 27, 34, 38, 65, 95-96, 97, 107, 124, 128, 130, 132, 137, 140, 153, 154, 155, 160, 191, 215, 249; and ageism 137

Accommodation Clearance Register 52, 115

Acts of Parliament:
    Civil Defence Act 1948 5, 11, 65, 168, 245
    Draft Emergency Powers (Defence) Bill 1958 and 1964 218, 220, 221
    Lunacy and Mental Treatment Act 37
    Mental Health Act 1959 219
    National (Armed Forces) Act 1939 62
    National Health Service Act 1946 4, 31, 245

'Acute' hospitals 98-99, 116, 119, 121, 129, 153, 154, 159

Ahern, Col Timothy 125-26

Allen, Sir Phillip 224-26

Alverstoke Naval College 41, 203

Ambulance and hospital trains 23-24

Ambulance Section (Civil Defence Corps) 31, Plate 10, Plates 17-22; as Ambulance and Casualty Collection Section 34, 35, 105-06, 120-21, 129; training vehicles for 40-41, 55, 107, 115-16; new ambulances for 106; decline of 105, 107; as Ambulance and First Aid Section 115-16, 123, 131, 184, 216, 217, 224

Ambulances, shortage and poor state of 10, 31-32, 40, Plate 23; use of converted coaches as 23, 59, 115; ambulance cars 26; comforting symbolism of 31, 32, 33, 122, Plates 9-10; converted lorries as 31; use of 33, 34, 91, 121, 127; impeded by debris 34, 59; increasingly unnecessary in nuclear attack 225

Armed Forces, medical establishment of and requirement for doctors 24-25, 62, 63, 64, 68, 69, 70, 71, 198, 206, 208; integration with civil facilities 70-71, 99, 123

Armer, Sir Frederick 52, 201

Army Medical Services 70

Army School of Health 232

Association of Municipal Corporations 228

Atomic bomb and warfare 8, 13-14, 20, 25, 27, 28, 59, 77, 83, 93, 206; UK weapons programme disclosed 1; Phases I-III (1949-57) 12-13, 17, 19, 20, 25, 38; rearmament from 1951 50

Atomic Energy Commission, US 91
'Atomic Warfare' manual 2
Attlee, Clement 172, 244
Auxiliary Fire Service 5, 106, 168, 243
'Auxiliary' hospitals 98-99, 121, 138, 159

Bainbridge, Maj-Gen 87
Baird, Sir Douglas 242
'Base' hospitals 21, 36
Bath 127
Berenbaum, Morris 126, 247
Berlin, blockade of, airlift and Berlin Wall 1, 9-10, 77, 110, 114, 151, 197, 216, 217, 218
Bevan, Aneurin 9, 69, 72, Plate 1
Beveridge Report 81
Bikini Atoll 91
Birmingham 98, 120, 150, 193
Bishop, 'Freddie', and Bishop Committee 113-14, 116, 151, 224
Blood, and Blood Transfusion Service 15, 41-44, 46-47, 50-51, 55, 118, 128, 250, Plate 26; dried plasma 42-43, 50-51, 128; Regional centres 44
Brecknock, Countess of 194
Bristol 90, 94, 126, 127, 150, 234, 235, 244, 248, Plate 8, Plate 25; Bishop of 237
Britain, possible destruction of 4, 19, 59; rebuilding state after nuclear war 45, 94, 215, 227; making 'bombproof' 45, 101; 'Blitz' spirit 60, 97; nuclear capability 94, 112; social collapse and public control during nuclear war 95, 157, 159, 218, 221, 223; spending out of control 102-03; new 'secret state' and state control 218-20, 247; greater transparency on nuclear matters 224, 225; local government key to rebuilding 227-29, 233-34, 235, 236
British Dental Association 198
British Medical Association (BMA) 72, 73, 74, 80-88 passim, 111, 125, 134, 197, 198, 203, 205, 206, 210-11, 212, 215, 231, 245, 246, 248, Plate 11, Plate 51; strike threatened 80; relaxes attitude towards government 200-01 *see also* General practice and practitioners
British Medical Guild 81, 213
British Oxygen Co 54

British Red Cross Society 145, 167, 168, 170, 171, 174, 180, 182, 184, 185, 187, 188, 190, 194, Plates 30-31; links with NHS severed 195
Brook, Norman 52, 56, 59, 76-77, 78, 79, 102, 110, 113, 218
Bryans, Dame Anne 194
Bunkers against nuclear attack 4, 5, 30, 89-90, 229
Burial arrangements during nuclear war 160-65, 227 *see also* Coffins
Butler, Richard ('Rab') 50, 109, 110-11, 113, 114, 218

Campaign for Nuclear Disarmament (CND) 7, 216, 217; 'Telling Britain' plan (1963) 7
Canada 24
Capital punishment 221, 222, 223
Carling, Sir Ernest Rock 9, 11, 15, 18, 20, 22, 28, 31, 32, 38, 55, 61, 66, 78, 96, 167, Plate 4
Casualties, treatment of 8; sorting of 121-22, 125-33 passim, 137, 139, 197, 244; 'casualty chain' 28, 34, 112, 120, 124, 137, 216, 246, 249
Casualties Union 181-82
'Casualty Collection Points' 121
'Casualty Filter Unit' 127-28
Censorship 141
Central Emergency Register, of doctors 200, 202
Central Medical Recruitment Committee 209, 211, 213, 215
Central/Local Medical War Committees 63, 74, 82, 87
Central/Local Recruitment Committees 82-86 passim, 88
Children, in nuclear war 6, 64-65, 114-15, 154, 155, 221, Plates 36-37
China 45, 225
Church, role in nuclear war and involvement in civil defence 238-40; 'Clergy at War', manual 238
Churchill, Sir Winston 53, 55, 56, 57, 60, 72, 112, Plate 41
Civil defence: precautions 12; expenditure on 45-46, 50, 52-56 passim, 102, 103, 109-11, 112, 242, 245; deficiencies of 47; 'deterrence' factor of 58, 111, 113, 247, 249; control centres 89, 90, 138; affected by advent of hydrogen bomb 91; crisis of public confidence in 217; ad hoc arrangements 218; new approach 224
Civil Defence (Burial) Regulations 1949 160
Civil Defence (Public Protection) Regulations 1967 229

Civil Defence Corps 5, 33, 43, 56, 113, 116, 161, 162, 168, 177, 184, 224, 226, Plates 38-40, Plate 52; demise of 243 *see also* Ambulance Section 31
Civil Defence Joint Planning Staff 9, 25, 26
Civil Defence Officers 17
Civil Defence Staff College, Sunningdale 2, 17, 21, 110, 120, 122, 129, 159, 204-06, 232, 235, 246, Plates 6-7
Civil Nursing Reserve 169, 185
Civilian War Dead Dept 160, 162, 163
Claxton, Dr Ernest 203
'Clergy in War', manual 238
Cockayne, Dame Elizabeth 186
Coffins, for mass burials 162-63, 165, Plates 32-34 *see also* Burial arrangements
Cold War 8, 19, 25, 38, 57, 91, 111, 129, 169, 198, 248, 249, 250; arms race 89, 91
County Councils Association 228
Coventry 90; rebellion by Council on civil defence matters 92-93, 111, 113
Cripps, Sir Stafford 69
Cuban Missile Crisis 114, 152, 197, 217, 218, 225
'Cushion' hospitals 20, 23, 28, 34, 36, 48
Cutler, Marian 178

Daley, Sir Allen 169
Danckerts, Justice 81
Defence (Administration of Justice) (England) Regulations 222
Defence (Public Security) Regulations 220
Defence Regulations 79, 80, 165, 220, 224, 225, 233, 236, 245
Defence Transition Committee 25, 52, 218
Defence White Paper, 1956 150
Dentists 198, 207
Dextran, synthetic blood substitute 43, 118
Dimond, Gen William 186
Director General of Medical Services 84
Disease and plague, danger of 233
Doctors *see* General practice and practitioners
Doctors, foreign, use of 24, 63, 219
Douglas, Sir William Scott 9, 82
Downes-Shaw, Sir Havergal 126

Drugs, supplies of 118-19
Drummond, Lt-Gen Sir Alexander 125

Ede, Chuter 47
Eden, Sir Anthony 103
Electricity supplies, disruption of 28, 38
'Emergency Home Nursing Service' 143
Emergency Medical Corps, proposed 203
Emergency Medical Services 5, 13, 41, 46, 61, 62, 63, 64
Ethics, medical, changes in 95, 97, 130, 132, 136, 138, 223
Evacuation ('dispersal') from hospitals/target areas 17, 18, 29, 32, 98, 119, 150, 151-55 passim, 197, 205, 232, Map 1
Executive Councils 5, 219; increasingly important role of 90-91
Exercises and Studies:
    'Britannia' (1949) 244
    'Exercise Minerva 65' (1965) 159
    'Exercise Savile' 177
    'Medical Caravan' (Sunningdale) 122-23, 127
    'NATO Exercise Civlog 65' 232, 233, 234
    'NATO Exercise Fallex 62' 216, 217
    'Operation Shuttlecock' (1959) 190
    'Reliance' (1958) 127-28, 130, 138, Plates 28-31
    'Study Bull Ring' (Birmingham) 120
    'Study Grass Seed' (Bristol) 234, 236
    'Study Janus 63' 227
    'Study Phoenix Five' (Sunningdale) 235, 236
    'Study Survival' (1967) 138

'Facade' of civil defence policies 3, 7, 35, 56, 57, 59, 60, 89, 100, 102, 108, 110-11, 112-13, 141, 197, 217, 224, 225, 240, 242, 243, 244, 249
Field Surgical Teams 15
First aid, responsibility of NHS 11; 'extended' 123, 131, 133; units 124, standard of 131; instruction in 147, 148-49, 173, 174, 190, 224-25, Plate 35; contents of kit 147-48
First World War, attitudes from 6, 244
Forward Medical Aid Units (FMAUs) 123-24, 127, 128, 129, 130, 132-40 passim, 157, 159, 189, 190-91, 192, 193, 204, 205, 216, 217, 232, 238, 240, 244, 249, Plate 31
Frankau, Sir Claude 9, 15, 16, 17, 78

Fuchs, Klaus 14
Fyfe, Sir David Maxwell 58, 90, 92

Gaitskell, Hugh 45
General Medical Council 212
General Medical Services Committee 210
General practice and practitioners, antipathy towards NHS 6, 28, 72, 212-13; centralised control during wartime, proposals for and opposition to 61-62, 65-68 passim, 72, 76, 78, 81, 82, 83, 86, 88, 197, 200-01, 202, 204, 205, 206, 207, 208, 215, 229, 245, 246, Plate 11, Plate 52; possible conscription or call-up of 62, 63, 68, 79, 86, 87, 197, 198; voluntary register of 79; retired doctors called on 199; terms of employment during war 201, 206; under control of MOH 202, 211, 213, 232; apparent resolution of control issue 208-11; failure of process 211-12, 223, 231 *see also* British Medical Association
Gleneagles golf club 22
'Green Goddess' fire engines 106
Greenline coaches 23

Harkness, Captain 163
Headmasters' Conference 115
Hersey, John 1, 2
Hill, Dr Charles 72-73, 74
Hiroshima 1, 4, 10, 12, 13, 14, 20, 41, 59, Plate 8
Hodsoll, Wg Cdr Sir John 142
'Home Cover' hospitals 98
Home Defence (Review) Committees 59, 110; 1960 114, 154, 165
'Home Defence' 102
Home nursing concept 143-44, 146, 149-50, 173, 174, 234
Hood, Lt-Gen Sir Alexander 9, 16, 66-67, 69, 73, Plate 5
Hornsby-Smith, Pat 175-76, Plate 15
'Hospital Evacuation Area' sector 98
Hospital organisation, post-war 10
Hospital plan 10, 18, 19, 24, 27, 38, 38, 45, 59, 94, 107, 108, 114, 119, 150, 154, 167, 204, 216
Hospital ships, proposed 44
Hospitals: beds, provision of 13-16 passim, 19, 21, 44, 51-52, 107, 108; food 119-20; as 'nuclear oasis' 120; 'home nursing' as an alternative 146; as 'human shields' 151; resistance to radiation 157; staff increasing involved in civil defence 167

Hospitals, hutted annexes to 46-47, 48, 50, 51, 108-09
Hydrogen bomb, different characteristics of 4, 36, 89, 91-94 passim, 97, 99, 100, 114, 120, 121, 125, 141, 143, 167, 183, 200, 206, 236, 240

Ince, Sir Godfrey 76, 77
Industrial Civil Defence Service 5
'Initial Phase of War, The', report 59
Inter-hospital transfers 23, 91, 115
Isle of Man Civil Defence Corps 243

Jenkins, Roy 226
Joint Consultants Committee 210

Kersley, George 125
Khrushchev, Nikita 110, 126
Kirkman, Sir Sidney Chevalier 111
Kleinsorge, Father 1-2
Korean War 8, 18, 38, 45, 53, 77, 80, 81, 86, 172, 173, 176, 199

Lapp, Ralph 91
Law enforcement during nuclear war 221-23, 235
Leamington Spa 173
Lichfield, Bishop of 239-40
Lloyd George, Maj Gwilym 101-02
Local Health Authorities 4, 35; antipathy towards NHS 6
London 12, 211; hospitals 36-37
'London Tactical Study' 34

Macdonald, Dr Peter 74
Macdonald, Mary 188
Macleod, Iain 57-58, Plate 15, Plate 42
Macmillan, Harold 103, 113
Macrae, Dr Angus 81, 83, 87
Main Churches Committee 238
'Main Hospital Area' sector 98
Mass casualties, concept of 1, 128, 129
'Mass compassion', concept of 4, 6, 10, 22, 28, 34, 40, 65, 97, 112, 121, 124, 128, 129, 140, 142, 151, 155, 166, 197, 215, 236, 243, 246, 249

Maternity and midwifery provision in nuclear war 35-36, 153, 155, 219, 240-42
Matthews, General 204
Maude Report 81
Medical aspects working party 66-67
Medical Association for the Prevention of War 93, 247
'Medical manpower in wartime', control of 61, 64, 66, 72, 73, 201, 210
Medical Officers of Health (MOH) 4, 34, 65, 67, 160, 197, 201, 202, 211, 213, 229, 232, 235, 242, 245, 246, Plate 41; loss of status in NHS 6; College of 73; become medical 'supremos' 202, 211, 230, 231-32, 234, 236, 246
Medical Priority Committee 63, 67, 74, 77; becomes National Manpower Committee 82
Medical Services Co-ordinating Committee 69
Medical Women's Federation 74
Middlesbrough 161
Military hospitals 99-100
Ministry of Agriculture, Fisheries and Food 120
Ministry of Health 17, 21, 25, 28, 40, 46, 48, 50, 51, 61, 63, 67, 68, 73, 74, 78, 81, 83, 84-86, 97, 99, 100, 104, 106, 108, 118, 130, 131, 132, 140, 143, 144, 148, 151, 153, 155, 158, 167, 168, 169, 172, 177, 179, 181, 184, 186, 188, 189, 193, 194, 195, 201, 203, 204, 205, 206, 209, 211, 215, 241; unprecedented spending by 48-49
Ministry of Housing and Local Government 163, 227
Ministry of Labour and National Service 75, 76, 78, 79, 86, 87; distrust of medical profession 77
Ministry of Public Buildings and Works 115
Ministry of Transport 119
Mobile First Aid Units (MFAUs) 29, 30, 33, 34, 55, 65, 122, 177, 182, 185, 192, 198, Plates 15-16
Mobile medical and surgical teams 15, 23, 25-26, 28, 61
Monkton, Sir Walter 103
Moran, Lord 72-73
Morgenthau, Hans J. 244
Mountbatten, Lady Louis 170, 173

Nagasaki 10, 20, 27, 59
Nash, Gilbert 75
National Health Service (NHS) 8, 11, 28, 46, 49, 68, 69, 88, 89, 100, 111, 209, 218, 245, 250; establishment of 1, 4, 21, 47, 61, 170,

246, Plates 2-3; as part of civil defence 9, 61, 62, 89, 100, 167; 'stretch' capability of 14, 16, 17, 19, 96; need to support military casualties 46, 48, 99, 100; high cost of 78, 80, 103, 214; negotiations over pay and conditions 80; plan to completely reshape legislation 218-19, 234

National Hospital Service Reserve (NHSR) 5, 29, 148, 167-69, 170, 172ff, 233, 245, 249, Plate 24, Plates 42-45, Plates 48-49; recruitment to 168, 174-75, 178, 179, 191; uniforms 180-81; 'Minister's Challenge Cup competition 181, 192; membership thrown open 185, 187, 188; demise of 196

National Insurance 50

National Medical Advisory Committee, proposed 73

National Medical Corps, proposed 66, 70, 74, 75, 79, 198, 203; proposed name change to Emergency Medical Corps 203

National and Local Medical Committees 67, 202, 205, 207, 208, 209, 211

National Medical Manpower Committee 77, 203, 209, 215

National Nursing Reserve 170, 171, 172

National Service 24, 176, 198, 206

National Union of Teachers 115

Newling, John, and Newling Committee 69, 71, 74, 75, 77

Northampton 159

Northern Ireland 42, 44, 53, 62, 103-04, 122

'Nuclear health service' 18, 20, 38, 49, 60, 89, 92, 111, 141, 205, 215, 223, 236, 242, 244; end of 243

Nuclear war: positive messages and reassurance regarding 2, 20, 27, 191-92, Plates 13-14; prospects of survival 2, 113, 126, 136, 140, 217, 226, 236; management of public fears 3, 147, 155, 225; propaganda 3, 167; shrinking early warning times 12, 24, 45, 95, 116, 152, 154, 239; risk of exposure of true nature of 25, 94, 129, 139, 150, 154, 159-60, 216, 226, 245, 248; 'normalisation' of 26, 28, 35, 125, 146; importance of maintaining public morale 31, 33, 38, 45, 48, 57-58, 60, 95, 101, 110, 113, 114, 122, 124, 132, 139-40, 141, 143, 159; nuclear 'home front' 3, 11, 31, 47, 65, 102, 226; prevention of 57, 58, 93, 247, 248; 'nuclear battleground', representation of 125, 177, 181; shortage of doctors 199; post-attack aftermath 216, 230-31, 233; law enforcement during 221-23, 235

Nurses 29, 123, 145, 146, 167, 168, 169, 185, Plate 27, Plate 41, Plate 48 *see also* National Hospital Service Reserve